Clinical Applications of Diffusion Imaging of the Brain

Guest Editor

L. CELSO HYGINO DA CRUZ JR, MD

NEUROIMAGING CLINICS OF NORTH AMERICA

www.neuroimaging.theclinics.com

Consulting Editor
SURESH K. MUKHERJI, MD

February 2011 • Volume 21 • Number 1

SAUNDERS an imprint of ELSEVIER, Inc.

W.B. SAUNDERS COMPANY
A Division of Elsevier Inc.

1600 John F. Kennedy Boulevard • Suite 1800 • Philadelphia, Pennsylvania 19103-2899

http://www.theclinics.com

NEUROIMAGING CLINICS OF NORTH AMERICA Volume 21, Number 1
February 2011 ISSN 1052-5149, ISBN 13: 978-1-4557-0468-2

Editor: Joanne Husovski
Developmental Editor: Donald Mumford

Neuroimaging Clinics of North America (ISSN 1052-5149) is published quarterly by Elsevier Inc., 360 Park Avenue South, New York, NY 10010-1710. Months of issue are February, May, August, and November. Business and editorial offices: 1600 John F. Kennedy Blvd., Suite 1800, Philadelphia, PA 19103-2899. Business and editorial offices: 6277 Sea Harbor Drive, Orlando, FL 32887-4800. Periodicals postage paid at New York, NY, and additional mailing offices. Subscription prices are USD 314 per year for US individuals, USD 436 per year for US institutions, USD 158 per year for US students and residents, USD 363 per year for Canadian individuals, USD 546 per year for Canadian institutions, USD 461 per year for international individuals, USD 546 per year for international institutions and USD 226 per year for Canadian and foreign students and residents. To receive student/resident rate, orders must be accompanied by name of affiliated institution, date of term, and the *signature* of program/residency coordinator on institution letterhead. Orders will be billed at individual rate until proof of status is received. Foreign air speed delivery is included in all *Clinics* subscription prices. All prices are subject to change without notice. POSTMASTER: Send address changes to *Neuroimaging Clinics of North America*, Elsevier Health Sciences Division, Subscription Customer Service, 3251 Riverport Lane, Maryland Heights, MO 63043. Telephone: 1-800-654-2452 (U.S. and Canada); 314-447-8871 (outside U.S. and Canada). Fax: 314-447-8029. E-mail: journalscustomerservice-usa@elsevier.com (for print support); journalsonlinesupport-usa@elsevier.com (for online support).

Reprints. For copies of 100 or more of articles in this publication, please contact the Commercial Reprints Department, Elsevier Inc., 360 Park Avenue South, New York, NY 10010-1710. Tel.: 212-633-3812; Fax: 212-462-1935; E-mail: reprints@elsevier.com.

Neuroimaging Clinics of North America is covered by *Excerpta Medical/EMBASE,* the RSNA Index of Imaging Literature, *MEDLINE/PubMed (Index Medicus),* MEDLINE/MEDLARS, SciSearch, Research Alert, and Neuroscience Citation Index.

Printed and bound by CPI Group (UK) Ltd, Croydon, CR0 4YY

Transferred to Digital Print 2011

GOAL STATEMENT

The goal of *Neuroimaging Clinics of North America* is to keep practicing radiologists and radiology residents up to date with current clinical practice in radiology by providing timely articles reviewing the state of the art in patient care.

ACCREDITATION

The *Neuroimaging Clinics of North America* is planned and implemented in accordance with the Essential Areas and Policies of the Accreditation Council for Continuing Medical Education (ACCME) through the joint sponsorship of the University of Virginia School of Medicine and Elsevier. The University of Virginia School of Medicine is accredited by the ACCME to provide continuing medical education for physicians.

The University of Virginia School of Medicine designates this educational activity for a maximum of 15 *AMA PRA Category 1 Credits*™ for each issue, 60 credits per year. Physicians should only claim credit commensurate with the extent of their participation in the activity.

The American Medical Association has determined that physicians not licensed in the US who participate in this CME activity are eligible for a maximum of 15 *AMA PRA Category 1 Credits*™ for each issue, 60 credits per year.

Credit can be earned by reading the text material, taking the CME examination online at http://www.theclinics.com/home/cme, and completing the evaluation. After taking the test, you will be required to review any and all incorrect answers. Following completion of the test and evaluation, your credit will be awarded and you may print your certificate.

FACULTY DISCLOSURE/CONFLICT OF INTEREST

The University of Virginia School of Medicine, as an ACCME accredited provider, endorses and strives to comply with the Accreditation Council for Continuing Medical Education (ACCME) Standards of Commercial Support, Commonwealth of Virginia statutes, University of Virginia policies and procedures, and associated federal and private regulations and guidelines on the need for disclosure and monitoring of proprietary and financial interests that may affect the scientific integrity and balance of content delivered in continuing medical education activities under our auspices.

The University of Virginia School of Medicine requires that all CME activities accredited through this institution be developed independently and be scientifically rigorous, balanced and objective in the presentation/discussion of its content, theories and practices.

All authors/editors participating in an accredited CME activity are expected to disclose to the readers relevant financial relationships with commercial entities occurring within the past 12 months (such as grants or research support, employee, consultant, stock holder, member of speakers bureau, etc). The University of Virginia School of Medicine will employ appropriate mechanisms to resolve potential conflicts of interest to maintain the standards of fair and balanced education to the reader. Questions about specific strategies can be directed to the Office of Continuing Medical Education, University of Virginia School of Medicine, Charlottesville, Virginia.

The faculty and staff of the University of Virginia Office of Continuing Medical Education have no financial affiliations to disclose.

The authors/editors listed below have identified no professional/financial affiliations for themselves or their spouse/partner:
Frederik Barkhof, MD, PhD; Raquel Ribeiro Batista, MD; Rafael F. Cabral, MD; L. Celso Hygino da Cruz, Jr, MD (Guest Editor); Antonio José da Rocha, MD, PhD; Romeu C. Domingues, MD; Roberto C. Domingues, MD; Emerson L. Gasparetto, MD, PhD; P. Ellen Grant, MD; Bruno Vasconcelos Sobreira Guedes, MD; Joanne Husovski, (Acquisitions Editor); Jared Isaacson, BS; Ademar Lucas, Jr, MD; Antonio Carlos Martins Maia, Jr, MD, PhD; Elias R. Melhem, MD, PhD; Paolo G. Nucifora, MD, PhD; Katyucia Rodrigues, MD; Fernanda C. Rueda Lopes, MD; Lubdha M. Shah, MD (Test Author); Isabela Garcia Vieira, MD; and Edward Yang, MD, PhD.

The authors listed below have identified the following professional/financial affiliations for themselves or their spouse/partner:
R. Gilberto González, MD, PhD is an industry funded research/investigator for Penumbra, Inc.
Suresh K. Mukherji, MD (Consulting Editor) is a consultant for Philips.
James Provenzale, MD is a consultant for Millenium Pharmaceuticals and Theradex, Inc, is an industry funded research/investigator for GE Healthcare and Bayer Pharmaceuticals, Inc., and is on the Advisory Board for Bayer Pharmaceuticals, Inc.
Albert J. Yoo, MD is an industry funded reseach/investigator for Penumbra, Inc.

Disclosure of Discussion of Non-FDA Approved Uses for Pharmaceutical Products and/or Medical Devices.
The University of Virginia School of Medicine, as an ACCME provider, requires that all faculty presenters identify and disclose any off-label uses for pharmaceutical and medical device products. The University of Virginia School of Medicine recommends that each physician fully review all the available data on new products or procedures prior to clinical use.

TO ENROLL

To enroll in the Neuroimaging Clinics of North America Continuing Medical Education program, call customer service at 1-800-654-2452 or sign up online at ***http://www.theclinics.com/home/cme***. The CME program is available to subscribers for an additional annual fee of USD 196.

Neuroimaging Clinics of North America

THE CLINICS ARE NOW AVAILABLE ONLINE!

Access your subscription at:
www.theclinics.com

Contributors

CONSULTING EDITOR

SURESH K. MUKHERJI, MD, FACR
Professor and Chief of Neuroradiology and
Head & Neck Radiology; Professor of
Radiology, Otolaryngology Head Neck
Surgery, Radiation Oncology, Periodontics and
Oral Medicine, University of Michigan Health
System, Ann Arbor, Michigan

GUEST EDITOR

L. CELSO HYGINO DA CRUZ Jr, MD
Radiologist, Clinics CDPI and Multi-Imagem;
Radiologist, Clinic IRM; Department of
Radiology, Federal University of Rio de
Janeiro, Rio de Janeiro, Brazil

AUTHORS

FREDERIK BARKHOF, MD, PhD
Department of Radiology, Vrije University
Medical Centre, Amsterdam, The Netherlands

RAQUEL RIBEIRO BATISTA, MD
Radiologist, Clínica de Diagnóstico por
Imagem, Rio de Janeiro, Brazil

RAFAEL F. CABRAL, MD
Department of Radiology, University Federal of
Rio De Janeiro; CDPI - Clinica De Diagnóstico
por Imagem, Rio De Janeiro, Brazil

L. CELSO HYGINO DA CRUZ Jr, MD
Radiologist, Clinics CDPI and Multi-Imagem;
Radiologist, Clinic IRM; Department of
Radiology, Federal University of Rio de
Janeiro, Rio de Janeiro, Brazil

ANTONIO JOSÉ DA ROCHA, MD, PhD
Section of Neuroradiology, Centro de Medicina
Diagnostica Fleury and Santa Casa de
Misericórdia de São Paulo, Paraíso, São Paulo,
Brazil

ROMEU C. DOMINGUES, MD
Radiologist, Clinics CDPI and Multi-Imagem,
Rio De Janeiro, Brazil

ROBERTO CORTES DOMINGUES, MD
Radiologist, Department of Radiology,
CDPI – Clínica de Diagnóstico por Imagem,
University of Rio de Janeiro, Rio de Janeiro,
Brazil

EMERSON L. GASPARETTO, MD, PhD
Department of Radiology, University Federal
of Rio De Janeiro; CDPI - Clinica De
Diagnóstico por Imagem, Rio De Janeiro, Brazil

R. GILBERTO GONZÁLEZ, MD, PhD
Neuroradiology Division, Professor of
Radiology, Harvard Medical School; Chief of
Neuroradiology, Massachusetts General
Hospital, Boston, Massachusetts

P. ELLEN GRANT, MD
Director of the Fetal-Neonatal Neuroimaging
and Developmental Science Center; Division
of Newborn Medicine, Department of
Medicine, Division of Neuroradiology,
Department of Radiology, Children's Hospital
Boston; Associate Professor of Radiology,
Harvard Medical School, Boston,
Massachusetts

BRUNO VASCONCELOS SOBREIRA GUEDES, MD
Fellow in Neuroradiology, Santa Casa de Misericórdia de São Paulo, São Paulo, Brazil

JARED ISAACSON, BS
Duke University School of Medicine, Durham, North Carolina

ADEMAR LUCAS Jr, MD
Fellow in Neuroradiology, Santa Casa de Misericórdia de São Paulo, São Paulo, Brazil

ANTONIO CARLOS MARTINS MAIA Jr, MD, PhD
Section of Neuroradiology, Centro de Medicina Diagnostica Fleury and Santa Casa de Misericordia de São Paulo, Paraíso, São Paulo, Brazil

ELIAS R. MELHEM, MD, PhD
Wallace T. Miller, Sr. Professor of Radiology and Chief, Division of Neuroradiology, Department of Radiology, University of Pennsylvania School of Medicine, Hospital of the University of Pennsylvania, Philadelphia, Pennsylvania

PAOLO G. NUCIFORA, MD, PhD
Assistant Professor, Division of Neuroradiology, Department of Radiology, University of Pennsylvania School of Medicine, Hospital of the University of Pennsylvania; Veterans Affairs Medical Center, Philadelphia, Pennsylvania

JAMES PROVENZALE, MD
Department of Radiology, Duke University Medical Center, Durham, North Carolina; Departments of Radiology, Oncology and Biomedical Engineering, Emory University School of Medicine, Atlanta, Georgia

KATYUCIA RODRIGUES, MD
Multi-Imagem/CDPI Clinics, Rio de Janeiro, Brazil

FERNANDA C. RUEDA LOPES, MD
CDPI – Clínica de Diagnóstico por Imagem; Department of Radiology, University of Rio de Janeiro, Rio de Janeiro, Brazil

ISABELA GARCIA VIEIRA, MD
Radiologist, Clinics CDPI and Multi-Imagem, Rio de Janeiro, Brazil

EDWARD YANG, MD, PhD
Fellow, Division of Neuroradiology, Department of Radiology, University of Pennsylvania School of Medicine, Hospital of the University of Pennsylvania, Philadelphia, Pennsylvania

ALBERT J. YOO, MD
Instructor of Radiology, Divisions of Diagnostic and Interventional Neuroradiology, Harvard Medical School; Director of Acute Stroke Intervention, Massachusetts General Hospital, Boston, Massachusetts

Contents

From their origin as simple techniques primarily used for detecting acute cerebral ischemia, diffusion MR imaging techniques have rapidly evolved into a versatile set of tools that provide the only noninvasive means of characterizing brain microstructure and connectivity, becoming a mainstay of both clinical and investigational brain MR imaging. In this article, the basic principles required for understanding diffusion MR imaging techniques are reviewed with clinical neuroradiologists in mind.

For over 20 years, conventional MR imaging has been used for assessing brain tumors. However, conventional MR imaging tends to underestimate the extent of the tumor, perhaps leading to suboptimal treatment. New MR imaging tools have been widely used to determine the grade, heterogeneity, and extent of brain tumors. Diffusion-weighted imaging has been studied extensively, helping in tumor grading, differential diagnosis, and postoperative evaluation. Diffusion tensor imaging can apparently delineate more accurately the tumor versus the infiltrating tumor between the peritumoral edema and the normal brain parenchyma. This article shows the main clinical applications of these sequences.

Diffusion magnetic resonance imaging is the best imaging tool for detecting acute ischemic brain injury. Studies have shown its high accuracy for delineating irreversible tissue damage within the first few hours after stroke onset; however, the true value of any diagnostic tool is whether it can be used to guide clinical management. This review discusses the role of diffusion imaging in the evaluation of the patient with acute ischemic stroke, and how this role is influenced by other important stroke-related variables, including the level of vessel occlusion and the clinical deficit. The review focuses on decision-making for intravenous and intra-arterial reperfusion therapies.

Multiple sclerosis (MS) is considered the most common inflammatory autoimmune neurologic disorder and the most frequent cause of nontraumatic neurologic disability in young and middle-age adults. This article reviews the basic features of its magnetic resonance (MR) imaging lesions and, primarily, the use of diffusion MR imaging, which is increasingly applied to assess patients with MS, not only to investigate plaques but also the normal-appearing white matter, gray matter, optic nerve, and spinal cord, because of its ability to detect and quantify disease-related pathologic conditions of the central nervous system.

resonance is a major advance in the continuing evolution of MR imaging. It provides contrasts and characterization between tissues at a cellular level that may imply differences in function as well as framework and have contributed to a better understanding of the pathophysiological mechanisms of several diseases.

Magnetic resonance (MR) imaging has been used by investigators and clinicians to assess the development of the brain in childhood to understand both patterns of normal growth and patterns by which a maturing brain may deviate from normal. Advanced MR techniques such as diffusion tensor imaging (DTI) have gained prominence as a means of assessing brain development. This review explains the sequence of brain maturation and the means by which DTI can be used to assess it in normal children.

Preface
MRI Diffusion Imaging in Daily Practice

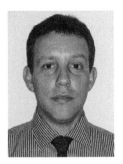

L. Celso Hygino da Cruz Jr, MD
Guest Editor

The intent of this issue of *Neuroimaging Clinics of North America* is to provide the readers an update about the current clinical applications of diffusion imaging, or those that may soon have mainstream clinical application. The review articles are addressed not only to the neuroradiologist, but also are applicable to most of the radiology community. Thus, the topics were selected in order to provide an overview of the technical and clinical issues related to the role of diffusion imaging in neuroradiology.

Currently, MRI diffusion imaging is part of daily practice and is used to achieve the majority of neurologic applications. Moreover, its applications have been continuously improving. As the acquisition techniques have evolved alongside the implementation of more powerful, homogeneous and linear gradients, with greater stability, higher quality diffusion imaging is the result.

New insights surround diffusion imaging, enabling one to get functional and even microstructural information through new forms of acquisition and postprocessing of the diffusion imaging, such as diffusion tensor imaging and tractography. To date, the clinical applications of diffusion imaging have been increased. Currently, this sequence can provide information for diagnosis, staging of disease, treatment planning, and treatment response that can direct overall patient management.

In this publication, we also point out exciting new applications in the neurological scenario, such as brain development, neoplasm, multiple sclerosis, trauma, and infection. From the data presently available, one may conclude that diffusion imaging has a vast application in clinical neurology. Nevertheless, there are many challenges still unresolved. It is precisely these challenges that keep us moving ahead to seek answers and advance technologically.

The topics published are devoted to achieve information that could benefit physicians in different clinical practice scenarios and in the academic field. The articles, presented by a variety of experienced radiologists, address topics with clinical applications of most relevance to daily practice.

I hope the readers find these articles informative, entertaining, provocative, and helpful in daily practice.

I do not have words to express my thankfulness to all of the authors for their invaluable contribution to make this issue a reality. I wish to express my sincere gratitude to the consulting editor, Suresh Mukherji, MD, for the opportunity and privilege to lead this project. Thanks also must be given to the series editor, Joanne Husovski, for

Neuroimag Clin N Am 21 (2011) xi–xii
doi:10.1016/j.nic.2011.03.002

guidance, patience, support, and encouragement throughout the process of preparation of this issue.

Last, and by no means least, I want to dedicate this conquest to my parents, Luiz Celso and Leonice, as well as to my wife, Simone, for their support and understanding during the process of my preparing this work.

L. Celso Hygino da Cruz Jr, MD

Multi-Imagem Clinic
Rua Saddock de Sá 266
Ipanema, Rio de Janeiro, Brazil
CEP: 22411 040

E-mail address:
celsohygino@hotmail.com

Diffusion MR Imaging: Basic Principles

Edward Yang, MD, PhD[a], Paolo G. Nucifora, MD, PhD[a,b],
Elias R. Melhem, MD, PhD[a],*

KEYWORDS

- MRI • Diffusion MRI • Diffusion tensor imaging
- Clinical neurology

Since the first descriptions of nuclear magnetic resonance (MR) in the 1950s, there has been interest in using MR to measure the diffusion properties of water.[1] With the advent of MR imaging scanners in the 1980s, it was natural for investigators to develop diffusion MR imaging techniques for imaging of the brain,[2–4] along the way demonstrating applications that are now familiar, such as restricted diffusion in acute cerebral ischemia[5] and measurement of the directional dependence (anisotropy) of water diffusion in cerebral white matter.[6] Once rapid single-shot echo planar imaging (SS-EPI) sequences became available in the early 1990s, diffusion MR imaging techniques were quickly adopted by many clinical radiologists and basic science investigators. As a result, there has been a rapid increase in knowledge of diffusion MR imaging techniques and their application to the study of brain pathology since that time: at last count, there were more than 8000 citations for brain diffusion MR imaging in the literature, approximately 2272 articles published in 2009 alone.

In this article, the basic principles required for understanding diffusion MR imaging techniques are reviewed with the clinical neuroradiologist in mind, setting the stage for detailed review of specific clinical applications in articles elsewhere in this issue. This article begins with a consideration of how diffusion MR imaging techniques exploit the random movements of water molecules to infer diffusion rates. It also considers the different methods for assessing anisotropic diffusion with emphasis on the most widely used model, known as diffusion tensor imaging (DTI). After reviewing current best practices in diffusion MR imaging acquisition, some of the common analytic methods used for diffusion MR imaging data are described, including advanced methods, such as tractography. Throughout, examples from the literature are used to illustrate the types of questions that can be addressed with diffusion techniques.

PHYSICAL BASIS OF DIFFUSION IMAGING
The Phenomenon of Brownian Motion

As commonly used in the physical sciences, the term, *diffusion*, carries two meanings. The classical meaning of the term refers to net molecular movement or flux down a concentration gradient. The Fick first law formalizes this concept and is familiar from medical school descriptions of respiratory physiology.[1] Diffusion also refers, however, to the random displacement of molecules of uniform concentration in solution. This phenomenon is known as brownian motion, after the botanist Robert Brown, who noted its role in the displacement of pollen particles in solution.

Brownian motion of water molecules is the key physical process that is measured in diffusion MR imaging experiments. According to theoretic models of brownian motion, the trajectory of a single molecule can be envisioned as a series of random collisions with surrounding molecules, all of which are agitated by thermal energy (Fig. 1). Over time, any given molecule is displaced outward with radial location governed by a gaussian probability distribution

[a] Division of Neuroradiology, Department of Radiology, University of Pennsylvania School of Medicine, Hospital of the University of Pennsylvania, 3400 Spruce Street, Philadelphia, PA 19104, USA
[b] Veterans Affairs Medical Center, Philadelphia, PA, USA
* Corresponding author.
E-mail address: Elias.melhem@uphs.upenn.edu

Neuroimag Clin N Am 21 (2011) 1–25
doi:10.1016/j.nic.2011.02.001

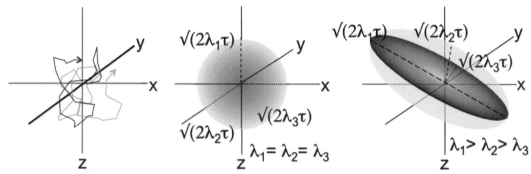

Fig. 1. Anisotropy as described by the DTI model. Hypothetical random paths of two molecules (red and blue) experiencing brownian motion are depicted (*left*). Representations of diffusion probability distributions (PDFs) for isotropic diffusion (*middle*) and anisotropic diffusion (*right*). For isotropic diffusion, there is equal likelihood of diffusion from the origin in all directions, resulting in a spherical PDF. With anisotropic diffusion, there is unequal diffusion, and under the DTI model, this anisotropy is described using 3 orthogonal gaussian distributions with magnitudes (eigenvalues) λ_1, λ_2, and λ_3, resulting in a diffusion ellipsoid PDF. The actual magnitude of the diffusion in each of the principal directions is proportional to the square root of the product of the eigenvalue for that direction and the time of diffusion τ. (*Data from* Basser PJ, Mattiello J, LeBihan D. MR diffusion tensor spectroscopy and imaging. Biophys J 1994;66(1):259–67.)

(ie, a spherical shell with thickness determined by the variance of the gaussian distribution). Einstein is credited with formalizing this relationship by suggesting the mean squared displacement, $<x^2>$, from an initial point source takes the form (Equation 1):

$$<x^2> = 6D\Delta t \qquad (1)$$

where D is the diffusion constant/coefficient that is dependent on temperature, molecular size, and solvent viscosity, and Δt represents the time elapsed from the initial position. Because the mean displacement, $<x>$, for a random process is zero, the variance (ie, square of the SD) is equal to this mean squared displacement.[7] At physiologic temperatures, the constant D for water has a value of approximately 3×10^3 mm^2 per second. Thus, over the 50- to 100-millisecond interval typically used in diffusion MR imaging experiments, the root mean squared displacement of water is on the order of a cell diameter, or approximately 10 mm.[1,8]

The Diffusion MR Experiment

In the context of an imaging experiment, the challenge is to sensitize the MR signal to the diffusion of water (as described by Equation 1) while retaining the positional information used to identify each voxel in the image. In a typical pulsed gradient spin-echo diffusion-weighted sequence, this task is accomplished through the application of motion-sensitizing gradients just before and after the 180° refocusing pulse (**Fig. 2**). Although the diffusion gradients are applied in the same

direction in the MR pulse diagram, the effect of the gradients on spin phase is opposite because of the intervening refocusing/inversion pulse. Water protons that maintain their initial position between the application of the two gradient pulses experience no diffusion-related dephasing because the two lobes of the diffusion gradient negate each other. Diffusion away from the initial starting point, however, results in incomplete reversal of diffusion-related dephasing and proportionate loss of phase coherence (ie, signal). The loss of phase coherence is identical if the diffusion gradient is applied in the inverse direction (eg, the −x direction instead of the +x direction), and the aggregate behavior of the innumerable protons within any given voxel determines the degree of signal loss. Although the overall phase coherence is decreased by the presence of diffusion, the phase encoding itself remains unperturbed: the degree of phase offset by the phase-encoding gradient remains the same as for the diffusion gradient-free case, and the positional information is still recoverable by a standard 2-D Fourier transform.

This process has been formalized mathematically. First, it must be appreciated that the signal of any given voxel in a spin-echo sequence without a diffusion gradient takes the form as described in Equation 2:

$$S_o \propto PD \times \left(1 - e^{-TR/T1}\right) \times e^{-TE/T2} \qquad (2)$$

where PD is proton density, T1 and T2 are tissue properties, and echo time (TE) and repetition time (TR) are set by the instrument operator.[9] These parameters are unchanged by the

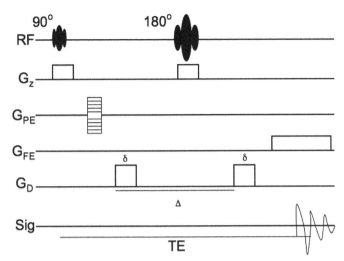

Fig. 2. Pulsed gradient spin-echo MR sequence for DWI. The typical elements of a spin-echo sequence are present, including a 180° refocusing pulse with readout/frequency-encoding gradient, G_{FE}; phase-encoding gradient, G_{PE}; and slice selection gradient, G_z. The motion-sensitizing (ie, diffusion) gradient, G_D, is applied before and after the refocusing pulse with duration, δ, and interval, Δ, as discussed in the text.

introduction of a diffusion gradient to the standard spin-echo sequence. There is exponential loss of signal (ie, dephasing), however, that occurs in the presence of a pulsed diffusion gradient, determined by the rate of diffusion in the direction of the diffusion gradient and strength/duration of the diffusion gradients. The relationship between the diffusion gradient, diffusion constant, initial signal, and diffusion-sensitized signal is described by the Stejskal-Tanner equation (Equation 3):

$$S_n = S_o \times e^{-b \times ADC_n} \tag{3}$$

where S_n represents the signal measured after application of a gradient in direction n, S_o represents the intrinsic signal without diffusion gradients, and ADC_n is the apparent diffusion coefficient (ADC) of water in the direction of the applied gradient.[10] The ADC is "apparent" in the sense that the diffusion constant may reflect macroscopic obstacles (eg, cell membranes or organelles) rather than the intrinsic mobility of water in the interrogated voxel.[11] For this reason, the ADC in living tissues is typically lower than that measured for water solutions (discussed previously), approximately 1×10^3 mm^2/s.[12] The value, b, is a measure of the diffusion weighting, factoring in both strength and duration of the diffusion gradient. For a typical, rectangular gradient pulse, it is defined as in Equation 4:

$$b = \gamma^2 G^2 \delta^2 \left(\Delta - \frac{\delta}{3} \right) \tag{4}$$

where γ represents the gyromagnetic ratio (1/(Tesla*sec)), G the strength of the diffusion

gradient (tesla/mm), δ the duration of the diffusion gradient (seconds), and Δ the interval between the start of each diffusion gradient (seconds). The units of b are seconds per m^2, and typically b has values of 500 to 1000 s/mm^2 in most clinical sequences.

From Equations 2–4, diffusion MR imaging contrast (ie, difference between gradients on and off) is most efficiently increased through the application of strong diffusion gradients (G) that, therefore, result in large b values. Increasing the duration of the diffusion gradient (δ) also has a large effect on the b value and is another means of achieving sufficiently high diffusion weighting, although at the potential cost of increasing the TE. Increasing δ is most useful when operating near the Food and Drug Administration limitations placed on maximal gradient strength for human-rated MR scanners.[8,13]

Solving for the ADC

In Equation 3, there are two unknown variables (S_o and ADC_n), one experimentally measured value (S_n), and one operator-specified value (b). Using basic algebra, the two unknown variables are readily solved by measuring S_n at two values of b, typically $b = 0$ and $b = 1000$ s/mm^2 (eg, **Fig. 3**A, C). Because $b = 0$ s/mm^2 yields $S_n = S_o$, it is simple to solve for the ADC_n value (Equation 5):

$$ADC_n = -\ln(S_n/S_o)/(b = 1000 \ s/mm^2) \tag{5}$$

On some instruments, a third b value may be chosen between these two values to increase

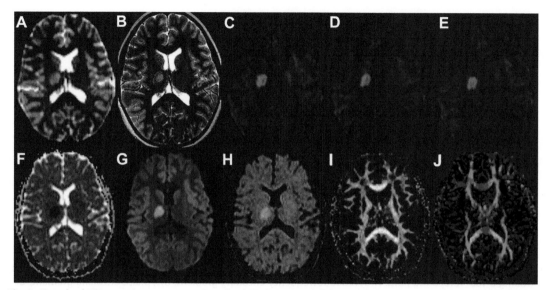

Fig. 3. Standard DTI experiment output. Standard 30-direction DTI was performed on a 10-year-old girl 15 hours after onset of left hemiparesis. The *b* = 0 (*A*) and T2-weighted (*B*) images demonstrate T2 hyperintensity in the posterior limb of the right internal capsule. DWI data from individual pulsed gradient directions (*C–E*) demonstrate sensitivity of white matter and, in particular, the corpus callosum to direction of the applied gradient. ADC (*F*) and DWI (*G*) demonstrate restricted diffusion in the right internal capsule lesion, consistent with acute infarction. Although not necessary in this instance, the exponential diffusion map (*H*) confirms that T2 shine-through does not significantly alter the DWI map. FA (*I*) and colored FA (*J*) maps show decrease in FA at the site of the infarct and also show relationship of the lesion to the internal capsule. Standard colored FA encoding is used: green (anteroposterior), blue (craniocaudad), and red (left-right) anisotropy.

accuracy of the regression, but the concept is identical. One caveat to this calculation is that it assumes monoexponential decay of the diffusion-weighted signal, something that is not always observed in biologic specimens. There is usually an asymptotic deviation from monoexponential decay with large measured displacements (ie, *b* values), a phenomenon attributed to macromolecular barriers, such as cell membranes.[12] At the *b* values typically encountered in a clinical diffusion MR imaging experiment, the deviations from monoexponential decay are relatively modest, but deviations from this assumption may have to be considered as diffusion gradient strength is increased, for example in diffusion spectrum imaging (DSI) or q-ball imaging (QBI) techniques (**Table 1**).[12,14,15] A second problem with calculations using Equation 5 is that it assumes isotropic diffusion of water throughout the brain. Because this is a fallacy in many regions of the brain (discussed later), it is standard practice to improve accuracy of the ADC measurement using values derived from 3 orthogonal directions, usually the X, Y, and Z axes relative to the scanner. Thus, the value of any given voxel in the ADC or diffusion-weighted images (DWI) reviewed by

a radiologist represents the averaged values of at least 3 gradient directions (Equations 6 and 7):

$$ADC_{xyz} = (ADC_x + ADC_y + ADC_z)/3 \qquad (6)$$

$$DWI_{xyz} = S_o \times e^{-b \times ADC_{xyz}} \qquad (7)$$

The ADC_{xyz} and DWI_{xyz} measurements from the 3-direction diffusion MR imaging experiment constitute the basic information available from a standard clinical MR sequence obtained for evaluation of stroke, and a study acquired in this way is referred to as a DWI experiment in this article.

The underlying SS-EPI spin-echo sequence is T2 weighted even on *b* = 1000 s/mm² images where the cerebrospinal fluid signal is dephased due to diffusion effects (see **Fig. 3**). This T2 weighting is necessary because of the interval required for the application of the diffusion gradient (longer TE)[16] and is valuable because it helps increase the conspicuity of lesions through combined effects of T2 and diffusion weighting.[8] In instances where DWI signal is questioned as a shine-through artifact from the underlying T2 weighting, the T2

Table 1
Imaging techniques

	DWI	DTI	QBI	DSI	Hemi-q-Space DSI	DKI
Encoding	SS-EPI-SE	SS-EPI-SE	SS-EPI-SE	2× Refocused SS-EPI-SE	SS-EPI-SE	2× Refocused SS-EPI-SE
Directions[a]	3	55	55	515 Points in q-space	129 Points in q-space	30
Matrix	160 × 136	128 × 128	128 × 128	128 × 128	112 × 112	128 × 128
Resolution	1.3 × 1.1 mm	1.8 × 1.8 mm	2.2 × 2.2 mm	2.0 × 2.0 mm	2.0 × 2.0 mm	2.0 × 2.0 mm
B Values (s/mm^2)	0, 500, 1000	1 q Radius (10) 1000	1 q Radius (30) 3000	5 q Radii, up to 17,000	5 q Radii, up to 12,000	0, 500, 1000, 1500, 2000, 2500
TE (ms)	92	63	82	154	89	108
TR (ms)	5500	14,000	16,400	3000	4200	2300
NEX	1	1	1	1	1	2
Acceleration Factor	1	2	2	NR	3	2
Acquisition Time (minutes)	30″	13′	16′	48′*	18′	12′
References	211	211	211	45,47	46	52

[a] Local protocol.
Abbreviations: NR, not reported; SE, spin echo; *, estimated from published acquisition parameters.

component can be removed computationally by dividing DWI_{xyz} by S_o, the latter representing the T2-weighted $b = 0$ s/mm^2 image. The resulting (DWI_{xyz}/S_o) image is known as the exponential image (see **Fig. 3H**).[17]

Diffusion Anisotropy

In the basic DWI experiment (described previously), water is assumed to diffuse equally in all directions (ie, isotropically), something that is demonstrably false in many locations in the brain. The tendency of water to diffuse preferentially in certain directions is known as anisotropy and is highly correlated with the presence of coherent fiber bundles in brain tissue. Anisotropy was first demonstrated through comparison of ADC values obtained with application of diffusion gradients perpendicular to and parallel to long white matter tracts.[18-22] The biophysical basis of this phenomenon remains somewhat uncertain. Measurements of unmyelinated neurons and neurons exposed to microtubule depolymerizing agents, however, still exhibit strong diffusion anisotropy, arguing against a primary role of the myelin sheath or cytoskeletal protein structure, respectively.[12,23-25] Rather, much of the measured anisotropy is attributed to the cell membranes of the axons themselves.[15] Therefore, anisotropic diffusion is commonly interpreted as coherent diffusion along the cell membranes of nerve fascicles as they traverse a voxel.

Because nerve fascicle orientation and trajectory cannot be noninvasively probed with any other method, measurement of diffusion anisotropy has attracted intense interest. The most widespread method for measuring diffusion anisotropy uses a model that assumes water diffusion at each voxel can be described by 3 orthogonal gaussian distributions with diffusion coefficients of magnitude λ_1, λ_2, and λ_3.[6] The relative magnitudes of the 3 diffusion coefficients determine the shape of the resulting probability distribution for water displacement/diffusion over the timescale of the applied diffusion gradient: if $\lambda_1 = \lambda_2 = \lambda_3$, the diffusion probability distribution for the voxel is spherical; if $\lambda_1 >> \lambda_2$, λ_3, the probability distribution takes on an elongated/ellipsoid shape (see **Fig. 1**, middle vs right panel). Because the set of 3 vectors (eigenvectors) corresponding to magnitudes λ_1, λ_2, and λ_3 (eigenvalues) specify a mathematical object known as a tensor, this model-based approach to measuring diffusion anisotropy is called DTI.

To determine the tensor for any given voxel, the diffusion coefficients along each of the 3 principal axes (X, Y, and Z) must be determined with respect to each of the other axes for a total of 9 values in a diffusion matrix:

$$\begin{bmatrix} D_{xx} & D_{xy} & D_{xz} \\ D_{yx} & D_{yy} & D_{yz} \\ D_{zx} & D_{zy} & D_{zz} \end{bmatrix} \tag{8}$$

As discussed previously, diffusion gradients applied in opposite directions (eg, D_{xy} and D_{yx}) cause the same resulting degree of dephasing. Therefore, only 6 unique diffusion measurements are required to fill the matrix in Equation 8. After performing a $b = 0$ measurement to solve S_o, Equation 5 is solved for each of these 6 directions to populate the diffusion tensor matrix. Using basic linear algebra to multiply matrix 8 by the eigenvector matrix, the eigenvalues λ_1, λ_2, and λ_3 can be readily determined. Although more than 6 direction-encoding gradients may be used (discussed later), it is assumed under the DTI model that there is still gaussian diffusion in 3 orthogonal directions (ie, diffusion tensor comprised of 3 eigenvectors) regardless of the number of direction-encoding gradients used. As expressed in terms of the eigenvalues, the mean diffusivity (MD) and the average diffusion-weighted signal (DWI_{avg}) in each voxel are defined as in Equations 9 and 10:

$$MD = (\lambda_1 + \lambda_2 + \lambda_3)/3 \tag{9}$$

$$DWI_{n=6} = S_o \times e^{-\sum_{n=1}^{6} b \times ADC_n} \tag{10}$$

A useful composite measure of the degree of anisotropy is known as fractional anisotropy (FA) and is defined as in Equation 11:

$$FA = \sqrt{\frac{3}{2}}$$
$$\times \frac{\sqrt{(\lambda_1 - MD)^2 + (\lambda_2 - MD)^2 + (\lambda_3 - MD)^2}}{\sqrt{\lambda_1^2 + \lambda_2^2 + \lambda_3^2}} \tag{11}$$

The FA has a value of zero when diffusion is equal in all 3 directions ($\lambda_1 = \lambda_2 = \lambda_3$) and a value close to 1 when diffusion in the principal direction greatly exceeds that in the other two dimensions of the tensor ($\lambda_1 >> \lambda_2$, λ_3).

Standard outputs of a DTI experiment include the raw data from each of the gradient sensitized SS-EPIs, the ADC image, the DWI image, the FA image, and a colored FA image (see **Fig. 3**). The colored FA image is an intuitive means of viewing information about anisotropic diffusion for the whole brain, where the anisotropy along the X, Y, and Z scanner axes are coded red, green, and blue, respectively; the intensity of the colors is modulated based on the magnitude of the underlying FA value.[26] As a result, major white matter tracts become conspicuous even without advanced postprocessing methods (described later).

Higher-Fidelity Representations of Diffusion Anisotropy

The major limitation of the DTI model is that it assumes the probability distribution function (PDF) of water in any brain voxel is defined by a gaussian probability function for each of 3 orthogonal planes. Many regions of the brain, however, contain crossing white matter tracts (eg, pons and centrum semiovale) with PDFs that cannot be accurately approximated using one of the tensor-based diffusion geometries. Therefore, FA measurements and tractography in these regions can be highly inaccurate using the DTI model.[27–30] Smaller voxel size can correct for this accuracy only to a limited extent[31] and does so at the cost of poor signal-to-noise ratio (SNR).

To properly model the PDF in these regions, advanced variants of diffusion imaging have been devised that require no a priori assumption of the shape of the PDF. All these approaches rely on the fact that the PDF is related by Fourier transform to the observed diffusion MR signal, S (q_i), where the vector, q_i ($q = \gamma\delta G$ using the same nomenclature from Equation 4), represents one of many diffusion vectors needed to solve the PDF. The relationship between signal distributed in q-space S(q_i) q_i, and the PDF is analogous to the relationship between signal distributed in k space S(k_x, k_y), phase-encoding gradient k_y, and the actual distribution of signal in space S(x,y) in structural MR imaging. This model-free approach to determining the PDF is, therefore, known as q-space imaging (QSI) and has a long history in the physical chemistry literature.[32,33] Initial biologic studies applied this technique to the study of metabolite or water diffusion as part of in vitro experiments,[34–37] including applications to more accurate measurements of diffusion coefficients of brain or spinal cord specimens.[37–39] Voxel-by-voxel determination of the PDF in a 3-D brain image with whole-brain coverage, however, has become possible only recently.[40,41]

In QSI with coverage of the whole brain, experimental data space can be envisioned as a 6-D space specified by a 3-D diffusion weighted image at each sampled region of the 3-D q-space specified by q_x, q_y, and q_z axes representing the strength of magnetic field applied in the X, Y, and Z directions in physical space.[41,42] QSI approaches all attempt to sample q-space more systematically than DTI (which samples as few as 7 points in q-space) so that the PDF can be accurately rendered. In the case of DSI, a cloud of q-space values of varying strength and direction is required (**Fig. 4**A), typically more than 100 diffusion gradient directions with 5 different q values (synonymous with 5 different b values).[43–47] Although the number of studies that have used DSI is relatively modest at present, it is currently the only technique that fully reconstructs the PDF and allows depiction of diffusion geometries that would obscured by reduction to the DTI model (**Fig. 5**). An alternative approach, known as QBI or high angular resolution diffusion imaging (HARDI),[48] samples only along the surface of a shell of fixed q. Using a mathematical theorem known as Funk-Radon transform,[43] QBI yields

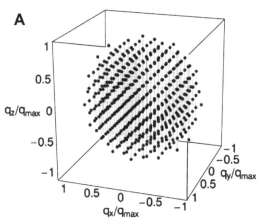
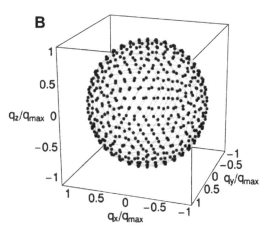

Fig. 4. Differences between DSI and QBI sampling of q-space. Whereas QSI (*A*) samples numerous points in q-space with varying q values and diffusion gradient directions (515 in the shown example), QBI (*B*) samples along the surface of a shell in q-space with fixed q. (*From* Tuch DS, Reese TG, Wiegell MR, et al. Diffusion MRI of complex neural architecture. Neuron 2003;40(5):885–95; with permission.)

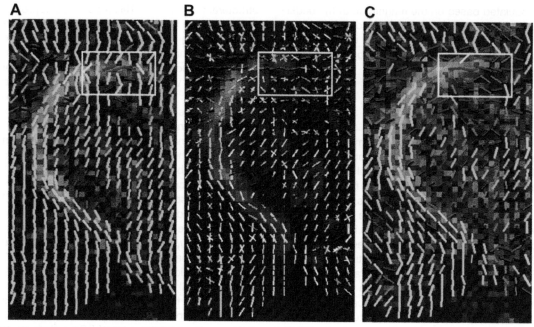

Fig. 5. Comparison of DTI and DSI data. A coronal slice of rat brain at the level of the optic tracts was analyzed using DTI and DSI techniques. The first eigenvector of the diffusion tensor (A), the ODF derived from the DSI experiment (B), and the primary orientation of the PDF/ODF from the DSI experiment (C) were plotted. In the boxed region in the vicinity of the superior colliculus, crossing fibers are resolved by DSI but are obscured by DTI. Concordance of DTI and DSI data, however, is good for the optic tract (white curvilinear superior-inferior tract visualized using manganese contrast) where fiber orientation is less complex. (*From* Lin CP, Wedeen VJ, Chen JH, et al. Validation of diffusion spectrum magnetic resonance imaging with manganese-enhanced rat optic tracts and ex vivo phantoms. Neuroimage 2003;19(3):482–95; with permission.)

a version of the PDF stripped of magnitude information, known as the orientational distribution function (ODF), and also has symmetry properties that may obscure some fiber geometries. These limitations may degrade the accuracy of FA or average diffusivity determined from QBI, but its ability to detect multidirectional diffusion geometries still far outperforms DTI in regions with crossing fibers (Fig. 6). Both QBI and DSI require higher b values than those used in typical DTI or clinical DWI (see Table 1).

One alternative to deriving the entire ODF or PDF is to quantify only the degree of deviation from normal gaussian behavior implicit in the DTI model, in mathematical terms, the excess kurtosis of the diffusion probability distribution.[49] This excess kurtosis is a direct result of nongaussian diffusional geometries (described previously), and, therefore, high excess kurtosis is interpreted as high microstructural complexity. Diffusion kurtosis images (DKIs) can be derived from DSI experiments, or they can be obtained using shorter, purpose-built diffusion MR imaging

sequences.[50] In the latter case, Equation 10 is modified to fit a nongaussian term (Equation 12):

$$DWI_n = S_o \times e^{\sum_{n=1}^{30} \left(-b \times ADC_n + \left(\frac{1}{6} \times b^2 \times (ADC_n)^2 \times K_n\right)\right)}$$

(12)

where K_n represents the apparent excess diffusional kurtosis for direction n. The mean kurtosis (MK) is then defined as the average of the K_n values for all diffusion gradient directions (30 in the Equation 12). Differences in MK have been used to separate low-grade from high-grade primary brain tumors[51] and to gauge age-related changes in the cerebral white matter.[52] However, the unique advantage of using MK compared with more traditional measures such as FA/MD awaits further research.

ACQUISITION OF DIFFUSION IMAGES

Given the exquisite sensitivity of diffusion MR imaging to small movements of protons, minimizing bulk (ie, patient) motion becomes of

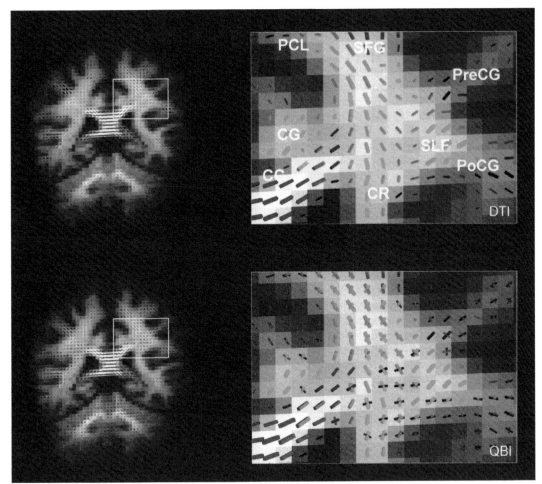

Fig. 6. Comparison of DTI to QBI. Comparison of voxelwise PDFs derived from DTI (*top row*) and low-frequency QBI (*bottom row*) for the centrum semiovale. Color encoding for each lobe of the PDF is according to standard color FA map convention. (*From* Tuch DS, Reese TG, Wiegell MR, et al. Diffusion MRI of complex neural architecture. Neuron 2003;40(5):885–95; with permission.)

paramount concern and has determined the choice of acquisition schemes for DWI and DTI experiments. SS-EPI sequences form the basis of most diffusion MR imaging protocols because they acquire an entire image slice in approximately 100 ms while offering improved SNRs compared with other rapid imaging sequences, such as SS fast spin-echo (SS-FSE).[53,54] SS-EPI sequences are typically performed with bipolar diffusion gradients or dual spin-echo–based sequences to minimize diffusion gradient-induced eddy currents that cause image distortion.[55,56] Further reduction in acquisition time is achieved using partial *k*-space reconstruction techniques that decrease the number of phase encodes required for image formation[57] and/or through multiplexed stimulation schemes enabling multiple slices to be interrogated simultaneously by SS-EPI.[58] Navigator-based SS-EPI sequences have been advocated

to correct for motion artifact[59] although seldom used in practice.

Scanner hardware must also be chosen with acquisition speed in mind. The strongest/fastest possible gradient coils are used to minimize the duration of the diffusion gradient and to obtain the best possible image resolution within the field of view (typically approximately 128 to 196 voxels or 1.5 to 2.0 mm). Parallel imaging techniques, such as sensitivity encoding (SENSE), array spatial sensitivity encoding technique (ASSET), and generalized auto-calibrating partially parallel acquisitions (GRAPPA), reduce acquisition time, and because the TE required is also decreased, there is the added benefit of reduction in the T2* susceptibility artifacts encountered in SS-EPI.[60,61] Although multichannel head coils used in parallel imaging improve SNR, SNR declines with increasing acceleration factors, and acceleration factors of 2 to 3 seem optimal.[57,62] In addition to intrinsically higher SNR,[63,64] higher field strength magnets improve the speed of parallel imaging acquisitions while limiting SNR loss with higher acceleration factors.[65,66] Tissue pulsation secondary to the cardiac cycle can be minimized through the use of cardiac gating although inclusion of gating does prolong overall acquisition time.[67,68]

There are a few special considerations for acquisition of DTI data. Although a minimum of 6 diffusion directions is required to solve the for the diffusion tensor, the SNR obtained with a number of excitations (NEX) = 1 is generally poor.[69] Because repeat acquisitions are required, many investigators have advocated using additional diffusion gradient directions (at least 20–30) rather than higher NEX values to achieve improved SNR, because they may also improve the reliability of the resulting MD/FA/tractography data.[13,70–72] There are dissenting opinions, however, on this issue.[73] Isotropic voxels of the smallest possible size are advocated for studies destined for tractography analysis to minimize the size of voxels containing crossing fibers (ie, volume averaging effect) and to avoid apparent image distortion.[27,74]

Although SS-EPI is the most widespread pulse sequence in use for diffusion MR imaging, other acquisition schemes have been proposed to address the deficiencies of SS-EPI. In particular, multishot fast spin-echo–based techniques, such as periodically rotated overlapping parallel lines with enhanced reconstruction (PROPELLER), have been advocated for their ability to correct for patient motion, decreased sensitivity to magnetic susceptibility effects, insensitivity to eddy current effects, and higher spatial resolution.[53,75,76] More recent modifications have reduced the longer acquisition time and higher specific absorption rate associated with these multishot techniques,[77,78] making them more competitive with SS-EPI–based methods. There is evidence that such FSE-based techniques may detect infarcts more sensitively[79] and yield more accurate DTI measures in the subcortical white matter[80] compared with SS-EPI techniques.

Examples of acquisition parameters for different types of diffusion MR imaging experiments are summarized in **Table 1**.

ANALYSIS OF DIFFUSION MR IMAGING DATA

Once a diffusion MR imaging experiment is completed, there are two types of data referenced to each voxel in the brain: scalar data (eg, FA and MD) and directional information, such as diffusion

tensor or PDF/ODF. These data provide a wealth of information about brain microstructure and connectivity. Although multiple types of scalar and fiber orientation analyses may be performed together in any single experiment, these analytic techniques are examined separately for clarity.

Scalar Data

Histogram analysis
The most straightforward type of diffusion MR imaging analysis is histogram analysis of whole-brain FA and MD data. The diffusion parameters are simply plotted against frequency, and because these parameters typically have near-normal distribution, parametric statistics (eg, t statistic) can be applied. This method is highly reproducible[81] and in its simplest form requires no preprocessing (eg, spatial normalization/registration) or a priori knowledge of the sites of disease. Whole-brain histogram analysis is best suited for diffuse-brain diseases that extensively involve white and/or gray matter structures. For example, histogram analysis has been used to demonstrate global increases in cerebral white matter MD as well as increased skew and variance in white matter FA/ADC with aging.[82–84] These histogram-derived measures correlate with decrease in cognitive, motor, and visual skills associated with aging.[85–89] Analogous work in patients with multiple sclerosis has demonstrated increased MD and decreased FA compared with normal controls, trends that correlate with disability scales.[90–92]

Region of interest analysis
Histogram analysis provides insight into global microstructural integrity. It overlooks, however, known brain circuits or radiographically demonstrable lesions. Therefore, analysis of specific of regions of interest (ROIs) is often required. In the simplest case, large enhancing or space-occupying lesions can be used as masks to select for relevant ROIs in the diffusion weighted images. Using such a strategy, investigators have identified MD values that discriminate poor from good responders to therapy in cases of primary CNS lymphoma[93] and recurrent glioblastoma.[94] Likewise, multiple sclerosis plaques identified on conventional imaging have been used to define ROIs for analysis (both for the lesion and contralateral normal-appearing white matter), establishing that the FA/MD abnormalities described for the whole brain are most severe at sites of MS plaques and are also present in normal-appearing white matter.[92,95–97]

The primary limitation of the ROI approach is consistent selection of ROIs, particularly when using normal anatomic landmarks for reference rather than lesions identified on conventional imaging.[98] Probabilistic segmentation[99,100] and deformation-based morphometry[101] approaches can automate and make more consistent the ROI selection process. However, transformations between conventional imaging space and diffusion imaging space can be affected by geometric distortion even within the same subject.[102] One possible solution to the problem of ROI selection lies in using the white matter tracts identified on color FA maps and tractography for anatomic reference,[76,103,104] a strategy shown to improve measurement reproducibility.[105] In one example of this approach to a group of amyotrophic lateral sclerosis (ALS) patients, the posterior limb of the internal capsule was identified for ROI analysis using tractography of the coroticospinal tract, allowing reproducible demonstration of decreased FA and increased MD in upper motor neurons.[106]

Tract-based spatial statistics

One of the more widespread algorithms for using white matter tract–based ROI selection is known as tract-based spatial statistics (TBSS), available as a module within the free Functional MRI of the Brain Analysis Group (FMRIB) Software Library (FSL) image analysis package. After an affine or nonlinear registration process and eddy current correction, TBSS constructs a skeleton consisting of the center point of the aggregated FA map for all subjects in the analysis. By analyzing white matter diffusivity within a specified radius of this skeleton (Fig. 7), grouped FA values demonstrate greatly reduced deviation from nongaussian behavior, enabling standard parametric statistics to be more reliably applied.[107,108] The approach has been successfully applied to investigations of normal aging, psychiatric disease, multiple sclerosis, neurodegenerative disease, and correlations between cognitive function and white matter structure.[109–124] Other similar techniques using white matter tract reference points have also been published, enabling determination of FA for entire tracts or regions surrounding white matter tracts.[125,126]

Voxel-based analysis

Voxel-based analysis (VBA) uses techniques first developed for group analysis of structural brain images and now is also widely used in functional MR imaging experiments.[127–129] In brief, VBA places group analysis subjects into a common 3-D space (ie, spatial normalization or registration), making analysis of any particular voxel theoretically comparable between subjects using standard parametric statistics, such as are available through widely used software packages, like FSL or SPM. Although typically registration is performed using affine (linear) spatial transformations on diffusion weighted images, FA template-based[130] or nonlinear deformation-based morphometry

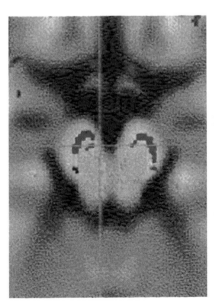
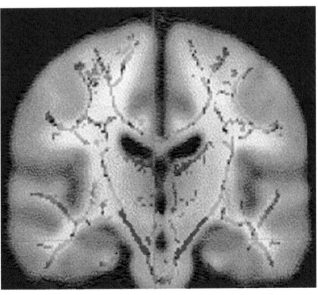

Fig. 7. TBSS results for comparison of 13 ALS patients with 20 controls. Axial (*left*) and coronal (*right*) images of the brain demonstrate the mean FA skeleton (*green*) with areas of FA decrease in ALS shown in blue and areas where FA inversely correlates with disease progression shown in red. Corticospinal tract structures are disproportionately affected as expected. (*From* Smith SM, Jenkinson M, Johansen-Berg H, et al. Tract-based spatial statistics: voxelwise analysis of multi-subject diffusion data. Neuroimage 2006;31(4):1487–505; with permission.)

techniques can also be used.[101,131–134] The VBA approach has been used to successfully aggregate subject data, for example, demonstrating hemispheric asymmetry of FA in normal subjects and loss of this asymmetry in subjects diagnosed with schizophrenia.[135,136] Potential pitfalls with VBA techniques include the variable degrees of geometric distortion secondary to magnetic susceptibility (eg, paranasal sinuses) present in different subjects as well as the fact that the size of the gaussian kernel used to blur the registered diffusion images can bias the underlying results.[137]

DTI atlases: reference values and automated ROI selection

As the number of studies reporting FA and MD abnormalities has grown, so has the need for reliable reference values for diffusion metrics specific to particular regions of the brain. Initial efforts along these lines focused on studying values in selected ROIs.[138,139] More recently, a DTI atlas was created using 81 normal subjects' DTI data and affine transformation of subject diffusion images (average of all diffusion weighted images for each subject) and associated tensor fields into standard International Consortium for Brain Mapping (ICBM)-152 space.[140] The ICBM DTI-81 atlas can generate normal reference values for FA throughout the brain, and future atlases may serve as reference guides to white matter connectivity and fiber tract measures too.

Because an atlas contains representative data from many subjects, it can also serve as a reference for performing automated white matter ROI selection. When new subjects' diffusion brain MR images were warped to ICBM DTI-81 space using nonlinear registration, the FA measures within computationally specified ROIs had good agreement with manual specification of the same regions. This approach was later extended to the subcortical white matter tracts.[141] The resulting 176 white matter regions parcellated by the ICBM DTI-81 atlas have been used to characterize both morphometric and diffusivity changes in the developing brains of children[142] (Fig. 8) and can theoretically be applied to other patient populations with grossly normal brains (eg, psychiatric patients, patients with mild traumatic brain injury, and so forth). The ICBM DTI-81 atlas also allows automated selection of ROIs for performing deterministic tractography (discussed later).[143]

Atlasing DTI data relies on accurate registration of tensor fields obtained for each subject, and the spatial transformation of a tensor field differs fundamentally from transformation of purely scalar data. In addition to displacement of voxel intensity, reorientation of the tensor's component eigenvectors is required at each voxel. The initial attempts at solving this reorientation problem have yielded satisfactory results,[144–146] but higher-precision deformable/nonlinear registration techniques for DTI data are in development,[147] for example, by devising rotationally invariant descriptors of the tensor field that can then be warped.[148]

Tractography

Tractography is the inference of nerve fascicle trajectories from DTI data and is analogous to similar procedures first developed for fluid mechanics.[27] It involves both postprocessing and comparison of summary statistics.

Deterministic tractography

The earliest and still most commonly used approach for performing DTI-based tractography

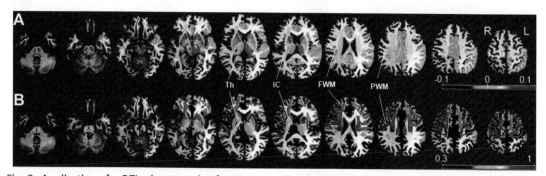

Fig. 8. Application of a DTI atlas to study of patient populations. The ICBM DTI-81 reference atlas was used to parcellate ROIs for FA measurements of 35 children between 2 and 18 years of age. The slopes (*A*) and R² values (*B*) were plotted for relationship of FA to subject age for each of 176 ROIs. A larger, positive, time dependence is observed in the brainstem, the thalamus (Th), the anterior limb of the internal capsules (IC), and the frontal and parietal white matter (FWM and PWM, respectively). (*From* Faria AV, Zhang J, Oishi K, et al. Atlas-based analysis of neurodevelopment from infancy to adulthood using diffusion tensor imaging and applications for automated abnormality detection. Neuroimage 2010;52:415–28; with permission.)

is known as deterministic or streamline tractography.[27,149–152] Perhaps the most widely used algorithm for deterministic tractography is known as fiber assignment by continuous tracking (FACT) and is included in the freely available DTIstudio package.[151,153] In this algorithm, a seed point is selected from the center of a starting voxel, and using the principal eigenvector for that voxel, the seed is displaced to the outer boundary of the voxel (**Fig. 9**A). Provided that the neighboring voxel does not exceed user specified cutoff criteria (typically FA <0.2 or turning angle >40°), the seed

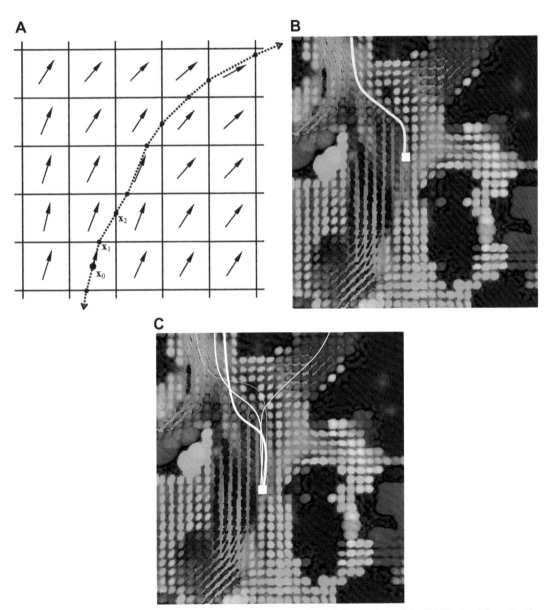

A

B

C

Fig. 9. Streamline/deterministic versus probabilistic tractography. (A) Illustration of the FACT algorithm. Starting from seed point, x_0, the path of a fiber tract (*dashed line*) is determined using the principal eigenvectors, denoted by the arrows. Once the fiber tract reaches a voxel boundary at x_1, the direction of the fiber tract is changed to that of the new voxel, subject to FA and turning angle criteria specified by the user. (B) Deterministic tractography algorithms produce a single best estimate of fiber trajectory through a given voxel. (C) In contrast, probabilistic algorithms model multiple possible trajectories through a voxel, which can be combined to produce a probability estimate for connectivity to other voxels. (*Reproduced from* Jiang H, van Zijl PC, Kim J, et al. DtiStudio: resource program for diffusion tensor computation and fiber bundle tracking. Comput Methods Programs Biomed 2006;81(2):106–16; with permission.)

is again displaced using the neighboring voxel's principal eigenvector to the neighboring voxel's border. This process is repeated until cutoff criteria are met, and by tracing the reverse direction from the original seed point, a complete tract is determined. In DTIstudio, this process is performed for all voxels in the experiment, and the resulting fiber tracts are stored. The user then specifies one or more ROIs (typically hand drawn) through which the tract of interest should or should not pass, using Boolean logic to decide which pathways are displayed (see **Fig. 9**B); constraining the fiber tracts by at least two ROIs has been shown to increase reproducibility of results.[154] The fiber tracts satisfying the user-specified constraints are then summarized by statistics (eg, mean length, fiber volume, and fiber count) and overlaid on the b0 diffusion image or any other structural MR imaging of the user's choice.

Deterministic tractography has been used in a wide variety of clinical and basic science applications. The most commonly encountered clinical application is delineation of the relationship of an intracranial mass lesion to major white matter tracts, such as the corticospinal tract,[155,156] arcuate fasciculus,[157] and optic radiations.[158,159] Use of tractography assists in selection of surgical approach, and there is evidence that it reduces operative time.[160] In cases of severely distorted underlying anatomy, the constraining ROI has been selected using activated voxels from functional MR imaging experiments.[161] When correlated with intraoperative cortical mapping, tractography of the corticospinal spinal tract has proved accurate within 1 cm.[155] Deterministic tractography has also proved useful in investigating disease processes previously inaccessible in living subjects. For instance, tractography investigations of periventricular leukomalacia have demonstrated relative preservation of the corticospinal tract and damage to other fiber tracts, including the retrolental internal capsule and the posterior thalamic radiations.[162,163] Deterministic tractography has also enabled basic investigations of white matter organization, for example, demonstrating asymmetry of white matter tracts in the brain.[164,165] As discussed previously, tractography data can be used to direct ROI-based analysis.

Probabilistic tractography

Deterministic tractography is unable to depict branching fiber tracts and forces an all-or-none choice for propagating a fiber tract, depending on FA/turning angle constraints specified by the user. The latter limitation is particularly problematic in areas of intrinsically abnormal white matter,

such as might be encountered in demyelinating or neurodegenerative disorders. Probabilistic tractography quantifies the connectivity between any two voxels using either fast marching methods[166,167] or inference of the PDF from the DTI data (eg, the algorithm used in the FDT module of the FSL software package).[168,169] Then, propagation of fiber tracts from initial seed points is repeated thousands of times using the connectivity information to statistically sample potential trajectories. Thus, multiple fiber trajectories can traverse a single voxel (see **Fig. 9**C), and the likelihood of connectivity between any two voxels can be quantified. Importantly, an FA cutoff value does not need to be specified, allowing inclusion of brain regions with microstructural abnormality.

Given the lack of strict FA cutoff criteria, probabilistic tractography is an obvious choice for delineating fiber tracts in areas of diseased white matter, and it has been applied to multiple sclerosis[170] and ALS.[171] The most popular application of probabilistic tractography, however, has been quantifying connectivity between brain ROIs. For example, it has been used to explore brain connectivity in normal subjects,[168,172] premature neonates,[173] and psychiatric patients.[174,175]

DSI/QBI-based tractography

As discussed previously, crossing fibers are poorly depicted by DTI techniques and more faithfully depicted using QBI/HARDI or DSI approaches. Although DSI and QBI techniques derive the PDF and ODF directly, tractography based on DSI/QBI experiments has so far relied primarily on adaptation of streamline rather than probabilistic tractography techniques.[46,47,176–178] As implemented in the TrackVis software package, DSI/QBI tractography is similar to FACT except that, for each directional component of the PDF/ODF, a fiber tract is displaced from the center to the edge of the seeding voxel (although in at least one published experiment, 30 seed points were randomly chosen within the starting voxel to increase accuracy[46]). At the edge of the voxel, the component of the neighboring voxel's ODF/PDF with diffusion direction closest to the original direction is chosen for propagation, subject to turning angle cutoff and optionally an MD cutoff criteria. Because the PDF/ODF is not limited to a diffusion ellipsoid, crossing fibers can be depicted (**Fig. 10**). Using automated brain parcellation techniques, whole-brain connectivity maps can then be derived. Although these connectivity maps do not quantify connectivity in the same way as probabilistic tractography, network analysis does provide a measure of "strength" of connection (ie, number of fiber tracts) between

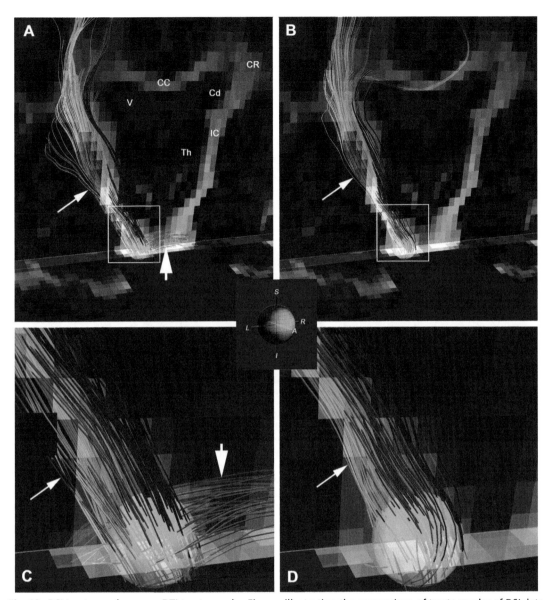

Fig. 10. DSI tractography versus DTI tractography. Figures illustrating the comparison of tractography of DSI data in low and high magnification (*A, C*) and DTI data (*B, D*) in the basis pontis of human brain in vivo. The intersections of the descending corticofugal fibers (*long stem arrow*) and transverse pontocerebellar fibers (*short stem arrow*) are seen with the DSI reconstruction, but not with DTI. CC, corpus callosum; Cd, caudate nucleus; CR, corona radiata; IC, internal capsule; Th, thalamus; V, lateral ventricle. (*From* Wedeen VJ, Wang RP, Schmahmann JD, et al. Diffusion spectrum magnetic resonance imaging [DSI] tractography of crossing fibers. Neuroimage 2008;41(4):1267–77; with permission.)

key gray matter nodes (**Fig. 11**).[46] This approach also allows individual versus group comparisons of white matter connectivity.

Groupwise analysis of tractography data
In most experiments using tractography, comparison of fiber tract metrics (volume, MD, and FA) from multiple subjects is necessary. As the number of subjects increases, the selection of constraining ROIs for tractography becomes an onerous task and subject to possible error. To automate this process and improve the reliability of summary statistics obtained for each subject, spatial normalization into a common space has been performed using reference atlases[143,179–182] or control samples.[183,184] Using the ICBM DTI-81 atlas (discussed previously),[143,185] choice of standardized ROIs on the template can be transferred

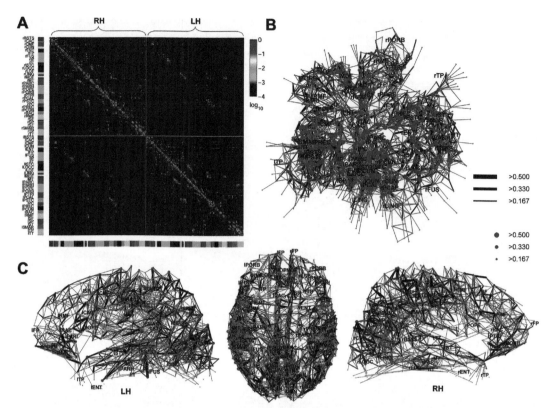

Fig. 11. DSI connectivity networks. DSI was used determine connectivity between 998 ROIs parcellated by deformation-based morphometry. (A) Matrix of fiber densities (connection weights) between all pairs of n = 998 ROIs. ROIs are plotted by cerebral hemispheres, with right-hemispheric ROIs in the upper left quadrant, left-hemispheric ROIs in the lower right quadrant, and interhemispheric connections in the upper right and lower left quadrants. The color bars at the left and bottom of the matrix correspond to the colors of 66 anatomic regions. All connections are symmetric and displayed with a logarithmic color map. (B) Kamada-Kawai force-spring layout of the connectivity backbone. Labels indicating anatomic subregions are placed at their respective centers of mass. Nodes (individual ROIs) are coded according to strength and edges are coded according to connection weight (see legend). (C) Dorsal and lateral views of the connectivity backbone. (From Hagmann P, Cammoun L, Gigandet X, et al. Mapping the structural core of human cerebral cortex. PLoS Biol 2008; 6(7):e159; with permission.)

automatically to subject brains for deterministic tractography. Conversely, subject data can be transformed into a common template space, allowing comparison of fiber tract morphology (eg, smoothness) in addition to underlying scalar data such as FA/MD.[179] As discussed previously, these approaches rely on accurate reorientation of the tensor field and will hopefully improve as deformable tensor registration techniques mature.[186,187]

Reproducibility and Validity of DTI Data

Reproducible measurements are essential for diffusion MR imaging to be a useful tool, particularly in large, multisite studies. For scalar measures, such as FA and MD, early studies established small coefficients of variation (CVs) for these measurements when obtained on the same

instrument on different days and slightly greater CVs for data obtained on different scanners.[188,189] In a recent multisite experiment using an optimized 3T protocol (cardiac-gated, 8-channel head coil, 32-direction DTI), the FA CV was less than 2% for both intersite and intrasite comparisons.[190] This study also demonstrated increased reproducibility (decreased CVs) when deformable registration or TBSS were used to select ROIs as opposed to rigid body registration of the FA map.

For tractography, it has been shown that white matter tracts have highly reproducible FA/MD measurements but less reliable tract fiber volume measurements.[190–192] In the case of the 3T experiment (discussed previously), the CVs for the FA and tract volume measured at three initial seeding ROIs were approximately 3% and 7.5%, respectively. Manual ROI placement is potentially a major source of error in tractography experiments where automation is not used, and as expected, different operators degrade the reproducibility of deterministic[193] and probabilistic[191,192] tractography. The CV is still less than 4%, however, for whole-tract FA measurements obtained by different operators.[191] Following probabilistic tractography, network measures, such as node strength and node cluster, coefficient have also been found fairly reproducible with CVs of less than a few percentage points.[194] Statistical sampling methods, such as bootstrapping, have also been introduced to improve inference of FA/MD values[195,196] and tensor orientation, including at sites of crossing fibers.[176,197–199]

The validity of tractography has been established through three lines of investigation. First, fiber tracts in the cerebrum and brainstem inferred from diffusion MR imaging experiments have been compared with gross neuroanatomic dissection from cadavers.[200–202] These studies have confirmed the connectivity of small fiber tracts, such as those connecting the inferior-superior frontal lobes and the complex morphology of

the optic radiations seen in tractography experiments.[202] Second, tracer studies have been performed using both histologic markers and MR contrast agents, such as manganese. Although dependent on anterograde transport of the marker from the site of injection, the tracer studies have established the validity of tractography in the optic pathway,[203,204] corticospinal tract,[205] corticothalamic tracts, and cortical association fibers, including to the contralateral hemisphere.[206] As expected, the degree of agreement was found to vary depending on user-specified criteria for tractography, such as FA and turning angle cutoff criteria. Third, detailed histologic analysis of myelinated fiber tracts was recently performed in concert with DSI. The accuracy of the resulting PDF was found to fall within 5.4° to 6.2°of the corresponding myelinated fiber, even in regions of the brain that contained crossing fiber tracts (Fig. 12).[207] Although the relationship of a fiber tract inferred from tractography to an actual fiber bundle remains uncertain, new diffusion MR imaging techniques have been

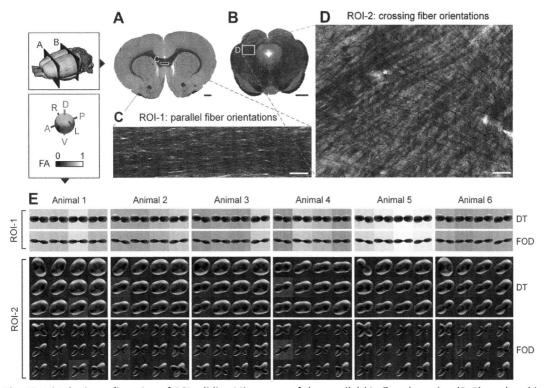

Fig. 12. Histologic confirmation of DSI validity. Microscopy of the parallel (*A, C*) and crossing (*B, D*) myeloarchitecture in two regions of the rat brain (ROI-1 and ROI-2) after myelin histologic staining. (*E*) Comparison of 3D DTI and DSI reconstructions from ROI-1 and ROI-2 across six rat specimens. Reconstructions are overlaid on a gray scale map of FA values. Scale bars, 1 mm (*A,C*) and 100 μm (*C,D*). Crossing fibers suggested by DSI data for ROI-2 are confirmed histologically. (*From* Leergaard TB, White NS, de Crespigny A, et al. Quantitative histologic validation of diffusion MRI fiber orientation distributions in the rat brain. PLoS One 2010;5(1):e8595; with permission.)

developed to quantify the distribution of axonal sizes within an ROI,[208,209] and the accuracy of these techniques has been confirmed using electron microscopy.[210]

SUMMARY

Whether used for clinical care or basic science investigation, the choice of a particular diffusion MR imaging technique and interpretation of the results relies on an understanding of the basic physical principles of the diffusion MR imaging experiment and the options for analyzing the resultant data. The authors have reviewed how application of motion-sensitizing gradients enables quantitative characterization of water diffusion in vivo. Through the application of the tensor model or through use of QSI techniques, reliable scalar measures of diffusivity and faithful representations of the water diffusion PDF can be obtained. Although comparison of scalar data is the simplest means for examining group DTI data, direct comparison of tractography and connectivity data is becoming increasingly feasible due to advances in postprocessing techniques and the availability of standardized templates for comparing subjects. These advanced techniques have become widely accessible to basic science and clinician investigators, creating new knowledge about the brain in health and disease, some of which are discussed in articles elsewhere in this issue.

REFERENCES

1. Basser PJ. Diffusion and diffusion tensor MR imaging fundamentals. In: Atlas SW, editor. Magnetic resonance imaging of the brain and spine. 4th edition. Philadelphia: Lippincott, Williams, Wilkins; 2008. p. 1752–67.

2. Le Bihan D, Breton E, Lallemand D, et al. MR imaging of intravoxel incoherent motions: application to diffusion and perfusion in neurologic disorders. Radiology 1986;161(2):401–7.

3. Thomsen C, Henriksen O, Ring P. In vivo measurement of water self diffusion in the human brain by magnetic resonance imaging. Acta Radiol 1987; 28(3):353–61.

4. Le Bihan D, Breton E, Lallemand D, et al. Separation of diffusion and perfusion in intravoxel incoherent motion MR imaging. Radiology 1988; 168(2):497–505.

5. Moseley ME, Kucharczyk J, Mintorovitch J, et al. Diffusion-weighted MR imaging of acute stroke: correlation with T2-weighted and magnetic susceptibility-enhanced MR imaging in cats. AJNR Am J Neuroradiol 1990;11(3):423–9.

6. Basser PJ, Mattiello J, LeBihan D. MR diffusion tensor spectroscopy and imaging. Biophys J 1994;66(1):259–67.

7. Savin T. Available at: http://web.mit.edu/savin/Public/.Tutorial_v1.2/Concepts.html. Accessed June 9, 2010, 2010.

8. Mukherjee P, Berman JI, Chung SW, et al. Diffusion tensor MR imaging and fiber tractography: theoretic underpinnings. AJNR Am J Neuroradiol 2008;29(4):632–41.

9. Bushberg JT, Seibert JA, Leidholdt EMJ, et al. Nuclear magnetic resonanace. The essential physics of medical imaging. 2nd edition. Philadelphia: Lippincott Williams & Wilkins; 2002. p. 373–413.

10. Stejskal EO, Tanner JE. Spin diffusion measurements: spin echoes in the presence of a time dependent field gradient. J Chem Phys 1965;42:288–92.

11. Le Bihan D. Looking into the functional architecture of the brain with diffusion MRI. Nat Rev Neurosci 2003;4(6):469–80.

12. Beaulieu C. The basis of anisotropic water diffusion in the nervous system—a technical review. NMR Biomed 2002;15(7–8):435–55.

13. Mukherjee P, Chung SW, Berman JI, et al. Diffusion tensor MR imaging and fiber tractography: technical considerations. AJNR Am J Neuroradiol 2008;29(5):843–52.

14. Mulkern RV, Gudbjartsson H, Westin CF, et al. Multi-component apparent diffusion coefficients in human brain. NMR Biomed 1999;12(1):51–62.

15. Beaulieu C, Allen PS. Water diffusion in the giant axon of the squid: implications for diffusion-weighted MRI of the nervous system. Magn Reson Med 1994;32(5):579–83.

16. Beauchamp NJ Jr, Ulug AM, Passe TJ, et al. MR diffusion imaging in stroke: review and controversies. Radiographics 1998;18(5):1269–83 [discussion: 1283–5].

17. Provenzale JM, Engelter ST, Petrella JR, et al. Use of MR exponential diffusion-weighted images to eradicate T2 "shine-through" effect. AJR Am J Roentgenol 1999;172(2):537–9.

18. Chenevert TL, Brunberg JA, Pipe JG. Anisotropic diffusion in human white matter: demonstration with MR techniques in vivo. Radiology 1990; 177(2):401–5.

19. Doran M, Hajnal JV, Van Bruggen N, et al. Normal and abnormal white matter tracts shown by MR imaging using directional diffusion weighted sequences. J Comput Assist Tomogr 1990;14(6):865–73.

20. Moseley ME, Cohen Y, Kucharczyk J, et al. Diffusion-weighted MR imaging of anisotropic water diffusion in cat central nervous system. Radiology 1990;176(2):439–45.

21. Turner R, Le Bihan D, Maier J, et al. Echo-planar imaging of intravoxel incoherent motion. Radiology 1990;177(2):407–14.

22. Moonen CT, Pekar J, de Vleeschouwer MH, et al. Restricted and anisotropic displacement of water in healthy cat brain and in stroke studied by NMR diffusion imaging. Magn Reson Med 1991;19(2): 327–32.

23. Beaulieu C, Allen PS. Determinants of anisotropic water diffusion in nerves. Magn Reson Med 1994; 31(4):394–400.

24. Norris DG. The effects of microscopic tissue parameters on the diffusion weighted magnetic resonance imaging experiment. NMR Biomed 2001;14(2):77–93.

25. Chin CL, Wehrli FW, Fan Y, et al. Assessment of axonal fiber tract architecture in excised rat spinal cord by localized NMR q-space imaging: simulations and experimental studies. Magn Reson Med 2004;52(4):733–40.

26. Pajevic S, Pierpaoli C. Color schemes to represent the orientation of anisotropic tissues from diffusion tensor data: application to white matter fiber tract mapping in the human brain. Magn Reson Med 1999;42(3):526–40.

27. Basser PJ, Pajevic S, Pierpaoli C, et al. In vivo fiber tractography using DT-MRI data. Magn Reson Med 2000;44(4):625–32.

28. Pierpaoli C, Barnett A, Pajevic S, et al. Water diffusion changes in Wallerian degeneration and their dependence on white matter architecture. Neuroimage 2001;13(6 Pt 1):1174–85.

29. Wiegell MR, Larsson HB, Wedeen VJ. Fiber crossing in human brain depicted with diffusion tensor MR imaging. Radiology 2000;217(3): 897–903.

30. Frank LR. Anisotropy in high angular resolution diffusion-weighted MRI. Magn Reson Med 2001; 45(6):935–9.

31. Pierpaoli C, Basser PJ. Toward a quantitative assessment of diffusion anisotropy. Magn Reson Med 1996;36(6):893–906.

32. Callaghan PT, Eccles CD, Xia Y. NMR microscopy of dynamic displacements: k-space and q-space imaging. J Phys E 1988;21:820–2.

33. Cory DG, Garroway AN. Measurement of translational displacement probabilities by NMR: an indicator of compartmentation. Magn Reson Med 1990;14(3):435–44.

34. Kuchel PW, Coy A, Stilbs P. NMR "diffusion-diffraction" of water revealing alignment of erythrocytes in a magnetic field and their dimensions and membrane transport characteristics. Magn Reson Med 1997;37(5):637–43.

35. Assaf Y, Cohen Y. Structural information in neuronal tissue as revealed by q-space diffusion NMR spectroscopy of metabolites in bovine optic nerve. NMR Biomed 1999;12(6):335–44.

36. Assaf Y, Cohen Y. Assignment of the water slow-diffusing component in the central nervous system using q-space diffusion MRS: implications for fiber tract imaging. Magn Reson Med 2000;43(2): 191–9.

37. Assaf Y, Mayk A, Cohen Y. Displacement imaging of spinal cord using q-space diffusion-weighted MRI. Magn Reson Med 2000;44(5):713–22.

38. King MD, Houseman J, Roussel SA, et al. q-Space imaging of the brain. Magn Reson Med 1994;32(6): 707–13.

39. King MD, Houseman J, Gadian DG, et al. Localized q-space imaging of the mouse brain. Magn Reson Med 1997;38(6):930–7.

40. Wedeen VJ, Reese TG, Tuch DS, et al. Mapping fiber orientation spectra in cerebral white matter with Fourier-transform diffusion MRI. Proc Intl Soc Magn Reson Med 2000;8:82.

41. Basser PJ. Relationships between diffusion tensor and q-space MRI. Magn Reson Med 2002;47(2): 392–7.

42. Hagmann P, Jonasson L, Maeder P, et al. Understanding diffusion MR imaging techniques: from scalar diffusion-weighted imaging to diffusion tensor imaging and beyond. Radiographics 2006; 26(Suppl 1):S205–23.

43. Tuch DS, Reese TG, Wiegell MR, et al. Diffusion MRI of complex neural architecture. Neuron 2003; 40(5):885–95.

44. Wedeen VJ, Hagmann P, Tseng WY, et al. Mapping complex tissue architecture with diffusion spectrum magnetic resonance imaging. Magn Reson Med 2005;54(6):1377–86.

45. Hagmann P, Kurant M, Gigandet X, et al. Mapping human whole-brain structural networks with diffusion MRI. PLoS One 2007;2(7):e597.

46. Hagmann P, Cammoun L, Gigandet X, et al. Mapping the structural core of human cerebral cortex. PLoS Biol 2008;6(7):e159.

47. Wedeen VJ, Wang RP, Schmahmann JD, et al. Diffusion spectrum magnetic resonance imaging (DSI) tractography of crossing fibers. Neuroimage 2008;41(4):1267–77.

48. Frank LR. Characterization of anisotropy in high angular resolution diffusion-weighted MRI. Magn Reson Med 2002;47(6):1083–99.

49. Jensen JH, Helpern JA. Quantifying non-Gaussian water diffusion by means of pulsed-field gradient MRI. Paper presented at 11th Annual Meeting of the ISMRM. Toronto, July 10–16, 2003.

50. Jensen JH, Helpern JA, Ramani A, et al. Diffusional kurtosis imaging: the quantification of non-gaussian water diffusion by means of magnetic resonance imaging. Magn Reson Med 2005; 53(6):1432–40.

51. Raab P, Hattingen E, Franz K, et al. Cerebral gliomas: diffusional kurtosis imaging analysis of microstructural differences. Radiology 2010; 254(3):876–81.

52. Falangola MF, Jensen JH, Babb JS, et al. Age-related non-Gaussian diffusion patterns in the prefrontal brain. J Magn Reson Imaging 2008; 28(6):1345–50.

53. Pipe JG, Farthing VG, Forbes KP. Multishot diffusion-weighted FSE using PROPELLER MRI. Magn Reson Med 2002;47(1):42–52.

54. Xu D, Henry RG, Mukherjee P, et al. Single-shot fast spin-echo diffusion tensor imaging of the brain and spine with head and phased array coils at 1.5 T and 3.0 T. Magn Reson Imaging 2004;22(6):751–9.

55. Alexander AL, Tsuruda JS, Parker DL. Elimination of eddy current artifacts in diffusion-weighted echo-planar images: the use of bipolar gradients. Magn Reson Med 1997;38(6):1016–21.

56. Reese TG, Heid O, Weisskoff RM, et al. Reduction of eddy-current-induced distortion in diffusion MRI using a twice-refocused spin echo. Magn Reson Med 2003;49(1):177–82.

57. Jaermann T, Pruessmann KP, Valavanis A, et al. Influence of SENSE on image properties in high-resolution single-shot echo-planar DTI. Magn Reson Med 2006;55(2):335–42.

58. Reese TG, Benner T, Wang R, et al. Halving imaging time of whole brain diffusion spectrum imaging and diffusion tractography using simultaneous image refocusing in EPI. J Magn Reson Imaging 2009;29(3):517–22.

59. Porter DA, Heidemann RM. High resolution diffusion-weighted imaging using readout-segmented echo-planar imaging, parallel imaging and a two-dimensional navigator-based reacquisition. Magn Reson Med 2009;62(2):468–75.

60. Bammer R, Auer M, Keeling SL, et al. Diffusion tensor imaging using single-shot SENSE-EPI. Magn Reson Med 2002;48(1):128–36.

61. Bammer R, Keeling SL, Augustin M, et al. Improved diffusion-weighted single-shot echo-planar imaging (EPI) in stroke using sensitivity encoding (SENSE). Magn Reson Med 2001;46(3):548–54.

62. Skare S, Newbould RD, Clayton DB, et al. Clinical multishot DW-EPI through parallel imaging with considerations of susceptibility, motion, and noise. Magn Reson Med 2007;57(5):881–90.

63. Guilfoyle DN, Suckow RF, Baslow MH. The apparent dependence of the diffusion coefficient of N-acetylaspartate upon magnetic field strength: evidence of an interaction with NMR methodology. NMR Biomed 2003;16(8):468–74.

64. Kuhl CK, Textor J, Gieseke J, et al. Acute and subacute ischemic stroke at high-field-strength (3.0-T) diffusion-weighted MR imaging: intraindividual comparative study. Radiology 2005;234(2):509–16.

65. Wiesinger F, Van de Moortele PF, Adriany G, et al. Parallel imaging performance as a function of field strength–an experimental investigation using electrodynamic scaling. Magn Reson Med 2004; 52(5):953–64.

66. Wiesinger F, Van de Moortele PF, Adriany G, et al. Potential and feasibility of parallel MRI at high field. NMR Biomed 2006;19(3):368–78.

67. Chien D, Buxton RB, Kwong KK, et al. MR diffusion imaging of the human brain. J Comput Assist Tomogr 1990;14(4):514–20.

68. Skare S, Andersson JL. On the effects of gating in diffusion imaging of the brain using single shot EPI. Magn Reson Imaging 2001;19(8):1125–8.

69. Basser PJ, Pierpaoli C. A simplified method to measure the diffusion tensor from seven MR images. Magn Reson Med 1998;39(6):928–34.

70. Batchelor PG, Atkinson D, Hill DL, et al. Anisotropic noise propagation in diffusion tensor MRI sampling schemes. Magn Reson Med 2003;49(6):1143–51.

71. Jones DK. The effect of gradient sampling schemes on measures derived from diffusion tensor MRI: a Monte Carlo study. Magn Reson Med 2004;51(4):807–15.

72. Ni H, Kavcic V, Zhu T, et al. Effects of number of diffusion gradient directions on derived diffusion tensor imaging indices in human brain. AJNR Am J Neuroradiol 2006;27(8):1776–81.

73. Landman BA, Farrell JA, Jones CK, et al. Effects of diffusion weighting schemes on the reproducibility of DTI-derived fractional anisotropy, mean diffusivity, and principal eigenvector measurements at 1.5T. Neuroimage 2007;36(4):1123–38.

74. Alexander AL, Hasan KM, Lazar M, et al. Analysis of partial volume effects in diffusion-tensor MRI. Magn Reson Med 2001;45(5):770–80.

75. Cheryauka AB, Lee JN, Samsonov AA, et al. MRI diffusion tensor reconstruction with PROPELLER data acquisition. Magn Reson Imaging 2004; 22(2):139–48.

76. Liu C, Bammer R, Kim DH, et al. Self-navigated interleaved spiral (SNAILS): application to high-resolution diffusion tensor imaging. Magn Reson Med 2004;52(6):1388–96.

77. Pipe JG, Zwart N. Turboprop: improved PROPELLER imaging. Magn Reson Med 2006; 55(2):380–5.

78. Wang FN, Huang TY, Lin FH, et al. PROPELLER EPI: an MRI technique suitable for diffusion tensor imaging at high field strength with reduced geometric distortions. Magn Reson Med 2005; 54(5):1232–40.

79. Forbes KP, Pipe JG, Karis JP, et al. Improved image quality and detection of acute cerebral infarction with PROPELLER diffusion-weighted MR imaging. Radiology 2002;225(2):551–5.

80. Gui M, Peng H, Carew JD, et al. A tractography comparison between turboprop and spin-echo echo-planar diffusion tensor imaging. Neuroimage 2008;42(4):1451–62.

81. Steens SC, Admiraal-Behloul F, Schaap JA, et al. Reproducibility of brain ADC histograms. Eur Radiol 2004;14(3):425–30.

82. Benedetti B, Charil A, Rovaris M, et al. Influence of aging on brain gray and white matter changes assessed by conventional, MT, and DT MRI. Neurology 2006;66(4):535–9.

83. Nusbaum AO, Tang CY, Buchsbaum MS, et al. Regional and global changes in cerebral diffusion with normal aging. AJNR Am J Neuroradiol 2001; 22(1):136–42.

84. Rovaris M, Iannucci G, Cercignani M, et al. Age-related changes in conventional, magnetization transfer, and diffusion-tensor MR imaging findings: study with whole-brain tissue histogram analysis. Radiology 2003;227(3):731–8.

85. Charlton RA, Barrick TR, McIntyre DJ, et al. White matter damage on diffusion tensor imaging correlates with age-related cognitive decline. Neurology 2006;66(2):217–22.

86. Charlton RA, Landau S, Schiavone F, et al. A structural equation modeling investigation of age-related variance in executive function and DTI measured white matter damage. Neurobiol Aging 2008;29(10):1547–55.

87. Charlton RA, Schiavone F, Barrick TR, et al. Diffusion tensor imaging detects age related white matter change over a 2 year follow-up which is associated with working memory decline. J Neurol Neurosurg Psychiatry 2010;81(1):13–9.

88. Grieve SM, Williams LM, Paul RH, et al. Cognitive aging, executive function, and fractional anisotropy: a diffusion tensor MR imaging study. AJNR Am J Neuroradiol 2007;28(2):226–35.

89. Della Nave R, Foresti S, Pratesi A, et al. Whole-brain histogram and voxel-based analyses of diffusion tensor imaging in patients with leukoaraiosis: correlation with motor and cognitive impairment. AJNR Am J Neuroradiol 2007;28(7):1313–9.

90. Cercignani M, Inglese M, Pagani E, et al. Mean diffusivity and fractional anisotropy histograms of patients with multiple sclerosis. AJNR Am J Neuroradiol 2001;22(5):952–8.

91. Nusbaum AO. Diffusion tensor MR imaging of gray matter in different multiple sclerosis phenotypes. AJNR Am J Neuroradiol 2002;23(6):899–900.

92. Rovaris M, Bozzali M, Iannucci G, et al. Assessment of normal-appearing white and gray matter in patients with primary progressive multiple sclerosis: a diffusion-tensor magnetic resonance imaging study. Arch Neurol 2002;59(9):1406–12.

93. Barajas RF Jr, Rubenstein JL, Chang JS, et al. Diffusion-weighted MR imaging derived apparent diffusion coefficient is predictive of clinical outcome in primary central nervous system lymphoma. AJNR Am J Neuroradiol 2010;31(1):60–6.

94. Pope WB, Kim HJ, Huo J, et al. Recurrent glioblastoma multiforme: ADC histogram analysis predicts response to bevacizumab treatment. Radiology 2009;252(1):182–9.

95. Rocca MA, Cercignani M, Iannucci G, et al. Weekly diffusion-weighted imaging of normal-appearing white matter in MS. Neurology 2000;55(6):882–4.

96. Rovaris M, Agosta F, Pagani E, et al. Diffusion tensor MR imaging. Neuroimaging Clin N Am 2009;19(1):37–43.

97. Werring DJ, Brassat D, Droogan AG, et al. The pathogenesis of lesions and normal-appearing white matter changes in multiple sclerosis: a serial diffusion MRI study. Brain 2000;123(Pt 8):1667–76.

98. Bilgili Y, Unal B. Effect of region of interest on inter-observer variance in apparent diffusion coefficient measures. AJNR Am J Neuroradiol 2004;25(1):108–11.

99. Anbeek P, Vincken KL, van Bochove GS, et al. Probabilistic segmentation of brain tissue in MR imaging. Neuroimage 2005;27(4):795–804.

100. Fischl B, Salat DH, Busa E, et al. Whole brain segmentation: automated labeling of neuroanatomical structures in the human brain. Neuron 2002; 33(3):341–55.

101. Klein A, Andersson J, Ardekani BA, et al. Evaluation of 14 nonlinear deformation algorithms applied to human brain MRI registration. Neuroimage 2009; 46(3):786–802.

102. Kumazawa S, Yoshiura T, Honda H, et al. Partial volume estimation and segmentation of brain tissue based on diffusion tensor MRI. Med Phys 2010; 37(4):1482–90.

103. Klein J, Stuke H, Rexilius J, et al. Towards user-independent DTI quantification. Proc SPIE 2008; 6914:E6911–8.

104. Jones DK, Travis AR, Eden G, et al. PASTA: pointwise assessment of streamline tractography attributes. Magn Reson Med 2005;53(6):1462–7.

105. Partridge SC, Mukherjee P, Berman JI, et al. Tractography-based quantitation of diffusion tensor imaging parameters in white matter tracts of preterm newborns. J Magn Reson Imaging 2005; 22(4):467–74.

106. Wang S, Poptani H, Woo JH, et al. Amyotrophic lateral sclerosis: diffusion-tensor and chemical shift MR imaging at 3.0 T. Radiology 2006;239(3):831–8.

107. Smith SM, Jenkinson M, Johansen-Berg H, et al. Tract-based spatial statistics: voxelwise analysis of multi-subject diffusion data. Neuroimage 2006; 31(4):1487–505.

108. Smith SM, Johansen-Berg H, Jenkinson M, et al. Acquisition and voxelwise analysis of multi-subject diffusion data with tract-based spatial statistics. Nat Protoc 2007;2(3):499–503.

109. Della Nave R, Ginestroni A, Tessa C, et al. Brain white matter tracts degeneration in Friedreich

ataxia. An in vivo MRI study using tract-based spatial statistics and voxel-based morphometry. Neuroimage 2008;40(1):19–25.

110. Della Nave R, Ginestroni A, Tessa C, et al. Brain white matter damage in SCA1 and SCA2. An in vivo study using voxel-based morphometry, histogram analysis of mean diffusivity and tract-based spatial statistics. Neuroimage 2008;43(1):10–9.

111. Giorgio A, Watkins KE, Douaud G, et al. Changes in white matter microstructure during adolescence. Neuroimage 2008;39(1):52–61.

112. Qiu D, Tan LH, Zhou K, et al. Diffusion tensor imaging of normal white matter maturation from late childhood to young adulthood: voxel-wise evaluation of mean diffusivity, fractional anisotropy, radial and axial diffusivities, and correlation with reading development. Neuroimage 2008;41(2):223–32.

113. Versace A, Almeida JR, Hassel S, et al. Elevated left and reduced right orbitomedial prefrontal fractional anisotropy in adults with bipolar disorder revealed by tract-based spatial statistics. Arch Gen Psychiatry 2008;65(9):1041–52.

114. Ciccarelli O, Behrens TE, Johansen-Berg H, et al. Investigation of white matter pathology in ALS and PLS using tract-based spatial statistics. Hum Brain Mapp 2009;30(2):615–24.

115. Roosendaal SD, Geurts JJ, Vrenken H, et al. Regional DTI differences in multiple sclerosis patients. Neuroimage 2009;44(4):1397–403.

116. Barrick TR, Charlton RA, Clark CA, et al. White matter structural decline in normal ageing: a prospective longitudinal study using tract-based spatial statistics. Neuroimage 2010;51(2):565–77.

117. Burzynska AZ, Preuschhof C, Backman L, et al. Age-related differences in white matter microstructure: region-specific patterns of diffusivity. Neuroimage 2010;49(3):2104–12.

118. Cheng Y, Chou KH, Chen IY, et al. Atypical development of white matter microstructure in adolescents with autism spectrum disorders. Neuroimage 2010;50(3):873–82.

119. Giorgio A, Palace J, Johansen-Berg H, et al. Relationships of brain white matter microstructure with clinical and MR measures in relapsing-remitting multiple sclerosis. J Magn Reson Imaging 2010;31(2):309–16.

120. Giorgio A, Watkins KE, Chadwick M, et al. Longitudinal changes in grey and white matter during adolescence. Neuroimage 2010;49(1):94–103.

121. Govindan RM, Makki MI, Wilson BJ, et al. Abnormal water diffusivity in corticostriatal projections in children with Tourette syndrome. Hum Brain Mapp 2010;31:1665–74.

122. Kochunov P, Coyle T, Lancaster J, et al. Processing speed is correlated with cerebral health markers in the frontal lobes as quantified by neuroimaging. Neuroimage 2010;49(2):1190–9.

123. Nave RD, Ginestroni A, Tessa C, et al. Regional distribution and clinical correlates of white matter structural damage in Huntington disease: a tract-based spatial statistics study. AJNR Am J Neuroradiol 2010;31:1675–81.

124. Raz E, Cercignani M, Sbardella E, et al. Clinically isolated syndrome suggestive of multiple sclerosis: voxelwise regional investigation of white and gray matter. Radiology 2010;254(1):227–34.

125. Hua K, Zhang J, Wakana S, et al. Tract probability maps in stereotaxic spaces: analyses of white matter anatomy and tract-specific quantification. Neuroimage 2008;39(1):336–47.

126. O'Donnell LJ, Westin CF, Golby AJ. Tract-based morphometry for white matter group analysis. Neuroimage 2009;45(3):832–44.

127. Ashburner J, Friston KJ. Voxel-based morphometry—the methods. Neuroimage 2000;11(6 Pt 1):805–21.

128. Jenkinson M, Bannister P, Brady M, et al. Improved optimization for the robust and accurate linear registration and motion correction of brain images. Neuroimage 2002;17(2):825–41.

129. Friston KJ, Ashburner J, Frith CD, et al. Spatial registration and normalization of images. Hum Brain Mapp 1995;3(3):165–89.

130. Abe O, Takao H, Gonoi W, et al. Voxel-based analysis of the diffusion tensor. Neuroradiology 2010;52:699–710.

131. Boardman JP, Counsell SJ, Rueckert D, et al. Abnormal deep grey matter development following preterm birth detected using deformation-based morphometry. Neuroimage 2006;32(1):70–8.

132. Verma R, Mori S, Shen D, et al. Spatiotemporal maturation patterns of murine brain quantified by diffusion tensor MRI and deformation-based morphometry. Proc Natl Acad Sci U S A 2005;102(19):6978–83.

133. Zollei L, Stevens A, Huber K, et al. Improved tractography alignment using combined volumetric and surface registration. Neuroimage 2010;51(1):206–13.

134. Ceritoglu C, Oishi K, Li X, et al. Multi-contrast large deformation diffeomorphic metric mapping for diffusion tensor imaging. Neuroimage 2009;47(2):618–27.

135. Buchel C, Raedler T, Sommer M, et al. White matter asymmetry in the human brain: a diffusion tensor MRI study. Cereb Cortex 2004;14(9):945–51.

136. Park HJ, Westin CF, Kubicki M, et al. White matter hemisphere asymmetries in healthy subjects and in schizophrenia: a diffusion tensor MRI study. Neuroimage 2004;23(1):213–23.

137. Jones DK, Symms MR, Cercignani M, et al. The effect of filter size on VBM analyses of DT-MRI data. Neuroimage 2005;26(2):546–54.

138. Shimony JS, McKinstry RC, Akbudak E, et al. Quantitative diffusion-tensor anisotropy brain MR imaging: normative human data and anatomic analysis. Radiology 1999;212(3):770–84.

139. Reich DS, Smith SA, Jones CK, et al. Quantitative characterization of the corticospinal tract at 3T. AJNR Am J Neuroradiol 2006;27(10):2168–78.

140. Mori S, Oishi K, Jiang H, et al. Stereotaxic white matter atlas based on diffusion tensor imaging in an ICBM template. Neuroimage 2008;40(2):570–82.

141. Oishi K, Zilles K, Amunts K, et al. Human brain white matter atlas: identification and assignment of common anatomical structures in superficial white matter. Neuroimage 2008;43(3):447–57.

142. Faria AV, Zhang J, Oishi K, et al. Atlas-based analysis of neurodevelopment from infancy to adulthood using diffusion tensor imaging and applications for automated abnormality detection. Neuroimage 2010;52:415–28.

143. Zhang W, Olivi A, Hertig SJ, et al. Automated fiber tracking of human brain white matter using diffusion tensor imaging. Neuroimage 2008;42(2):771–7.

144. Park HJ, Kubicki M, Shenton ME, et al. Spatial normalization of diffusion tensor MRI using multiple channels. Neuroimage 2003;20(4):1995–2009.

145. Alexander DC, Pierpaoli C, Basser PJ, et al. Spatial transformations of diffusion tensor magnetic resonance images. IEEE Trans Med Imaging 2001;20(11):1131–9.

146. Xu D, Mori S, Shen D, et al. Spatial normalization of diffusion tensor fields. Magn Reson Med 2003;50(1):175–82.

147. Zhang H, Yushkevich PA, Alexander DC, et al. Deformable registration of diffusion tensor MR images with explicit orientation optimization. Med Image Anal 2006;10(5):764–85.

148. Ingalhalikar M, Yang J, Davatzikos C, et al. DTI-DROID: diffusion tensor imaging-deformable registration using orientation and intensity descriptors. Int J Imaging Syst Technol 2010;20:99–107.

149. Conturo TE, Lori NF, Cull TS, et al. Tracking neuronal fiber pathways in the living human brain. Proc Natl Acad Sci U S A 1999;96(18):10422–7.

150. Jones DK, Simmons A, Williams SC, et al. Non-invasive assessment of axonal fiber connectivity in the human brain via diffusion tensor MRI. Magn Reson Med 1999;42(1):37–41.

151. Mori S, Crain BJ, Chacko VP, et al. Three-dimensional tracking of axonal projections in the brain by magnetic resonance imaging. Ann Neurol 1999;45(2):265–9.

152. Poupon C, Clark CA, Frouin V, et al. Regularization of diffusion-based direction maps for the tracking of brain white matter fascicles. Neuroimage 2000;12(2):184–95.

153. Jiang H, van Zijl PC, Kim J, et al. DtiStudio: resource program for diffusion tensor computation and fiber bundle tracking. Comput Methods Programs Biomed 2006;81(2):106–16.

154. Huang H, Zhang J, van Zijl PC, et al. Analysis of noise effects on DTI-based tractography using the brute-force and multi-ROI approach. Magn Reson Med 2004;52(3):559–65.

155. Berman JI, Berger MS, Chung SW, et al. Accuracy of diffusion tensor magnetic resonance imaging tractography assessed using intraoperative subcortical stimulation mapping and magnetic source imaging. J Neurosurg 2007;107(3):488–94.

156. Kamada K, Sawamura Y, Takeuchi F, et al. Functional identification of the primary motor area by corticospinal tractography. Neurosurgery 2007;61(Suppl 1):166–76 [discussion: 176–7].

157. Kamada K, Todo T, Masutani Y, et al. Visualization of the frontotemporal language fibers by tractography combined with functional magnetic resonance imaging and magnetoencephalography. J Neurosurg 2007;106(1):90–8.

158. Nilsson D, Starck G, Ljungberg M, et al. Intersubject variability in the anterior extent of the optic radiation assessed by tractography. Epilepsy Res 2007;77(1):11–6.

159. Okada T, Miki Y, Kikuta K, et al. Diffusion tensor fiber tractography for arteriovenous malformations: quantitative analyses to evaluate the corticospinal tract and optic radiation. AJNR Am J Neuroradiol 2007;28(6):1107–13.

160. Bello L, Gambini A, Castellano A, et al. Motor and language DTI Fiber Tracking combined with intraoperative subcortical mapping for surgical removal of gliomas. Neuroimage 2008;39(1):369–82.

161. Schonberg T, Pianka P, Hendler T, et al. Characterization of displaced white matter by brain tumors using combined DTI and fMRI. Neuroimage 2006;30(4):1100–11.

162. Hoon AH Jr, Lawrie WT Jr, Melhem ER, et al. Diffusion tensor imaging of periventricular leukomalacia shows affected sensory cortex white matter pathways. Neurology 2002;59(5):752–6.

163. Nagae LM, Hoon AH Jr, Stashinko E, et al. Diffusion tensor imaging in children with periventricular leukomalacia: variability of injuries to white matter tracts. AJNR Am J Neuroradiol 2007;28(7):1213–22.

164. Nucifora PG, Verma R, Melhem ER, et al. Leftward asymmetry in relative fiber density of the arcuate fasciculus. Neuroreport 2005;16(8):791–4.

165. Barrick TR, Lawes IN, Mackay CE, et al. White matter pathway asymmetry underlies functional lateralization. Cereb Cortex 2007;17(3):591–8.

166. Parker GJ, Haroon HA, Wheeler-Kingshott CA. A framework for a streamline-based probabilistic index of connectivity (PICo) using a structural

interpretation of MRI diffusion measurements. J Magn Reson Imaging 2003;18(2):242–54.

167. Parker GJ, Wheeler-Kingshott CA, Barker GJ. Estimating distributed anatomical connectivity using fast marching methods and diffusion tensor imaging. IEEE Trans Med Imaging 2002;21(5): 505–12.

168. Behrens TE, Johansen-Berg H, Woolrich MW, et al. Non-invasive mapping of connections between human thalamus and cortex using diffusion imaging. Nat Neurosci 2003;6(7):750–7.

169. Behrens TE, Woolrich MW, Jenkinson M, et al. Characterization and propagation of uncertainty in diffusion-weighted MR imaging. Magn Reson Med 2003;50(5):1077–88.

170. Cader S, Johansen-Berg H, Wylezinska M, et al. Discordant white matter N-acetylasparate and diffusion MRI measures suggest that chronic metabolic dysfunction contributes to axonal pathology in multiple sclerosis. Neuroimage 2007;36(1): 19–27.

171. Ciccarelli O, Behrens TE, Altmann DR, et al. Probabilistic diffusion tractography: a potential tool to assess the rate of disease progression in amyotrophic lateral sclerosis. Brain 2006;129(Pt 7): 1859–71.

172. Croxson PL, Johansen-Berg H, Behrens TE, et al. Quantitative investigation of connections of the prefrontal cortex in the human and macaque using probabilistic diffusion tractography. J Neurosci 2005;25(39):8854–66.

173. Counsell SJ, Dyet LE, Larkman DJ, et al. Thalamo-cortical connectivity in children born preterm mapped using probabilistic magnetic resonance tractography. Neuroimage 2007;34(3):896–904.

174. Price G, Cercignani M, Parker GJ, et al. Abnormal brain connectivity in first-episode psychosis: a diffusion MRI tractography study of the corpus callosum. Neuroimage 2007;35(2):458–66.

175. Gutman DA, Holtzheimer PE, Behrens TE, et al. A tractography analysis of two deep brain stimulation white matter targets for depression. Biol Psychiatry 2009;65(4):276–82.

176. Berman JI, Chung S, Mukherjee P, et al. Probabilistic streamline q-ball tractography using the residual bootstrap. Neuroimage 2008;39(1): 215–22.

177. Wahl M, Barkovich AJ, Mukherjee P. Diffusion imaging and tractography of congenital brain malformations. Pediatr Radiol 2010;40(1):59–67.

178. Wahl M, Strominger Z, Jeremy RJ, et al. Variability of homotopic and heterotopic callosal connectivity in partial agenesis of the corpus callosum: a 3T diffusion tensor imaging and Q-ball tractography study. AJNR Am J Neuroradiol 2009;30(2):282–9.

179. Pai D, Soltanian-Zadeh H, Hua J. Evaluation of fiber bundles across subjects through brain mapping and registration of diffusion tensor data. Neuroimage 2011;54:S165–75.

180. Clayden JD, Storkey AJ, Munoz Maniega S, et al. Reproducibility of tract segmentation between sessions using an unsupervised modelling-based approach. Neuroimage 2009;45(2):377–85.

181. Goodlett CB, Fletcher PT, Gilmore JH, et al. Group statistics of DTI fiber bundles using spatial functions of tensor measures. Med Image Comput Comput Assist Interv 2008;11(Pt 1):1068–75.

182. Goodlett CB, Fletcher PT, Gilmore JH, et al. Group analysis of DTI fiber tract statistics with application to neurodevelopment. Neuroimage 2009;45(Suppl 1): S133–42.

183. Ciccarelli O, Toosy AT, Parker GJ, et al. Diffusion tractography based group mapping of major white-matter pathways in the human brain. Neuroimage 2003;19(4):1545–55.

184. Avants BB, Cook PA, Ungar L, et al. Dementia induces correlated reductions in white matter integrity and cortical thickness: a multivariate neuroimaging study with sparse canonical correlation analysis. Neuroimage 2010;50(3):1004–16.

185. Zhang Y, Zhang J, Oishi K, et al. Atlas-guided tract reconstruction for automated and comprehensive examination of the white matter anatomy. Neuroimage 2010;52:1289–301.

186. Zhang H, Awate SP, Das SR, et al. A tract-specific framework for white matter morphometry combining macroscopic and microscopic tract features. Med Image Comput Comput Assist Interv 2009;12(Pt 2):141–9.

187. Yushkevich PA, Zhang H, Simon TJ, et al. Structure-specific statistical mapping of white matter tracts. Neuroimage 2008;41(2):448–61.

188. Cercignani M, Bammer R, Sormani MP, et al. Inter-sequence and inter-imaging unit variability of diffusion tensor MR imaging histogram-derived metrics of the brain in healthy volunteers. AJNR Am J Neuroradiol 2003;24(4):638–43.

189. Pfefferbaum A, Adalsteinsson E, Sullivan EV. Replicability of diffusion tensor imaging measurements of fractional anisotropy and trace in brain. J Magn Reson Imaging 2003;18(4):427–33.

190. Vollmar C, O'Muircheartaigh J, Barker GJ, et al. Identical, but not the same: intra-site and inter-site reproducibility of fractional anisotropy measures on two 3.0T scanners. Neuroimage 2010;51(4):1384–94.

191. Ciccarelli O, Parker GJ, Toosy AT, et al. From diffusion tractography to quantitative white matter tract measures: a reproducibility study. Neuroimage 2003;18(2):348–59.

192. Heiervang E, Behrens TE, Mackay CE, et al. Between session reproducibility and between subject variability of diffusion MR and tractography measures. Neuroimage 2006;33(3):867–77.

193. Wakana S, Caprihan A, Panzenboeck MM, et al. Reproducibility of quantitative tractography methods applied to cerebral white matter. Neuroimage 2007;36(3):630–44.

194. Vaessen MJ, Hofman PA, Tijssen HN, et al. The effect and reproducibility of different clinical DTI gradient sets on small world brain connectivity measures. Neuroimage 2010;51(3):1106–16.

195. Zhu T, Liu X, Connelly PR, et al. An optimized wild bootstrap method for evaluation of measurement uncertainties of DTI-derived parameters in human brain. Neuroimage 2008;40(3):1144–56.

196. Chung S, Pelletier D, Sdika M, et al. Whole brain voxel-wise analysis of single-subject serial DTI by permutation testing. Neuroimage 2008;39(4): 1693–705.

197. Jones DK. Determining and visualizing uncertainty in estimates of fiber orientation from diffusion tensor MRI. Magn Reson Med 2003;49(1):7–12.

198. Jones DK, Pierpaoli C. Confidence mapping in diffusion tensor magnetic resonance imaging tractography using a bootstrap approach. Magn Reson Med 2005;53(5):1143–9.

199. Lazar M, Alexander AL. Bootstrap white matter tractography (BOOT-TRAC). Neuroimage 2005; 24(2):524–32.

200. Stieltjes B, Kaufmann WE, van Zijl PC, et al. Diffusion tensor imaging and axonal tracking in the human brainstem. Neuroimage 2001;14(3):723–35.

201. Catani M, Howard RJ, Pajevic S, et al. Virtual in vivo interactive dissection of white matter fasciculi in the human brain. Neuroimage 2002;17(1):77–94.

202. Lawes IN, Barrick TR, Murugam V, et al. Atlas-based segmentation of white matter tracts of the human brain using diffusion tensor tractography and comparison with classical dissection. Neuroimage 2008;39(1):62–79.

203. Lin CP, Tseng WY, Cheng HC, et al. Validation of diffusion tensor magnetic resonance axonal fiber imaging with registered manganese-enhanced optic tracts. Neuroimage 2001;14(5):1035–47.

204. Yamada M, Momoshima S, Masutani Y, et al. Diffusion-tensor neuronal fiber tractography and manganese-enhanced MR imaging of primate visual pathway in the common marmoset: preliminary results. Radiology 2008;249(3):855–64.

205. Dauguet J, Peled S, Berezovskii V, et al. Comparison of fiber tracts derived from in-vivo DTI tractography with 3D histological neural tract tracer reconstruction on a macaque brain. Neuroimage 2007;37(2):530–8.

206. Dyrby TB, Sogaard LV, Parker GJ, et al. Validation of in vitro probabilistic tractography. Neuroimage 2007;37(4):1267–77.

207. Leergaard TB, White NS, de Crespigny A, et al. Quantitative histological validation of diffusion MRI fiber orientation distributions in the rat brain. PLoS One 2010;5(1):e8595.

208. Assaf Y, Blumenfeld-Katzir T, Yovel Y, et al. AxCaliber: a method for measuring axon diameter distribution from diffusion MRI. Magn Reson Med 2008; 59(6):1347–54.

209. Alexander DC, Hubbard PL, Hall MG, et al. Orientationally invariant indices of axon diameter and density from diffusion MRI. Neuroimage 2010;52: 1374–89.

210. Barazany D, Basser PJ, Assaf Y. In vivo measurement of axon diameter distribution in the corpus callosum of rat brain. Brain 2009;132(Pt 5): 1210–20.

211. Wahl M, Lauterbach-Soon B, Hattingen E, et al. Human motor corpus callosum: topography, somatotopy, and link between microstructure and function. J Neurosci 2007;27(45):12132–8.

Diffusion MR Imaging: An Important Tool in the Assessment of Brain Tumors

L. Celso Hygino da Cruz Jr, MD[a,b,c,*],
Isabela Garcia Vieira, MD[a], Romeu C. Domingues, MD[a,c]

KEYWORDS

• Brain tumors • Diffusion-weighted imaging
• Diffusion tensor imaging

In the United States, approximately 40,000 new cases of malignant and nonmalignant brain neoplasm are diagnosed annually, and it is estimated that brain tumors cause the deaths of 13,000 patients every year. The prevalence of primary neoplasms of the central nervous system (CNS) is around 15,000 to 17,000 new cases each year. Although this incidence annually represents only 1.3% of all new cases of cancer, brain tumors correspond to 2.3% of all deaths caused by cancer. Brain metastases occur in around 100,000 persons annually with malignancy elsewhere in the body, approximately 30% of all patients with disseminated cancer.[1] When metastatic lesions are included, brain tumors are estimated to cause the death of 90,000 patients every year.[2–4] Gliomas are the leading cause of primary CNS tumor, accounting for 40% to 50% of cases[5] and 2% to 3% of all cancers.[6] The mortality rate of primary malignant brain tumors is around 4 per 100,000 person-year.[7,8] Despite new treatment approaches, patient survival still remains very low, varying between 16 and 53 weeks.[9]

For more than 20 years, conventional MR imaging, typically T1- and T2-weighted imaging, has been used for assessing brain tumors including initial detection, diagnosis, guiding intervention, monitoring after therapy, and overall prognosis.[10] Surgical excision of the visible abnormality is often attempted, despite a consensus that conventional MR imaging has a tendency to underestimate the extent of the tumor, which in turn, many suspect, leads to suboptimal treatment.[11] In part this is because most primary brain neoplasms, especially high-grade gliomas, infiltrate the brain parenchyma out beyond the enhancing portion of the lesion. This infiltration appears to follow the main fiber bundles, possibly along the vessel channels, without disrupting the blood-brain barrier.[12] Many other imaging techniques are under development to attempt to address these and other issues.[13]

New advanced MR imaging tools have been widely used to determine the grade, heterogeneity, and extent of brain tumors. Diffusion-weighted imaging (DWI) has been studied extensively in the evaluation of brain tumors; helping, for example, in tumor grading, differential diagnosis, and postoperative evaluation. Diffusion tensor imaging (DTI) has the apparent ability to illustrate the relationship of a tumor with the nearby main fiber tracts, delineating more accurately the tumor versus the infiltrating tumor between the peritumoral edema

[a] Clinics CDPI and Multi-Imagem, Rua Saddock de Sá 266, Rio de Janeiro, Brazil
[b] Clinics IRM Rua Capitao Salomao 44, Rio de Janeiro, Brazil
[c] Department of Radiology, Federal University of Rio de Janeiro, Rio de Janeiro, Brazil
* Corresponding author. Avenue Pasteur 162/401, Rio de Janeiro, CEP 22290-240, Brazil.
E-mail address: celsohygino@hotmail.com

Neuroimag Clin N Am 21 (2011) 27–49
doi:10.1016/j.nic.2011.01.010
1052-5149/11/$ – see front matter © 2011 Elsevier Inc. All rights reserved.

and the normal brain parenchyma.[13] More recently, it has been suggested that DTI might be used to aid in surgical planning,[14] be helpful in radiotherapy planning,[15] and to monitor the tumor recurrence and tumor response to treatment.[16] A preoperative approach that maps, even imperfectly, the tumor and its relationship to nearby functional structures may facilitate the patient's outcome[17] because a complete-as-possible lesion resection that does not harm vital brain functions is always desired.[18,19] Although these new applications have not been proven or even widely studied in multicenter clinical trials, many individual practitioners are actively using DTI.

CLINICAL USE
Assessment of Extracranial Tumors

Epidermoid tumor
As the signal intensity of epidermoid tumor is frequently quite similar to cerebrospinal fluid on conventional T1- and T2-weighted images, its diagnosis can be challenging in clinical practice. Arachnoid cysts may have a similar appearance on conventional MR imaging, complicating the

differential diagnosis between these two extra-axial lesions.[20] DWI can be used as an effective way of differentiating an arachnoid cyst from epidermoid tumors.[21] Both lesions present the same T1 and T2 signal intensity characteristic of cerebrospinal fluid. On DWI, epidermoid tumors are hyperintense, because they are solidly composed (Fig. 1), whereas arachnoid cysts are hypointense, demonstrating high diffusivity (Fig. 2).[21] Apparent diffusion coefficient (ADC) values of epidermoid tumors are similar to those of the brain parenchyma or may be slightly reduced, impeded by tumor contents, such as keratinous debris.[22] Whereas ADC values of arachnoid cysts are similar to those of cerebrospinal fluid.[23] As a result, DWI can be used to better assess follow-up of surgically resected epidermoid tumors, proving efficacious in the detection of residual lesions.[24]

Meningioma
Most meningiomas, especially malignant and atypical samples, have a restricted diffusion (Fig. 3), displaying low ADC values, when

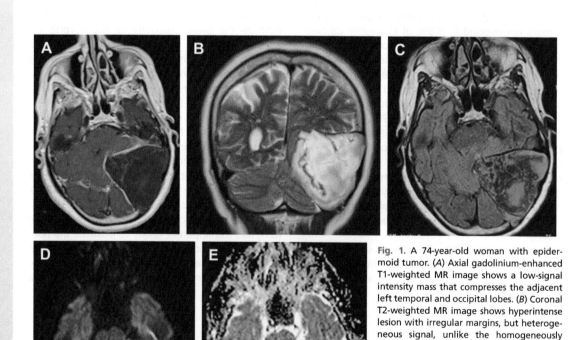

Fig. 1. A 74-year-old woman with epidermoid tumor. (A) Axial gadolinium-enhanced T1-weighted MR image shows a low-signal intensity mass that compresses the adjacent left temporal and occipital lobes. (B) Coronal T2-weighted MR image shows hyperintense lesion with irregular margins, but heterogeneous signal, unlike the homogeneously high-signal intensity of cerebrospinal fluid. (C) On axial fluid-attenuated inversion recovery (FLAIR) MR image, signal heterogeneity within the center of the mass is appreciated. (D) Axial DWI MR image reveals markedly high-signal intensity in the tumor and (E) apparent diffusion coefficient (ADC) map image shows signal intensity in the tumor is similar to the brain parenchyma.

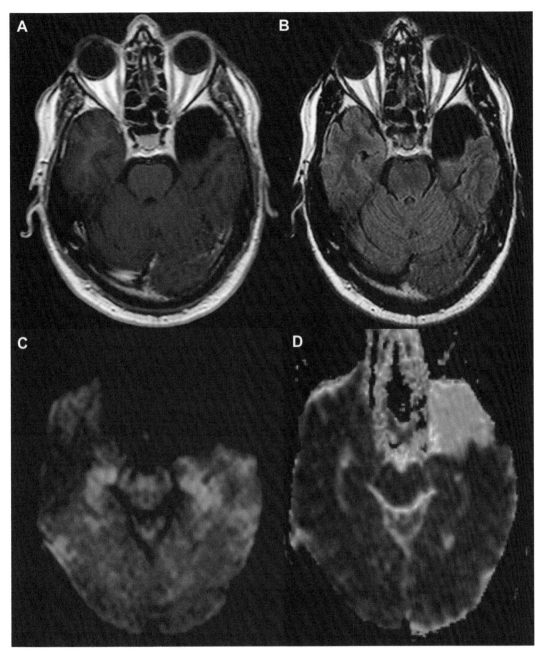

Fig. 2. A 40-year-old, man with arachnoid cyst. (A) Axial gadolinium-enhanced T1-weighted and (B) axial FLAIR MR images show an extra-axial lesion in the left middle fossa with signal intensity similar to that of cerebrospinal fluid, compressing the adjacent temporal lobe. (C) Axial DWI MR image and (D) apparent diffusion coefficient (ADC) map image reveals facilitated diffusion.

compared with typical meningiomas (**Fig. 4**).[25,26] Some aspects have been postulated to contribute to decrease ADC values in malignant and atypical meningiomas, including hypercellularity, a high nuclear-to-cytoplasmic ratio, prominent nucleoli, and decreased extracellular water.[26] The preoperative measurement of ADC values may predict the malignancy of meningiomas, which may be useful

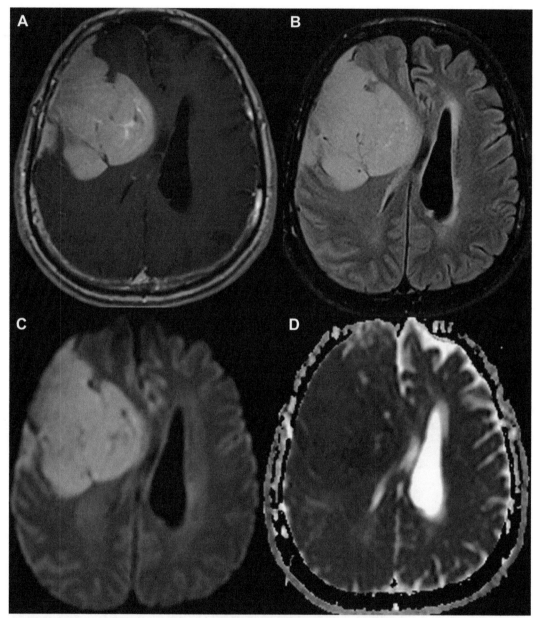

Fig. 3. A 52-year-old man with meningosarcoma. (*A*) Axial postcontrast T1-weighted image and (*B*) axial T2-weighted image show an extra-axial enhancing lesion in the right frontal region, compressing adjacent cerebral parenchyma, with restricted diffusion (*C, D*), probably caused by high cellularity.

to decide on the surgical strategy or to prescribe the adjunctive therapy. As a consequence, a more accurate prognosis may be obtained. A more recent report suggested that DTI could be also useful in such differentiation. The investigators demonstrated a significantly intratumoral microscopic disorganization in classic meningioma, based on lower fractional anisotropy (FA) and greater λ_2 and λ_3, when compared with atypical meningioma.[27]

Characterization of Intracranial Cystic Masses

DWI can also provide a sensitive and specific method for differentiating tumor from abscess in certain settings.[28–31] The abscesses have a high

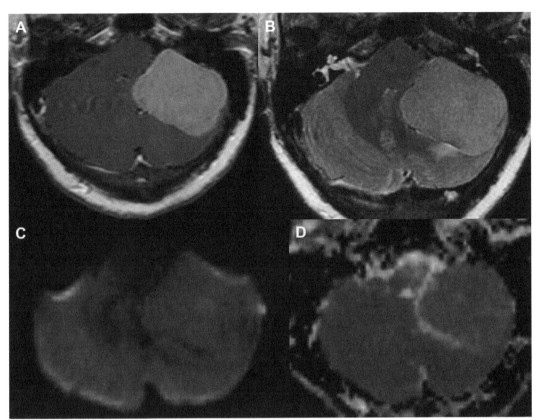

Fig. 4. A 64-year-old woman with typical meningioma. (*A*) Axial postcontrast T1-weighted image and (*B*) axial T2-weighted image show an extra-axial enhancing lesion in the left cerebellopontine angle cistern, compressing adjacent brainstem and cerebellum. (*C*) Axial diffusion-weighted image and (*D*) ADC map demonstrate isointense signal intensity suggesting cellularity similar to that of brain tissue.

signal on DWI and a reduced ADC within the cavity (**Fig. 5**). This restricted diffusion is probably related to the characteristic of the pus in the cavity. Because pus is a viscous fluid and may, in turn, lead to reduced water mobility, lower ADC, and bright signal on DWI.[32] On the other hand, necrotic and cystic tumors display a low signal on DWI with an increased ADC as well as isointense or hyperintense DWI signal intensity in the lesion margins (**Fig. 6**).[30] Although these findings can be helpful, they are of course not absolute: under certain conditions, restricted diffusion has been documented in hemorrhagic metastases, radiation necrosis, and cystic astrocytoma.[33]

Tumor Grading

Tumor grading is very important in treatment decision and evaluation of prognosis. In certain settings diffusion imaging appears to increase both the sensitivity and specificity of MR imaging in the evaluation of brain tumors by providing information about tumor cellularity, which may, in turn, improve the prediction of tumor grade (**Fig. 7**).[13,34–41] Free water molecules' diffusivity is restricted by cellularity increases present in high-grade lesions.[42,43] The reduction in extracellular space as well as the high nuclear-to-cytoplasmic ratios of some cancer cells causes a relative reduction in the ADC values.[44] A correlation between ADC values and tumor cellularity[25,43] has been described, with lower ADC values suggesting high-grade lesions.[25,45] In some studies, however, ADC values found in high- and low-grade gliomas have overlapped somewhat.[25] Thus, evaluation of tumor grade with diffusion image remains uncertain and still cannot be considered a reliable tool for this purpose.

DWI has also been shown to assist in assessing high cellularity of other brain neoplasms. In some studies, lymphoma, a highly cellular tumor,

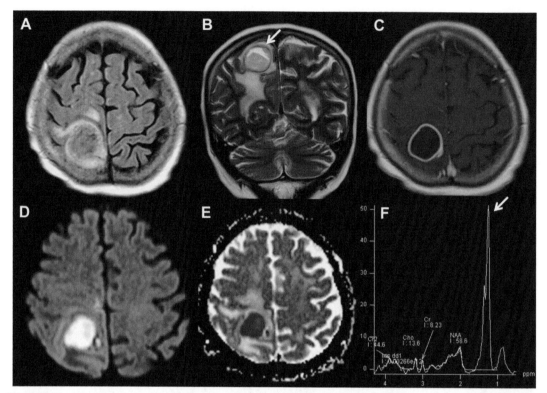

Fig. 5. A 67-year-old woman with pyogenic brain abscess. (A) Axial FLAIR MR image and (B) coronal T2-weighted MR image show a heterogeneous, slightly hyperintense lesion with surrounding vasogenic edema in the right frontoparietal region. Note also a hypointense rim (*arrow*) on T2-weighted image, suggesting a capsule. (C) Axial gadolinium-enhanced T1-weighted image shows a thick wall of enhancement of the late capsule stage abscess. (D) Axial diffusion-weighted image shows markedly high signal intensity within the abscess cavity and slightly isointense to hypointense surrounding edema. (E) ADC map reveals low signal intensity within the abscess cavity, representing restricted diffusion, and hyperintense areas surrounding the edema. (F) Single voxel proton MR spectroscopy (echo time 30 milliseconds) from the abscess cavity shows a lactate-lipid peak (1.3 ppm) (*arrow*).

has been found to present hyperintense signal intense on DWI and reduced ADC values (**Figs. 8** and **9**).[46]

DWI may also be helpful in distinguishing medulloblastoma, which displays a restricted diffusion (**Fig. 10**) from other pediatric brain tumors, also presumably because of the densely packed tumor cells and high nuclear-to-cytoplasmic ratio.[47,48] In one report, the solid enhancing portion of cerebellar hemangioblastomas on postcontrast T1-weighted images was, together with other posterior fossa neoplasms, the only one to demonstrate hypointensity on DWI (**Fig. 11**). The main explanation for the high ADC values in these tumors was suggested to be due to the rich vascular spaces present in hemangioblastomas.[49] Pilocytic astrocytoma usually does not present restricted or facilitated diffusibility.

ADC values seem to be similar to the brain parenchyma ADC values (**Fig. 12**).

DTI has also been used to attempt grading of brain neoplasms and seems to provide some utility by assessment of tumor cellularity. To date, the additional information provided by DTI has not yet been shown to correlate with tumor cellularity,[50] given that a high degree of fiber tract disorganization in the tumor core is thought to be present.[51] Nevertheless, one report has argued that FA can distinguish high-grade gliomas from low-grade gliomas.[52] This study found a significant difference between FA values when only the solid portion of the lesion was analyzed, avoiding the necrotic and cystic portions. The FA values in high-grade gliomas were higher than those in the low-grade gliomas, which was taken to suggest higher symmetry of histologic organization.

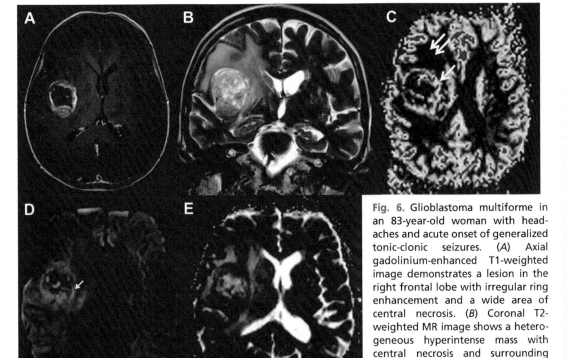

Fig. 6. Glioblastoma multiforme in an 83-year-old woman with headaches and acute onset of generalized tonic-clonic seizures. (*A*) Axial gadolinium-enhanced T1-weighted image demonstrates a lesion in the right frontal lobe with irregular ring enhancement and a wide area of central necrosis. (*B*) Coronal T2-weighted MR image shows a heterogeneous hyperintense mass with central necrosis and surrounding signal abnormality likely related to tumor extension and edema. (*C*) Axial relative cerebral blood volume color map shows elevated blood volume relative to contralateral white matter (*arrow*). Note the decreased blood volume in the white matter immediately surrounding the lesion, secondary to the space-occupying effects of vasogenic edema (*double arrows*). (*D*) Axial diffusion-weighted image shows a high signal in the periphery of the tumor, corresponding to its solid portion (*arrow*). (*E*) ADC map reveals low signal intensity in the periphery of the tumor, representing restricted diffusion.

However, these results are somewhat contradictory to the usual understanding of the microstructure of high-grade gliomas. The histologic characteristics of high-grade gliomas compared with those of low-grade gliomas typically reveal pleomorphologic structures and a regressive organization rather than an increase in parallel histologic organization.[52] A separate report found no differences between low- and high-grade gliomas with regard to FA values in the tumor center. This may be consistent with the disorganization of fiber tracts in the center of both entities, resulting in a loss of structural organization.[51]

Preoperative Planning and Peritumoral Margins

The goal of a surgical approach to the brain neoplasm is the complete resection of the tumor, coupled with minimum neurologic deficit.[53] Thus, the precise determination of the margins of the tumor is considered to be of the utmost importance to the management of brain tumors. Although a variety of approaches have been used, diffusion imaging has also been enlisted in the attempt to determine the margins of tumors in the brain. It is suggested that DWI can provide information about peritumoral neoplastic cell infiltration,[13,34–39] perhaps even help discriminate the boundaries between tumor, infiltrating tumor, peritumoral edema, and normal brain parenchyma.[13,34,54,55] However, not all studies have found DWI to be helpful in the evaluation of tumor extensions,[25,41,56] most likely because of the difficulty in finding the borders of some tumors, even on histopathology. Due to the challenges of obtaining a histologic standard of reference ("gold standard"), it is reasonable to question DWI's ability distinguish neoplastic cell infiltration beyond the enhancing portion of the lesion on the abnormal hyperintense T2-weighted image,

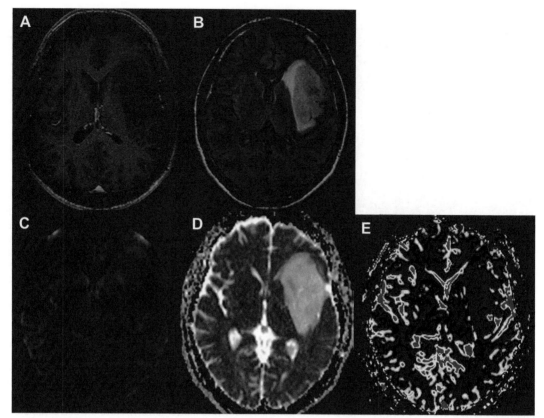

Fig. 7. A 52-year-old man with low-grade glioma. (*A*) Axial contrast-enhanced T1-weighted image demonstrates a nonenhancing left frontal mass. (*B*) Axial FLAIR MR image shows that mass is slightly hyperintense, with perilesional edema. (*C*) Axial diffusion-weighted image and (*D*) apparent diffusion coefficient map do not demonstrate restriction diffusion. (*E*) Axial relative cerebral blood volume color map does not show hyperperfusion areas within the lesion.

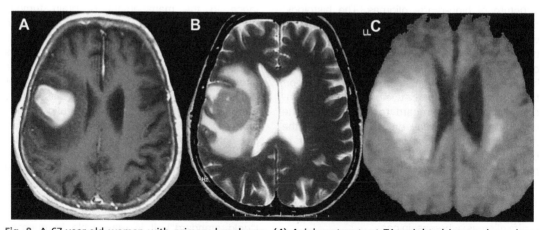

Fig. 8. A 67-year-old woman with primary lymphoma. (*A*) Axial postcontrast T1-weighted image shows large homogeneously enhanced lesion in the right frontal lobe with mass effect. (*B*) Axial T2-weighted image shows a homogeneous hypointense mass with surrounding vasogenic edema. (*C*) Axial diffusion-weighted image demonstrates markedly high signal intensity in this tumor, compatible with restricted diffusion.

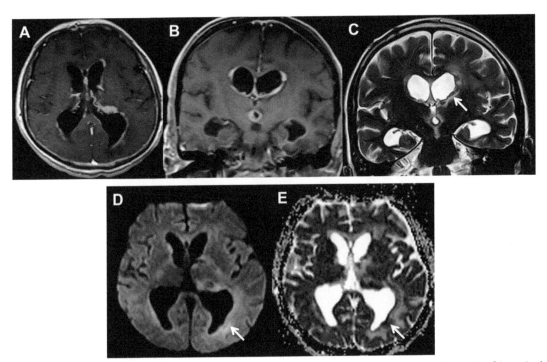

Fig. 9. Diffuse subependymal spread of lymphoma in a 76-year-old man with a previous diagnosis of intestinal lymphoma and presented with decreased level of consciousness and seizures. (*A*) Axial and (*B*) coronal contrast-enhanced T1 MR images show diffuse nodular enhancement subependymal of the lateral ventricles that has hypointense signal (*arrow*) on T2-weighted image, suggesting hypercellularity (*C*). (*D*) Axial diffusion-weighted image shows hyperintense periventricular signal (*arrow*). (*E*) ADC map corresponding to (*D*) reveals low signal intensity subependymal (*arrow*), representing restricted diffusion, commonly seen in lymphoma due to high cellularity.

which traditionally is thought to represent vasogenic edema with or without tumor invasion.

Some investigators believe that metastases with perilesion edema have higher ADC values than a primary brain tumor with peritumoral edema, and these investigators have suggested that higher ADC values may allow better differentiation between metastases and primary lesions.[36] In high-grade gliomas, the abnormal hyperintense T2-weighted image is thought to represent not only vasogenic edema but also infiltrative neoplasms cells. The normal white matter extracellular space contents a complex matrix, which restricts the free motion of water molecules.[57] Cell infiltration alters the integrity of extracellular matrix, reducing the obstruction for free water molecules to diffuse. However, this logic is somewhat speculative and vasogenic edema with neoplasm cells infiltration may be found in high-grade gliomas; whereas, in cases of meningiomas, metastases and low-grade gliomas vasogenic edema without neoplasm infiltration are seen—both with similar ADC values.

Although the specific biophysics of perilesional edema remains unclear, and ADC alone may not differentiate peritumoral edema with infiltration from peritumoral edema without infiltration, a number of investigators have reported that DTI can detect variations in FA values around lesions. This has led to speculation that these variations may be due to the presence of infiltrative tumor. However, it is not clear if an infiltrating tumor will destroy fibers and, therefore, result in lower FA, or if the tumor infiltrating along the fibers actually increases FA by having more ultrastructure aligned with the fibers. Any significant difference in the FA values of either the enhancing or nonenhancing portion of the two tumoral lesions was previously described,[58] whereas another report has verified that the periphery of low-grade gliomas, without abnormal hyperintense signal on the T2-weighted images, contains a considerable amount of preserved fiber tracts (high FA values), whereas most tracts are disarranged in high-grade gliomas (low FA values).[51] Diffusion-tensor imaging seems to demonstrate that the periphery of low-grade

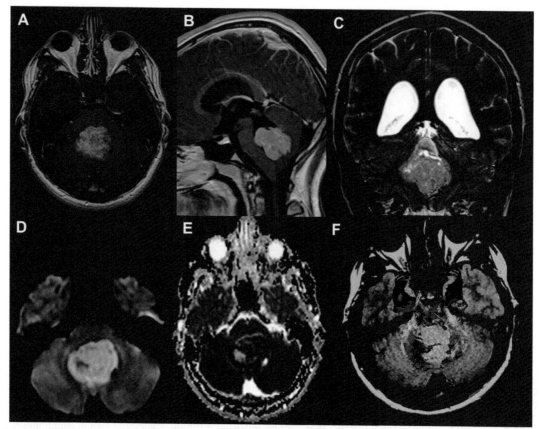

Fig. 10. A 15-year-old boy with medulloblastoma. (*A*) Axial and (*B*) sagittal contrast-enhanced T1-weighted images demonstrate strong and slightly heterogeneous enhancement of tumor, which expands the fourth ventricle. (*C*) Coronal T2-weighted image shows slightly heterogeneous, predominantly hyperintense mass without significant surrounding edema. (*D*) Axial diffusion-weighted image shows markedly high signal intensity in this lesion. (*E*) ADC map reveals that mass is hypointense to normal cerebellar parenchyma, consistent with restricted diffusion. (*F*) Tractography demonstrates displacement of the corticospinal tract and others adjacent tracts without clear evidence of invasion or disruption of these fibers.

gliomas contains preserved fiber tracts, whereas most tracts are disarranged in high-grade gliomas. However, the presence of edema can obscure fiber tracts that are present.

Patterns of white matter tracts involvement
The involvement of the white matter tracts can often be identified in brain tumor patients by using either FA maps or tractography. Based on DTI findings, resulting from studies of brain tumor patients, the white matter involvement by a tumor can be arranged into five categories[40]:

Displaced: maintained normal or slightly decreased anisotropy relative to the contralateral tract in the corresponding location but situated in an abnormal T2-weighted image signal intensity area or presented in an abnormal orientation (**Figs. 13** and **14**)

Invaded: reduced anisotropy; the main fiber tracts remained identifiable on orientated color-coded FA maps

Disrupted: marked reduced anisotropy; the main fiber tracts are unidentifiable on oriented color-coded FA maps (see **Fig. 14**)

Infiltrated: slightly reduced anisotropy without displacement of white matter architecture; the fibers remaining identifiable on orientation maps (**Fig. 15**)

Edematous: marked reduced anisotropy with normal anisotropy and normal orientated on color-coded FA maps, but located in an abnormal T2-weighted image signal intensity area.[50]

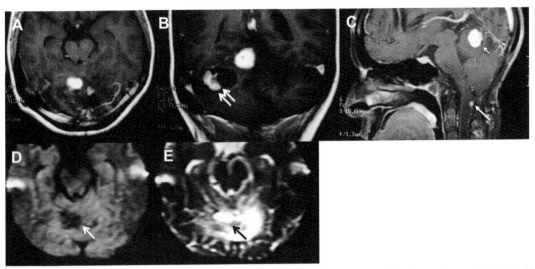

Fig. 11. A 34-year-old woman with cerebellar hemangioblastomas and von Hippel-Lindau syndrome. (*A*) Axial, (*B*) coronal, and (*C*) sagittal postcontrast T1-weighted images show a predominantly cystic lesion with a mural nodule (*double arrows*) in the right cerebellum and another solid lesion in the cerebellar vermis (*small arrow*) with strong enhancement of the solid component. A predominantly cystic lesion with a mural nodule in the upper aspect of the cervical spine (*large arrow*) is also demonstrated. (*D*) Axial diffusion-weighted image demonstrates low signal intensity in the solid lesion (*white arrow*). (*E*) ADC map reveals that lesion is very hyperintense compared with normal brain parenchyma, representing facilitated diffusion (*black arrow*).

Low-grade neoplasms are typically well-circumscribed lesions that do not cause invasion or destruction of fiber tracts. Such lesions tend to produce a displacement or deviation, rather than destruction, of surrounding white matter fibers.[15,59] Furthermore, displacement, rather than infiltration, of the adjacent white matter tracts has also been described in cerebral metastases (see **Fig. 13**)[15] and meningiomas.[60] Finally, in some cases of high-grade gliomas, the tumor could cause not only invasion and disruption of the main fiber tracts but also associated displacement. So while DTI can identify tracts and help determine the presence or absence of invasion versus displacement, the presence or absence of displacement does not appear to be highly diagnostic for high- or low-grade malignancy.

The anisotropy in the T2-weighted image hyperintense area that surrounds the tumor is typically reduced, either because of invasion of neoplastic cells or because of edema. One report noted that in patients with high-grade gliomas, but not with low-grade gliomas or cerebral metastases, the anisotropy is also low in the white matter areas adjacent to tumors that look normal on T2-weighted image, as compared

with the contralateral hemisphere.[15] The same situation has been reported in lymphomas. When compared with the abnormal white matter adjacent to metastases, decreased anisotropy in the abnormal white matter that surrounds the gliomas was demonstrated.[61] FA values decrease in the abnormal area that surrounds high-grade tumors on T2-weighted imaging. Again, this presumably happens because of increased water content and also tumor invasion.[16] This is not uniform: a certain number of studies have not found any difference in the analyses of abnormal white matter adjacent to high-grade gliomas and metastases.[16]

One important finding, the presence of tract disruption, is mostly found in high-grade tumors and is thought to be caused by a combination of peritumoral edema, tumor mass effect and tumor infiltration effect.[15,60] The main fiber tracts are infiltrated in cases of gliomatosis cerebri (see **Fig. 15**), which has a specific histopathologic behavior. In this lesion, the neoplastic cells form parallel rows among nerve fibers, preserving them. However, there is destruction of the myelin sheaths. Thus, the anisotropy is slightly reduced when compared with normal subjects but increased when compared with high-grade

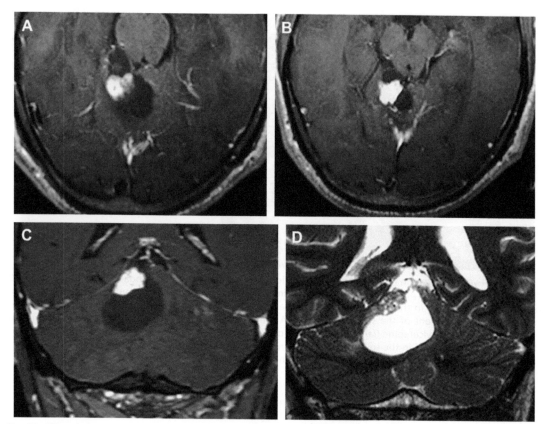

Fig. 12. Pilocytic astrocytoma in a 10-year-old boy with vomiting and headaches. (*A, B*) Axial and (*C*) coronal post-contrast T1-weighted images show a cystic-solid cerebellar mass, with homogeneous enhancement of the solid components. (*D*) Coronal T2-weighted image demonstrates a heterogeneous lesion, with solid portion showing slightly hyperintense compared with normal gray matter.

gliomas.[62] The main fiber tracts can remain identifiable on orientation maps and also on the tractography.

Metastatic lesions are surrounded by abnormal T2-weighted image that most likely consists of vasogenic edema. The edematous areas have reduced FA values. This fact is typically explained by an increase in water content rather than by destruction or invasion of nerve fibers to be consistent with neuropathologic findings. DTI has not been reported to help in differentiation of apparently normal white matter from edematous brain and enhancing peritumoral margins.[63] The drop in FA values of the area infiltrated by cell tumors is lower than that in the peritumoral edema.[2,14,50] DTI can distinguish edematous areas with intact fibers (mostly found in metastases) from disrupted fibers (mostly found in high-grade gliomas).[64]

Combination of DTI with functional MR imaging

Intracranial neoplasms may involve both the functional cortex and the corresponding white matter tracts. The preoperative identification of eloquent areas through noninvasive methods, such as blood-oxygen-level-dependent functional MR imaging (fMR imaging) and DTI tractography, offers some advantages. Not only can it reduce the time of surgery in some instances, but it may also minimize some intraoperative cortical stimulation methods, such as the identification of language cortex.[64] The combination of DTI tractography and fMR imaging might allow us to precisely map an entire functional circuit.[65] The fMR imaging can be an accurate and noninvasive method used to map functional cerebral cortex, identifying eloquent areas in the cortex and displaying their relationship to the lesion[19]; whereas

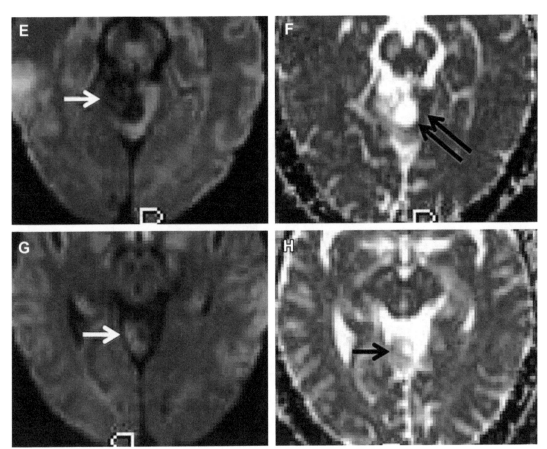

Fig. 12. (*E, G*) Axial diffusion-weighted image and (*F, H*) ADC demonstrate isointense signal intensity in the solid portion (*single arrows*) and facilitated diffusion in its cystic portion (*double arrows*).

DTI may be able to accurately identify the main fiber tracts to be avoided during surgery so as to safely guide the tumor resection.[2] As a result, neurosurgeons may have more information to inform the choice of surgical approach to be taken. This better evaluation of risks by neurosurgeons is possible if they can know the spatial relation between the tumor and major fiber tracts,[66] thereby avoiding postoperative neurologic deficit.[3,67] However, this remains to be proven in randomized trials.

Posttreatment Evaluation

Assessment of treatment response typically relies on the assessment of contrast enhancement on subsequent imaging studies within 24 to 48 hours after the surgical procedure[68] and later by the evaluation of tumor size weeks to months after conclusion of therapy.[69] The appearance of a new enhancing area often results in management alterations, leading frequently to adjuvant therapy. A recent report has observed the benefits of performing DWI in immediate postoperative MR imaging examinations.[68] Areas of restricted diffusion were described adjacent to low- or high-grade glioma tumor resection cavity. Follow-up MR imaging examinations revealed that these restricted diffusion areas resolved, and that contrast enhancing appears in the corresponding location. This enhancement subsequently regressed to form an area of encephalomalacia. Because conventional MR imaging examination at the time of the enhancement period is easily misdiagnosed as tumor recurrence (**Fig. 16**) or tumor progression, such findings can lead to erroneous interpretation of treatment failed and the initiation of a new adjuvant therapy. Investigators have concluded that a corresponding area of restricted diffusion almost always precedes the delayed contrast enhancement described, which invariably evolves

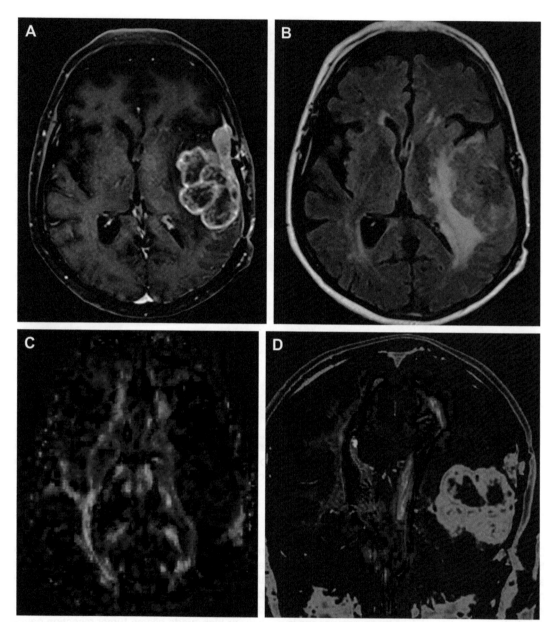

Fig. 13. Solitary cerebral metastasis from colonic cancer in a 65-year-old man with seizures. (*A*) Axial postcontrast T1-weighted MR image demonstrates a heterogeneously enhancing mass in the left temporal lobe with extensive surrounding edema. (*B*) Axial FLAIR image shows that lesion has predominantly isointense signal intensity compared with gray matter. Axial diffusion tensor imaging–FA map (*C*) and tractography (*D*) show dislocation of the anterior and posterior portions of the internal capsule.

into encephalomalacia or gliotic cavity on long-term follow-up studies, representing areas of infarct, ischemia, or even venous congestion, secondary to acute cellular damage.[44] Such findings are unlikely to represent early recurrence.

DWI might also be a marker for the response to therapy because changes in tumor water diffusibility may occur secondarily to changes in cell density (**Fig. 17**). In this setting, ADC appears to be a sensitive and an early predictor of therapeutic efficacy.[70] Specifically, investigators prospectively compared tumor diffusion values at 3 weeks after initiation of therapy with pretreatment images so as to measure ADC changes

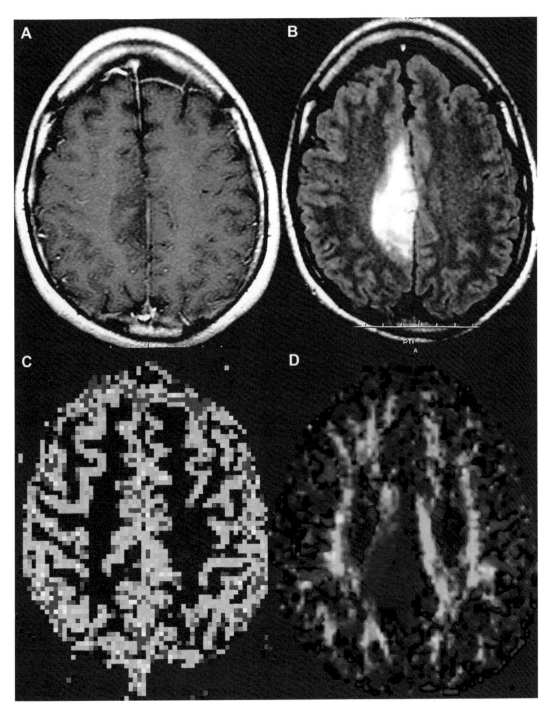

Fig. 14. A 40-year-old man with low-grade glioma. (*A*) Axial contrast-enhanced T1-weighted image shows a non-enhancing right cortico-subcortical frontal lesion and has hyperintense signal on FLAIR image (*B*). Relative cerebral blood volume map (*C*) does not demonstrate areas of hyperperfusion within the lesion. (*D*) Diffusion tensor imaging–FA map shows disruption of the posterior cingulate gyrus and displacement of the superior region of internal capsule.

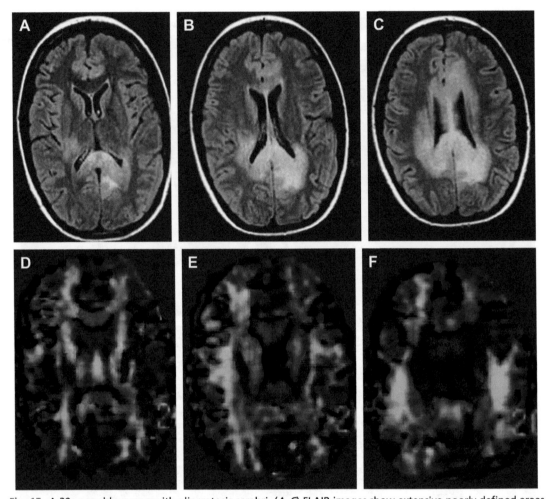

Fig. 15. A 39-year-old woman with gliomatosis cerebri. (*A–C*) FLAIR images show extensive poorly defined areas of hyperintensity involving both hemispheres, without enhancement on postcontrast T1-weighted images (not shown here). (*D–F*) Diffusion tensor imaging–FA maps demonstrate slightly reduced anisotropy in these areas with direction of the fiber tracts are preserved. This is probably explained by the fact that gliomatosis cerebri is a diffusely invading lesion that preserves the normal underlying cytoarchitectural pattern because it does not destroy the nerve fibers.

induced by therapy.[71] If this methodology holds up in multicenter trials, it would allow a lack of change in ADC values in the tumor to indicate a failure in therapy. This would, in turn, provide an opportunity to switch to a more beneficial therapy, minimizing the morbidity associated with a prolonged and inefficient treatment. The logic behind this methodology is that successful treatment will result in extensive cell damage, leading to a reduction in cell density. The neoplasm cell loss results in an increase in extracellular space that can raise free water molecule diffusibility. As increases in brain tumors ADC correspond to decreases in tumor volume in long-term follow-up studies,

DWI may, therefore, be an important surrogate marker for quantification of treatment response.

DTI may also play a role in the management of patients undergoing radiation therapy and chemotherapy. By adding information about the location of white matter tracts, DTI tractography might be successfully used alongside fMR imaging for radiosurgery planning. In theory, this should allow a reduction of the dose applied as well as the volume of normal brain irradiated with a high dose, hopefully reducing necrosis.[15] DTI may also help in the early detection of white matter injuries caused by chemotherapy and radiation therapy. A report showed a correlation

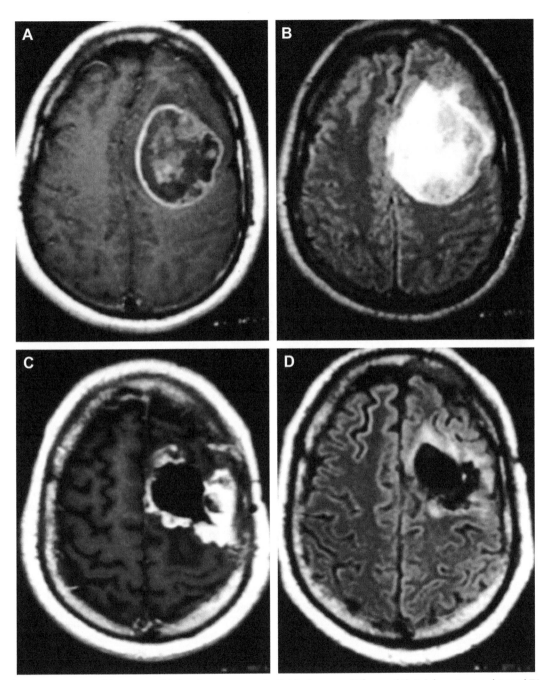

Fig. 16. A 65-year-old woman with local recurrence of glioblastoma multiforme. (*A*) Axial contrast-enhanced T1-weighted image demonstrates a lesion in the left frontal lobe with heterogeneous and predominantly irregular ring enhancement, and a wide area of central necrosis. (*B*) Axial FLAIR MR image shows a heterogeneous hyperintense mass with central necrosis and surrounding signal abnormality likely related to tumor extension and edema. On postcontrast T1-weighted image (*C*), the postsurgery cavity shows irregular peripheral enhancement, with slight hyperintense signal in correspondence on FLAIR MR image (*D*).

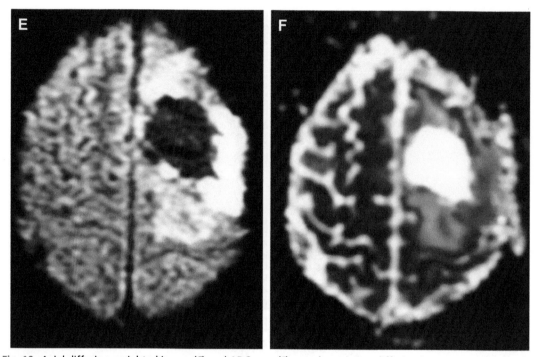

Fig. 16. Axial diffusion-weighted image (*E*) and ADC map (*F*) reveal restriction diffusion in some peripheral areas of the postsurgery cavity, representing tumoral recurrence.

between the reductions of FA values, young age at treatment, an increased interval since the beginning of treatment, and the poor intellectual outcome in patients with medulloblastoma.[72] The possibility of using FA or other DTI changes as a biomarker for neurotoxicity is enticing.

POTENTIAL FUTURE APPLICATIONS

Although DWI has been recently used to assess brain tumor diagnoses (**Fig. 18**) and treatments, to help in the preoperative planning, and to guide surgery intraoperatively, there are still a number of new areas and possibly future applications. These include therapy monitoring, monitoring radiation, or other treatments via quantitative assessment of white matter changes as a marker for toxicity; plasticity after surgery, radiation, or other treatment; and so on. However, many of these techniques will require improved image quality. Specifically, DWI is an echo-planar sequence that suffers from a low signal-to-noise ratio (SNR) due to the need for rapid acquisition approaches. The types of quantification of diffusibility or anisotropy that might allow these advanced applications are very sensitive to inadequate SNR. Mean diffusibility and FA values

may vary with different SNR. With the appropriate SNR, and if more powerful gradients could be used, a smaller voxel could be obtained in a clinically acceptable measurement time. The voxel size typically used in diffusion images is big enough to cause partial-volume effect and this makes the correct identification of the intersection fibers within the same voxel difficult. A smaller voxel size may be helpful in solving the problem of crossing fibers and can be useful to delineate small white matter structures. A better SNR in a 3.0 tesla scanner has been demonstrated. However, some challenges remain, including geometric distortions.[73] More importantly, for the future will be the move beyond the tensor representation of diffusion. This model fails to account for cases of intersection and dispersion of fibers in a same voxel.[74] Because insertion of fibers is the key event in linking white matter to gray matter and because so much of the brain is composed of regions of intersecting fibers, it seems highly likely that the method that goes beyond the tensor to so-called "supertensor" representations will become useful once the technology allows these techniques to be practical. One such approach is called diffusion spectrum imaging (DSI). Other

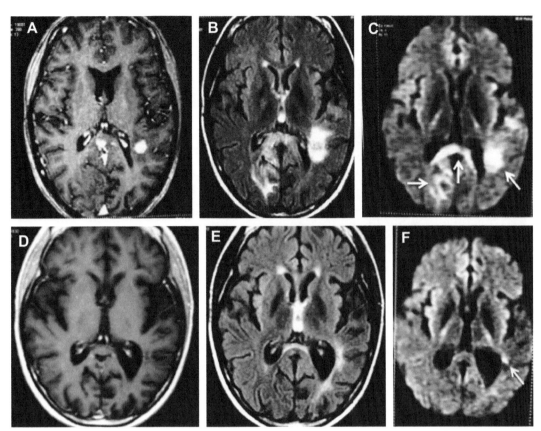

Fig. 17. A 25-year-old woman with B-cell lymphoma before and after treatment with chemotherapy. (*A–C*) Images obtained before treatment. (*A*) Axial contrast-enhanced T1-weighted image shows nodular enhancing lesions in the splenium of the corpus callosum and deep left parietal white matter. (*B*) Axial FLAIR image reveals that these lesions have hyperintense signal and the infiltrative lesion of the splenium of the corpus callosum extends to the right occipital white matter. There are also surrounding edema. (*C*) Axial diffusion-weighted image corresponding to (*B*) shows markedly high signal intensity in these lesions (*arrows*). (*D–F*) Images obtained 6 months after chemotherapy. (*D*) Axial contrast-enhanced T1-weighted, (*E*) axial MR imaging and (*F*) diffusion-weighted images show disappearance of enhancement in all lesions and significant reduction in the size of the left parietal lesion (*arrow*) and disappearance of infiltrative lesion of the corpus callosum. These findings can predict a good treatment response.

variants of this same approach go by other names (eg, high angular resolution diffusion imaging, or HARDI). However, the concept is the same: to move beyond the limitations of the tensor model. With the increasing popularity of DTI, its limitations will become familiar to more investigators and these more advanced methods will likely become the dominant approach for investigating the brain. The better understanding and assessment of both large and small fibers will almost certainly help in the evaluation of the relationship between brain neoplasm lesions and the underlying normal anatomy. Diffusional kurtosis (DK) imaging is a new technique that precisely defines diffusion metric, allowing the characterization of non-gaussian water diffusion behavior and is complimentary to ADC and FA. DK imaging can represent the microstructure of the tissue, as the non-gaussianity of water diffusion is thought to depend on cell membranes, organelles, and water compartments.[75] The mean kurtosis (MK) has some advantages over FA. For instance, MK can be used to characterize both gray and white matter and to resolve the crossing fiber tracts.[76] A recent report demonstrates that DK imaging was able to depict microstructural changes within glioma tissue

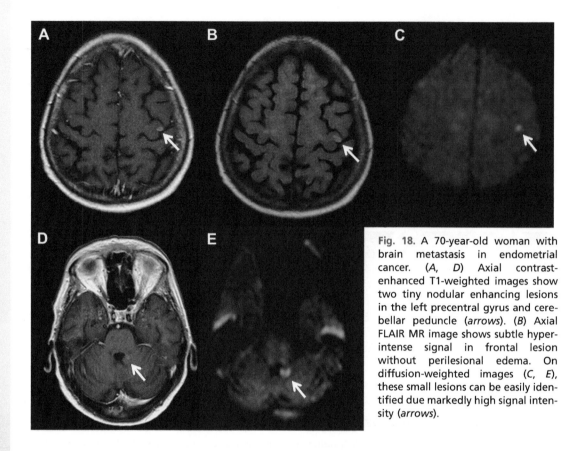

Fig. 18. A 70-year-old woman with brain metastasis in endometrial cancer. (*A, D*) Axial contrast-enhanced T1-weighted images show two tiny nodular enhancing lesions in the left precentral gyrus and cerebellar peduncle (*arrows*). (*B*) Axial FLAIR MR image shows subtle hyperintense signal in frontal lesion without perilesional edema. On diffusion-weighted images (*C, E*), these small lesions can be easily identified due markedly high signal intensity (*arrows*).

and could add information regarding the differentiation between different grades.[77]

SUMMARY

Although initial reports suggest advantages of DWI and DTI in the evaluation of patients with brain tumors, these reports are largely single-center, uncontrolled, preliminary findings. Therefore these results must be cautiously interpreted. Multicenter studies are sorely needed. There are difficulties in designing prospective studies that assess certain methods such as intraoperative MR imaging, where blinding is difficult and bias inevitably is present.

As suggested above, there remain substantial technical hurdles, even though the rapid evolution of MR imaging systems is making ever more powerful approaches possible. Improvements are particularly welcome given the limited SNR of diffusion overall. For example, the limited spatial resolution of echo planar imaging approaches may lead to reduced sensitivity. The method herein assessed is only capable of depicting the prominent fiber tracts[14] and more advanced approaches (eg, DSI) may be much more useful in the future. Susceptibility artifacts can cause image distortion that prevents DTI data from being accurately analyzed[14] and numerous other technical challenges remain.

Diffusion imaging seems to offer the possibility of adding important information to presurgical planning. Although experience is limited, DTI seems to provide useful local information about the structures near the tumor, and this appears to be useful in planning. In the future, DTI may provide an improved way to monitor intraoperative surgical procedures as well as their complications. Furthermore, evaluation of the response to treatment with chemotherapy and radiation therapy might also be possible. Although diffusion imaging has some limitations, it is an area of active investigation and implementation in clinical practice.

ACKNOWLEDGMENTS

The authors would like to thank A. Gregory Sorensen, PhD, for helping editing this manuscript.

REFERENCES

1. Knisely JP, Rockwell S. Importance of hypoxia in the biology and treatment of brain tumors. Neuroimaging Clin N Am 2002;12:525–36.
2. Landis SH, Murray T, Bolden S. Cancer statistics, 1998. CA Cancer J Clin 1998;48:6–29.
3. Berens ME, Rutka JT, Rosenblum ML. Brain tumor epidemiology, growth, and invasion. Neurosurg Clin N Am 1990;1:1–18.
4. Jemal A, Thomas A, Murray T, et al. Cancer statistics, 2002. CA Cancer J Clin 2002;52(1):23–47.
5. Koeller KK, Henry JM. Superficial gliomas: radiologic-pathologic correlation. Radiographics 2001;21:1533–56.
6. Hunt D, Treasure P. Year of life lost due to cancer in East Anglia 1990–1994. Cambridge (UK): East Anglian Cancer Intelligence Unit, Institute of Public Health; 1998.
7. Ries LAG, Eisner MP, Kosary CL, et al. editors. SEER cancer statistics review, 1973–1996. Bethesda (MD): National Cancer Institute. NIH Pub; 2000.
8. Jemal A, Clegg LX, Ward E, et al. Annual report to the nation on the status of cancer, 1975–2001, with a special feature regarding survival. Cancer 2004; 101(1):3–27.
9. Brain MRC Tumor Working Party. Prognostic factor for high-grade malignant glioma: development of a prognostic index. A report of the Medical Research Council Brain Tumor Working Party. J Neurooncol 1990;9:47–55.
10. Felix R, Schorner W, Laniado M, et al. Brain tumors: MR imaging with gadolinium-DPTA. Radiology 1985; 156:681–8.
11. Tovi M. MR imaging in cerebral gliomas analysis of tumor tissue components. Acta Radiol Suppl 1993; 384:1–24.
12. Knopp EA, Cha S, Johnson G, et al. Glial neoplasms: dynamic contrast-enhanced T2*-weighted MR imaging. Radiology 1999;211:791–8.
13. Brunberg JA, Chenevert TL, McKeever PE, et al. In vivo MR determination of water diffusion coefficients and diffusion anisotropy: Correlation with structural alteration in gliomas of the cerebral hemispheres. AJNR Am J Neuroradiol 1995;16:361–71.
14. Mori S, Frederiksen K, Van Zijl PCM, et al. Brain white matter anatomy of tumor patients evaluated with diffusion tensor imaging. Ann Neurol 2002;51:377–80.
15. Price SJ, Burnet NG, Donovan T, et al. Diffusion tensor imaging of brain tumors at 3T: a potential tool for assessing white matter tract invasion. Clin Radiol 2003;58:455–62.
16. Lu S, Ahn D, Johnson G, et al. Peritumoral diffusion tensor imaging of high-grade gliomas and metastatic brain tumors. AJNR Am J Neuroradiol 2003; 24:937–41.
17. Laundre BJ, Jellinson BJ, Badie B, et al. Diffusion tensor imaging of the corticospinal tract before and after mass resection as correlated with clinical motor findings: preliminary data. AJNR Am J Neuroradiol 2005;26:791–6.
18. Maldjian JA, Schulder M, Liu WC, et al. Intraoperative functional MRI using a real-time neurosurgical navigation system. J Comput Assist Tomogr 1997; 21:910–2.
19. Schulder M, Maldjian JA, Liu WC, et al. Functional image-guided surgery of intracranial tumors located in or near the sensorimotor cortex. J Neurosurg 1998;89:412–8.
20. Barboriak DP. Imaging of brain tumors with diffusion-weighted and diffusion tensor MR imaging. Magn Reson Imaging Clin N Am 2003;11:379–401.
21. Tsuruda JS, Chew WM, Moseley ME, et al. Diffusion-weighted MR imaging of the brain: value of differentiating between extra-axial cysts and epidermoid tumors. AJNR Am J Neuroradiol 1990;155:1049–65.
22. Tsuruda JS, Chew WM, Moseley ME, et al. Diffusion-weighted MR imaging of extraaxial tumors. Magn Reson Med 1999;9:352–61.
23. Chen S, Ikawa F, Kurisu K, et al. Quantitative MR evaluation of intracranial epidermoid tumors by fast fluid-attenuated inversion recovery imaging and echo-planar diffusion-weighted imaging. AJNR Am J Neuroradiol 2001;22(6):1089–96.
24. Laing AD, Mitchell PJ, Wallace D. Diffusion-weighted magnetic resonance imaging of intracranial epidermoid tumors. Australas Radiol 1999;43:16–9.
25. Kono K, Inoue Y, Nakayama K, et al. The role of diffusion-weighted imaging in patients with brain tumors. AJNR Am J Neuroradiol 2001;22:1081–8.
26. Filippi CG, Edgar MA, Ulug AM, et al. Appearance of meningiomas on diffusion-weighted images: correlation diffusion constants with histopathologic findings. AJNR Am J Neuroradiol 2001;22:65–72.
27. Toh CH, Castillo M, Wong AM, et al. Differentiation between classic and atypical meningiomas with use of diffusion tensor imaging. AJNR Am J Neuroradiol 2008;29:1630–5.
28. Guo AC, Provenzale JM, Cruz LC Jr, et al. Cerebral abscesses: investigation using apparent diffusion coefficient maps. Neuroradiology 2001;43:370–4.
29. Bergui M, Zhong J, Bradac GB, et al. Diffusion-weighted images of intracranial cyst-like lesions. Neuroradiology 2001;439(10):824–9.
30. Chang SC, Lai PH, Chen WL, et al. Diffusion-weighted MRI features of brain abscess and cystic or necrotic brain tumors: comparison with conventional MRI. Clin Imaging 2002;26(4):227–36.
31. Chan JH, Tsui EY, Chau LF, et al. Discrimination of an infected brain tumor from a cerebral abscess by combined MR perfusion and diffusion imaging. Comput Med Imaging Graph 2002;26(1):19–23.

32. Ebisu T, Tanaka C, Umeda M, et al. Discrimination of brain abscess from necrotic or cystic tumors by diffusion-weighted echo planar imaging. Magn Reson Imaging 1996;14(9):1113–6.

33. Hartmann M, Jansen O, Heiland S, et al. Restricted diffusion within ring enhancement is not pathognomonic for brain abscess. AJNR Am J Neuroradiol 2001;22(9):1738–42.

34. Tien RD, Feldesberg GJ, Friedman H, et al. MR imaging of high-grade cerebral gliomas: value of diffusion-weighted echo-planar pulse sequence. AJR Am J Roentgenol 1994;162:671–7.

35. Eis M, Els T, Hoehn-Berlage M, et al. Quantitative diffusion MR imaging of cerebral tumor and edema. Acta Neurochir Suppl (Wien) 1994;60:344–6.

36. Krabbe K, Gideon P, Wang P, et al. MR diffusion imaging of human intracranial tumours. Neuroradiology 1997;39:483–9.

37. Le Bihan D, Douek P, Argyropoulou M, et al. Diffusion and perfusion magnetic resonance imaging in brain tumors. Top Mang Reson Imaging 1993;5:25–31.

38. Tsuruda JS, Chew WM, Moseley ME, et al. Diffusion-weighted MR imaging of extraaxial tumors. Magn Reson Med 1991;19:316–20.

39. Yanaka K, Shirai S, Kimura H, et al. Clinical application of diffusion-weighted magnetic resonance imaging to intracranial disorders. Neurol Med Chir 1995;16:361–71.

40. Cruz LC Jr, Sorensen GS. Diffusion tensor magnetic resonance imaging of brain tumors. Neurosurg Clin N Am 2005;16:115–34.

41. Stadnik TW, Chaskis C, Michotte A, et al. Diffusion-weighted MR imaging of intrcerebral masses: comparison with conventional MR imaging and histologic findings. AJNR Am J Neuroradiol 2001;22:969–76.

42. Pierpaoli C, Jezzard P, Basser P, et al. Diffusion tensor MR imaging of the human brain. Radiology 1996;201:637–48.

43. Sugahara T, Korogi Y, Kochi M, et al. Usefulness of diffusion-weighted MRI with echo-planar technique in the evaluation of cellularity in gliomas. J Magn Reson Imaging 1999;9:53–60.

44. Cha S. Update on brain tumor imaging: from anatomy to physiology. AJNR Am J Neuroradiol 2006;27:475–87.

45. Noguchi K, Watanabe N, Nagayoshi T, et al. Role of diffusion-weighted echo-planar MRI in distinguishing between brain abscess and tumor: a preliminary report. Neuroradiology 1999;41:171–4.

46. Guo AC, Cummings TJ, Dash RC, et al. Lymphomas and high-grade astrocytomas: comparison of water diffusibility and histologic characteristics. Radiology 2002;224(1):177–83.

47. Gauvain KM, McKinstry RC, Mukherjee P, et al. Evaluating pediatric brain tumor cellularity with diffusion-tensor imaging. AJR Am J Roentgenol 2001;177:449–54.

48. Koetsenas AL, Roth TC, Manness WK, et al. Abnormal diffusion-weighted MRI in medulloblastoma: does it reflect small cell histology? Pediatr Radiol 1999;29:524–6.

49. Quadrery FA, Okamoto K. Diffusion-weighted MRI of haemangioblastomas and other cerebellar tumours. Neuroradiology 2003;45(4):212–9.

50. Witwer BP, Moftakhar R, Hasan KM, et al. Diffusion-tensor imaging of white matter tracts in patients with cerebral neoplasm. J Neurosurg 2002;97:568–75.

51. Goebell E, Paustenbach S, Vaeterlein O, et al. Low-grade and anaplastic gliomas: differences in architecture evaluated with diffusion-tensor MR imaging. Radiology 2006;239:217–22.

52. Inoue T, Ogasawara K, Beppu T, et al. Diffusion tensor imaging for preoperative evaluation of tumor grade in gliomas. Clin Neurol Neurosurg 2005;107:174–80.

53. Jellinson BJ, Field AS, Medow J, et al. Diffusion tensor imaging of cerebral white matter: a pictorial review of physics, fiber tract anatomy, and tumor imaging patterns. AJNR Am J Neuroradiol 2004;23:356–69.

54. Maier SE, Gudbjartsson H, Patz SL, et al. Line scan diffusion imaging: characterization in healthy subjects and stroke patients. Am J Roentgenol 1998;171:85–93.

55. Yoshiura T, Wu O, Zaheer A, et al. Highly diffusion-sensitized MRI of brain: dissociation of gray and white matter. Magn Reson Med 2001;45:734–40.

56. Castillo M, Smith JK, Kwock L, et al. Apparent diffusion coefficients in the evaluation of high-grade cerebral gliomas. AJNR Am J Neuroradiol 2001;22(1):60–4.

57. Giese A, Westphal M. Glioma invasion in the central nervous system. Neurosurgery 1996;39:235–52.

58. Tsuchiya K, Fujikawa A, Nakajima M, et al. Differentiation between solitary metastasis and high-grade gliomas by diffusion tensor imaging. Br J Radiol 2005;78:533–7.

59. Weishmann UC, Symms MR, Parker GJ, et al. Diffusion tensor imaging demonstrates deviation of fibers in normal appearing white matter adjacent to a brain tumour. J Neurol Neurosurg Psychiatry 2000;68:501–3.

60. Holodny AI, Ollenschleger M, Liu WC, et al. Identification of the corticospinal tracts achieved using blood-oxygen-level-dependent and diffusion functional MR imaging in patients with brain tumors. AJNR Am J Neuroradiol 2001;22(1):83–8.

61. Jellison NJ, Wu Y, Field AS, et al. Diffusion tensor imaging metrics for tissue characterization: discriminating vasogenic edema from infiltrating tumor. Paper presented at: American Society of Neuroradiology 41st Annual Meeting. Washington, DC, April 27 to May 2, 2003.

62. Akai H, Mori H, Aoki S, et al. Diffusion tensor tractography of gliomatosis cerebri: fiber tracking through

the tumor. J Comput Assist Tomogr 2005;29(1): 127–9.

63. Sha S, Bastin ME, Whittle IR, et al. Diffusion tensor MR imaging of high-grade cerebral gliomas. AJNR Am J Neuroradiol 2002;23:520–7.

64. Tummala RP, Chu RM, Liu H, et al. Application of diffusion-tensor imaging to magnetic-resonance-guided brain tumor resection. Pediatr Neurosurg 2003;39: 39–43.

65. Krings T, Reiges MH, Thiex R, et al. Functional and diffusion-weighted magnetic resonance images of space-occupying lesions affecting the motor system: imaging the motor cortex and pyramidal tracts. J Neurosurg 2001;95(5):816–24.

66. Mamata H, Mamata Y, Westin CF, et al. High-resolution line scan diffusion tensor MR imaging of white matter fiber tract anatomy. AJNR Am J Neuroradiol 2002;23:67–75.

67. Mamata Y, Mamata H, Nabavi A, et al. Intraoperative diffusion imaging on a 0.5 Tesla interventional scanner. J Magn Reson Imaging 2001;13:115–9.

68. Smith JS, Cha S, Catherine M, et al. Serial diffusion-weighted magnetic resonance imaging in case of glioma: distinguishing tumor recurrence from postresection injury. J Neurosurg 2005;103: 428–38.

69. James K, Eisenhauer E, Christian M, et al. Measuring response in solid tumors: unidimensional versus bidimensional measurement. J Natl Cancer Inst 1999;91:523–8.

70. Ross BD, Chenevert TL, Kim B, et al. Magnetic resonance imaging and spectroscopy: application to experimental neuro-oncology. Quart Magn Res Biol Med 1994;1:89–106.

71. Moffat BA, Chenevert TL, Lawrence TS, et al. Functional diffusion map: a noninvasive MRI biomarker for early stratification of clinical brain tumor response. Proc Natl Acad Sci U S A 2005;102(15):5524–9.

72. Khong PL, Kwong DL, Chan GC, et al. Diffusion-tensor imaging for the detection and qualification of treatment-induced white matter injury in children with medulloblastoma: a pilot study. AJNR Am J Neuroradiol 2003;24:734–40.

73. Hunsche S, Mosely ME, Stoeter P, et al. Diffusion-tensor MR imaging at 1.5T and 3.0T: initial observations. Radiology 2001;221:550–6.

74. Wiegell MR, Larsson HB, Wedeen VJ. Fiber crossing in human brain depicted with diffusion tensor MR imaging. Radiology 2000;217:897–903.

75. Jensen JH, Helpern JA, Ramani A, et al. Diffusional kurtosis imaging: the quantification of non-gaussian water diffusion by means of magnetic resonance imaging. Magn Reson Med 2005;53:1432–40.

76. Hui ES, Cheung MM, Qi L, et al. Towards better MR characterization of neural tissue using directional diffusion kurtosis analysis. Neuroimage 2008;42:122–34.

77. Raab P, Hattingen E, Franz K, et al. Cerebral gliomas: diffusional kurtosis imaging analysis of microstructural differences. Radiology 2010;254: 876–81.

Clinical Applications of Diffusion MR Imaging for Acute Ischemic Stroke

Albert J. Yoo, MD[a],*, R. Gilberto González, MD, PhD[b]

KEYWORDS

- Diffusion MR imaging • Acute ischemic stroke
- Intravenous reperfusion therapy
- Intra-arterial reperfusion therapy

Acute ischemic stroke (AIS) is the third leading cause of death and the leading cause of severe disability in adults. There are approximately 700,000 ischemic strokes annually in the United States.[1] Reperfusion therapy is the only proven treatment of AIS.[2–5] Current treatment approaches include intravenous tissue plasminogen activator (IV tPA), thrombolytic and/or mechanical intra-arterial therapies (IATs), and combined intravenous/intra-arterial (IV/IA) bridging therapy.

The randomized controlled trials (RCTs) that have validated reperfusion therapy (and guide current clinical practice) used noncontrast computed tomography (NCCT) criteria for assessment of parenchymal injury. Patients were excluded from therapy if they had infarcts that involved greater than one-third of the middle cerebral artery (MCA) territory or that resulted in severe edema or mass effect. However, it is widely believed that advanced neuroimaging methods including diffusion magnetic resonance (MR) imaging provide a better means of patient selection than NCCT, and may allow the treatment window to be extended for patients with AIS.

This article reviews the evidence for using diffusion MR imaging in the evaluation of patients with AIS, with a focus on extended window reperfusion therapies.

IMAGING THE INFARCT CORE USING DIFFUSION MR IMAGING

Within the first several hours after the occlusion of a cerebral vessel, the hypoperfused territory is composed of tissue that is irreversibly injured (the infarct core) and a surrounding region of threatened but viable tissue (the ischemic penumbra). The infarct core grows into the penumbra to an extent determined largely by the collateral circulation. Within the infarct core, cell death occurs via a variety of mechanisms, including excitotoxicity, oxidative/nitrosative stress, inflammation, apoptosis, and peri-infarct depolarization.[6] The loss of cellular energy metabolism causes a failure of membrane ionic pumps, resulting in cytotoxic edema and restricted diffusion of water, which is detectable on diffusion MR imaging (Fig. 1). The biophysical basis of this restricted diffusion is not clearly known, but proposed mechanisms include movement of water into the intracellular compartment,[7] cell swelling resulting in reduction of the extracellular space,[8] and increased cytoplasmic viscosity.[9]

Of the available MR imaging and computed tomography (CT) measurements, abnormalities detected on diffusion MR imaging are considered the most reliable estimate of the infarct core, and

Supported in part by NIH/NINDS grant NS050041 to RGG.

[a] Divisions of Diagnostic and Interventional Neuroradiology, Harvard Medical School, Massachusetts General Hospital, 55 Fruit Street, Gray 241, Boston, MA 02114, USA

[b] Neuroradiology Division, Harvard Medical School, Massachusetts General Hospital, 55 Fruit Street, Gray 241, Boston, MA 02114, USA

* Corresponding author.
E-mail address: ajyoo@partners.org

A   B   C   D

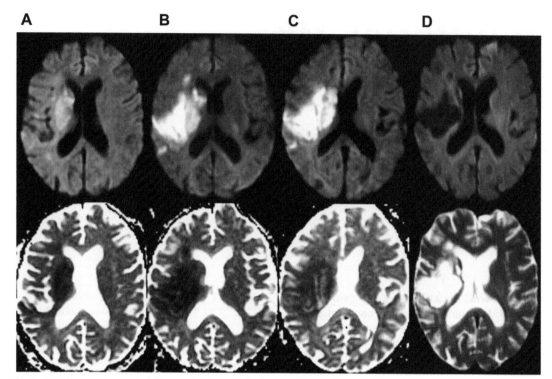

Fig. 1. DWI hyperintense signal may arise from T2 hyperintensity and/or restricted diffusion. Therefore, DWI (*top*) images must be interpreted in the context of ADC (*bottom*) images. Reduced ADC signal confirms restricted diffusion. In the setting of cerebral ischemia, restricted diffusion is visible within the first several hours of onset (*A*, 13 hours), peaks within 2 to 4 days (*B*, 39 hours), and starts to resolve by 1 week (*C*, 6 days). There is increased diffusion in chronic infarcts (*D*, 3 months).

are characterized by diffusion-weighted imaging (DWI) hyperintensity with associated reduction in apparent diffusion coefficient (ADC) signal. Diffusion imaging is highly sensitive (91%–100%) and specific (86%–100%) for the identification of early ischemic brain injury (within 6 hours of symptom onset),[10–12] and has similar accuracy for the prediction of cortical infarction as [11C]flumazenil positron emission tomography,[13] which is a reliable marker of neuronal integrity. In comparison, NCCT and nondiffusion MR imaging suffer from low sensitivity (20%–50%; **Fig. 2**).[11,14,15] Furthermore,

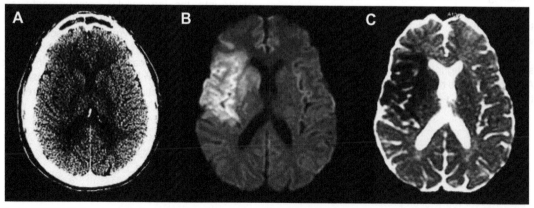

Fig. 2. NCCT (*A*) shows subtle hypodensity in the right putamen and insula. Concurrent MR imaging DWI (*B*) and ADC (*C*) images delineate a larger region of ischemic injury involving the right basal ganglia, insula, and frontal operculum.

because of its high image contrast,[11] DWI shows superior interreader agreement compared with NCCT and conventional MR imaging for lesion detection and estimation of infarct size.[11,16]

In the absence of therapy, ischemic diffusion abnormalities rarely reverse.[17] With early reperfusion, partial reversal of diffusion abnormalities can be observed,[18–22] with most rates ranging from 8% to 20% (Fig. 3). Brain regions that undergo reversal typically have mild ADC depression,[21] indicating that these areas have a mild reduction in blood flow,[23] or that it is early in the course of ischemia.[19,21] However, the volume of tissue with diffusion normalization is usually small (5.1–16 cm³),[13,18,20,21] and this normalization has not been shown to improve clinical outcomes.[21,24] Any clinical benefit associated with diffusion imaging reversal is likely related to the effects of accompanying tissue reperfusion, notably penumbral salvage. Moreover, delayed regrowth into a previously observed diffusion abnormality frequently occurs, a phenomenon termed late secondary ischemic injury.[18,19] Taken together, the evidence indicates that the signal abnormality observed on diffusion MR imaging is currently the best marker of the infarct core, an opinion supported by multiple expert panels (class I, level of evidence A).[25,26]

USING DIFFUSION MR IMAGING TO SELECT PATIENTS FOR IV THROMBOLYSIS

Numerous studies have examined the usefulness of diffusion MR imaging for selecting patients for IV therapies outside the 3-hour window. The major selection criterion has been a volumetric mismatch between the perfusion and diffusion imaging lesions (Fig. 4). This mismatch serves as an imaging surrogate of penumbral tissue.

Evidence Supporting the Mismatch Hypothesis

Until the ECASS-3 (European Cooperative Acute Stroke Study 3) results, previous studies that used NCCT-based selection failed to extend the time window for IV tPA beyond 3 hours. ATLANTIS

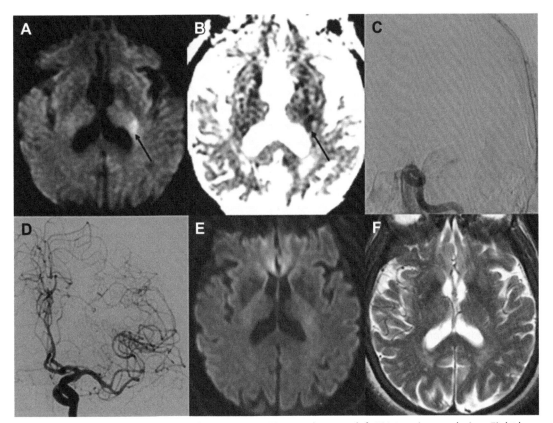

Fig. 3. 79-year-old woman presents with NIHSS score 22 secondary to a left ICA terminus occlusion. Eight hours after onset, there is a small focus of restricted diffusion adjacent to the atrium of the left lateral ventricle (A, B; arrows). Pretreatment (C) and posttreatment (D) angiograms show successful endovascular recanalization of the terminal ICA occlusion. DWI (E) and T2 (F) images at 40 hours after onset show near-complete lesion reversal.

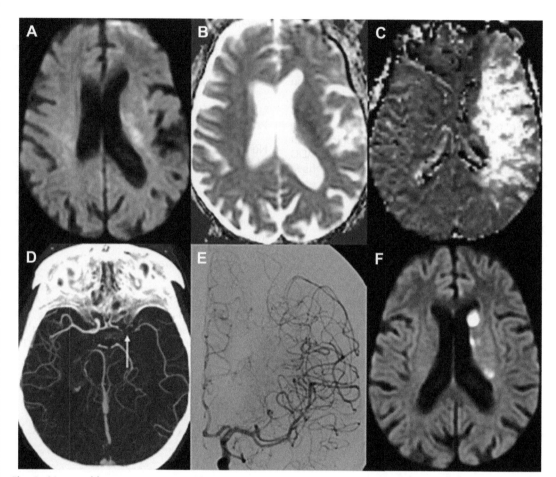

Fig. 4. 91-year-old woman presents with NIHSS score 22 secondary to left ICA terminus occlusion. MR imaging performed at 90 minutes after onset shows faint restricted diffusion in the left corona radiata (*A, B*). There is a larger region of MTT abnormality (*C*) consistent with a significant perfusion/diffusion mismatch. CTA shows the left ICA occlusion (*D, arrow*), which underwent successful endovascular revascularization (*E*). MR imaging performed 4 days later shows salvage of most of the mismatch territory (*F*). The patient had an independent outcome (mRS score 1) at 3 months.

(Alteplase Thrombolysis for Acute Noninterventional Therapy in Ischemic Stroke),[27,28] ECASS,[29] and ECASS-2[30] could not show a clinical benefit that outweighed treatment risk in the 5-hour to 6-hour window. In comparison, multiple studies using MR imaging perfusion/diffusion mismatch have shown positive clinical results for extended window treatment with IV tPA, and provide the strongest evidence for this imaging approach.

In large multicenter studies, patient selection using the perfusion/diffusion mismatch was shown to safely and effectively extend the treatment window for IV tPA up to 6 hours.[31–33] The most frequently used mismatch definition was a perfusion lesion at least 20% larger than the diffusion lesion. Furthermore, patients were excluded if they had extensive infarcts greater than one-third or one-half of the MCA territory. Patients with

a perfusion/diffusion mismatch treated with IV tPA beyond 3 hours appeared to do just as well as patients treated within the 3-hour window using traditional NCCT criteria.[31,33,34] In a multicenter study of 1210 patients,[31] there were no significant differences in favorable 3-month clinical outcome (modified Rankin scale [mRS] score 0–1; 35.4% vs 40.0%), symptomatic intracerebral hemorrhage (sICH) (5.3% vs 4.4%), and mortality (13.7% vs 13.3%) between patients treated within 3 hours using NCCT versus those treated beyond 3 hours based on a 20% perfusion/diffusion mismatch. Onset-to-treatment time (OTT) was not a predictor of safety or efficacy in univariate or multivariate analysis. The perfusion imaging techniques were heterogeneous among the centers and included nonthresholded mean transit time (MTT) maps and time-to-peak (TTP) maps with a delay of more than 4 seconds and without thresholding. Other studies have found similar results,[32–34] supporting the idea that a favorable cerebrovascular physiology may be more important than ischemic duration for extended window therapy.

Trials of IV Desmoteplase

Direct RCT evidence supporting the usefulness of mismatch-based selection was provided by trials of desmoteplase, a thrombolytic agent with high fibrin specificity and a long half-life.[35,36] In the randomized, placebo-controlled DIAS (Desmoteplase in Acute Ischemic Stroke) trial,[37] patients with OTT within 3 to 9 hours, a perfusion abnormality of 2 cm in diameter involving hemispheric gray matter, and a perfusion/diffusion mismatch of 20% or greater were included and randomized to 62.5 µg/kg, 90 µg/kg, 125 µg/kg, or placebo (part 2, n = 57 patients). Mismatch volumes were assessed by visual estimation. Compared with placebo (n = 27), the 125-µg/kg desmoteplase dose (n = 15) resulted in a higher reperfusion rate on MR imaging performed after 4 to 8 hours (71.4% vs 19.2%, P = .001) and higher rates of 90-day favorable clinical outcome (60% vs 22.2%, P = .009). As in other studies, OTT interval was not associated with reduced treatment effect. In a similar study design, the DEDAS (Dose Escalation of Desmoteplase for Acute Ischemic Stroke) trial[38] confirmed the clinical benefit of the 125-µg/kg desmoteplase dose relative to placebo in patients who fulfilled all MR imaging selection criteria, without a difference in sICH rate or mortality.

The Clinical Response of Mismatch Patients to Reperfusion

The beneficial clinical response of mismatch patients to documented reperfusion was shown in DEFUSE (Diffusion and Perfusion Imaging Evaluation for Understanding Stroke Evolution),[39] a phase II study examining 74 consecutive patients treated with IV tPA between 3 and 6 hours after stroke onset. Treatment selection was based on NCCT, not on an MR imaging mismatch. A total of 1020 patients were screened for 74 patients (7.2%). Patients with a baseline perfusion/diffusion mismatch (mismatch ratio ≥20%, and absolute mismatch ≥10 mL) who underwent early reperfusion (>30% reduction in perfusion lesion volume on MR imaging performed 3–6 hours after IV tPA treatment) had better outcomes than mismatch patients without reperfusion (odds ratio [OR] 5.4; 95% confidence interval [CI] 1.1–25.8). In addition, patients without a perfusion/diffusion mismatch did not seem to benefit from early reperfusion,

although there were only 11 patients without a mismatch in the study. Penumbral imaging used T_{max} with a 2-second delay.

The Limitations of the Mismatch Approach

Despite the favorable data in support of the mismatch hypothesis, there is no conclusive evidence that the mismatch alone identifies patients who respond to thrombolysis.[25,40–42] This uncertainty was recently highlighted by the results of the phase III DIAS-2 study,[43] which failed to confirm the DIAS and DEDAS findings.[37,38] In this study, patients with stroke with a 20% visual mismatch on either MR imaging or CT perfusion were randomized in a 1:1:1 fashion to 90 µg/kg IV desmoteplase, 125 µg/kg IV desmoteplase, and placebo. Among the low-dose, high-dose, and placebo groups, respectively, the rates of favorable clinical outcome at 90 days were 47%, 36%, and 46%; the rates of sICH were 3.5%, 4.5%, and 0%; and the mortality was 11%, 21%, and 6%. One-third of enrolled patients were evaluated with CT perfusion.

In addition, EPITHET (the Echoplanar Imaging Thrombolytic Evaluation Trial),[44] a phase II placebo-controlled, randomized trial of IV tPA administered 3 to 6 hours after stroke onset, failed to show any significant difference in the primary end point of infarct growth, or in reperfusion and clinical outcomes, between patients with a perfusion/diffusion mismatch (perfusion/diffusion ratio >1.2, and absolute mismatch volume ≥10 mL) and those without a mismatch, for both the IV tPA and placebo groups. As in DEFUSE, MR imaging findings were not used for patient selection or treatment allocation. These results are consistent with previous studies that have shown that the perfusion/diffusion mismatch does not predict infarct growth, and that lesion growth is equally common in patients with and without a mismatch.[45,46]

A recent meta-analysis of the DEDAS, DIAS, DIAS II, DEFUSE, and EPITHET trials analyzed the data from 502 mismatch patients who were treated with IV thrombolysis or placebo beyond 3 hours.[42] Although patients with an imaging mismatch showed higher rates of reperfusion with thrombolysis (adjusted OR [a-OR] 3.0; 95% CI 1.6–5.8), there was no significant improvement in favorable clinical outcome by thrombolytic therapy (a-OR 1.3; 95% CI 0.8–2.0). Furthermore, there was a significant increase in mortality and sICH after treatment, but these end points did not remain significant after exclusion of abandoned desmoteplase doses. These negative results suggest that the clinical and tissue response to reperfusion therapy may not be dependent strictly on the presence of a mismatch as it is currently defined.[47]

ALTERNATIVE APPROACHES TO IMAGING-BASED SELECTION

There are several challenges to the mismatch approach. First, the 20% mismatch threshold is an arbitrary value.[40,48,49] Post hoc analyses of DEFUSE and EPITHET have found more optimal definitions, but these require prospective validation.[50,51] Second, perfusion imaging methods and parameters are heterogeneous among different centers, a factor that has been shown to affect the size of the mismatch.[46] Third, mismatch assessment is based on visual estimation, which suffers from a high degree of error.[38,52] However, the most fundamental problem with the mismatch approach is that it provides a nonspecific assessment of stroke physiology.

Because a mismatch ratio is a relative measure, the same ratio can equate to different absolute tissue volumes and hence represent varying stroke severities. Despite identical imaging selection criteria for DIAS, DEDAS, and DIAS-2, baseline strokes in DIAS-2 were less severe across all study groups (average National Institutes of Health Stroke Scale [NIHSS] score of 9 vs 12 in DIAS and DEDAS). Similarly, diffusion lesion volumes and absolute mismatch volumes were significantly smaller in DIAS-2, despite the higher relative mismatch volume, and the rate of vessel occlusion was lower. The less severe stroke population in DIAS-2 helps to explain the high placebo response rate that contributed to the failure of this study. Likewise, despite similar imaging criteria between DEFUSE and EPITHET (eg, T_{max} threshold of 2 seconds), the DEFUSE cohort had lower baseline NIHSS scores (11.5 vs 13) and smaller baseline diffusion (10 vs 21 mL) and perfusion (48 vs 192 mL) lesion volumes.[53]

To address this problem, approaches based on absolute lesion volume have been proposed. In support of this concept, a post hoc analysis of EPITHET recently showed that diffusion and perfusion lesion volumes influence clinical response to IV tPA, whereas mismatch ratios do not.[54] This finding is reasonable when one considers that a small territory at risk likely results in a favorable clinical outcome even if the perfusion abnormality is 20% larger than the core infarct defined by diffusion imaging. Similarly, a significant neurologic deficit caused by a large core infarct is not influenced by improved perfusion in the surrounding tissue. It is the size and eloquence of the infarct and the territory at risk that are critical to outcome.

Diffusion MR imaging must be analyzed in the context of other important stroke-related variables, including the level of vessel occlusion and the clinical deficit.

The Importance of Vessel Imaging: Is There a Proximal Artery Occlusion Causing a Significant Stroke Syndrome?

When a patient presents with a significant clinical stroke syndrome reflected in an NIHSS score of 10 or greater, vessel imaging represents a critical early step in patient management because it quickly identifies patients who harbor a proximal artery occlusion (PAO) (Box 1).[55–59] Using clinical stroke severity alone to triage patients to vascular imaging is limited by a high degree of overlap in

---

Box 1
Is there a PAO?

Rationale for vessel imaging:

- There is significant overlap in NIHSS scores between patients with and without a proximal occlusion.
- Vessel imaging is a screening test for endovascular therapy: terminal internal carotid artery (ICA), MCA M1 or proximal M2 segment, and vertebrobasilar occlusions are the targets for IAT.
- Vessel status provides important prognostic information: more proximally located occlusions, particularly terminal ICA occlusions, have the worst outcomes following reperfusion therapy.

Imaging Approach:

- CT angiography (CTA) is the best noninvasive test, and has high accuracy for detecting proximal intracranial artery occlusions. Maximum intensity projection images facilitate lesion detection.
- MR angiography performs reasonably well in detecting major vessel occlusion, but is prone to patient motion and flow-related artifact. It is less sensitive for detecting M2 occlusions.

Recommendations:

- Noninvasive vessel imaging should be performed in all patients with suspected ischemic stroke.
- CTA is the test of choice.
- Imaging of the cervical vessels is helpful to detect steno-occlusive disease that may be the embolic source and that may need to be addressed during the endovascular procedure (eg, carotid stent placement).

NIHSS scores between patients with and without PAO.[55,59] Therefore, it is recommended that noninvasive vessel imaging with CT or MR angiography should be performed on all patients with suspected stroke or transient ischemic attack.[25]

The presence of a proximal occlusion is associated with significantly worse clinical outcomes. In a large prospective study of CTA in 735 patients with stroke or TIA at 2 major academic centers (the STOPStroke study[55]), patients with PAO, particularly involving the ICA, basilar artery, or MCA M1 and M2 segments had worse 6-month functional outcomes (OR 0.33; 95% CI 0.24–0.45) and higher mortality (OR 4.5; 95% CI 2.7–7.3) than those with normal CTA findings (**Fig. 5**). ICA or basilar artery occlusion was an independent predictor of functional outcomes (OR 0.44, $P = .04$). Another study of 480 patients showed that patients with major strokes secondary to PAO classified according to the Boston Acute Stroke Imaging Scale (BASIS) accounted for all the deaths, had longer ICU and hospital stays, and were more likely to be discharged to a rehabilitation facility (all outcomes, $P<.0001$).[60] Although major strokes comprised less than one-third of the cohort, they accounted for 60% of the total in-hospital costs.

On the other hand, if no arterial occlusion is seen, the prognosis is much improved. In a study of 35 patients with acute stroke who underwent MR angiography in the first 24 hours,[61] the average amount of infarct growth at 2 to 4 days in patients without a visible occlusion was only 1.7 cm³. Another study examined 283 consecutive patients with stroke who underwent catheter angiography for intended IAT.[62] The investigators found 28 patients without a visible occlusion, of whom 21 (75%) had a good 3-month outcome (mRS score ≤ 2). Twenty-seven patients had follow-up imaging: 5 normal scans, 8 lacunar strokes, 2 striatocapsular strokes, and 12 small/medium infarcts.

The precise location of the occlusion provides further information regarding prognosis and response to therapy. In general, arterial occlusions that arise more proximally are associated with worse outcomes, with terminal ICA occlusions having the poorest outcomes among anterior circulation strokes.[55,63,64] A major reason is that such occlusions are associated with greater clot burden,[65] which in turn hinders the degree and speed of recanalization for both IV[66] and IA[65,67,68] therapies. In 1 study of 135 patients with AIS who underwent IAT, patients with large thrombus (>2 vessel diameters) had lower rates of recanalization (50% vs 61%, $P = .22$) with significantly longer times to recanalization (median, 113 vs 74 minutes, $P<.001$).[65] Large thrombus was an independent predictor of poor outcome (OR 2.4; 95% CI 1.06–5.57) and mortality (OR 4.0; 95% CI 1.2–13.2).

Furthermore, the territory at risk expands with occlusion of more proximal branch points. As one would expect, a larger amount of lesion growth is observed with M1 (MCA stem) versus M2 (post-MCA bifurcation) occlusions, despite similar recanalization rates.[69] In addition, within the M1 segment itself, a proximal clot occludes the lenticulostriate arteries, leading to early infarct extension into the basal ganglia.[70] For terminal ICA occlusions, there are 2 factors that promote worse outcomes: involvement of both the anterior cerebral artery (ACA) and MCA territories, and a marked impairment of the collateral circulation. Occlusion of the ACA A1 (precommunicating) segment results in a variable reduction of flow into the distal ACA territory, which is dependent on the caliber of the anterior communicating artery (ACOM) and the contralateral A1 segment. An isolated hemisphere is rare,[71] and leads to rapid infarction of the ACA and MCA territories (**Fig. 6**). However, even with the presence of an ACOM, in many cases the occlusion of antegrade flow through the ipsilateral

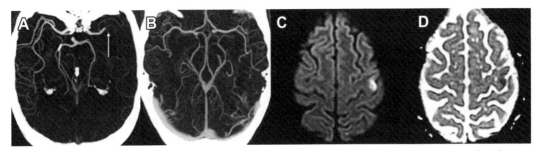

Fig. 5. The patient in (*A*) had a left distal M1 occlusion (*arrow*) with NIHSS score 20. He was treated with IV tPA but he died. The patient in (*B*), (*C*), and (*D*) had no visible occlusion on CTA (*B*). MR imaging showed small foci of restricted diffusion in the left precentral gyrus (*C, D*). She had an independent outcome (mRS score 0) at 3 months.

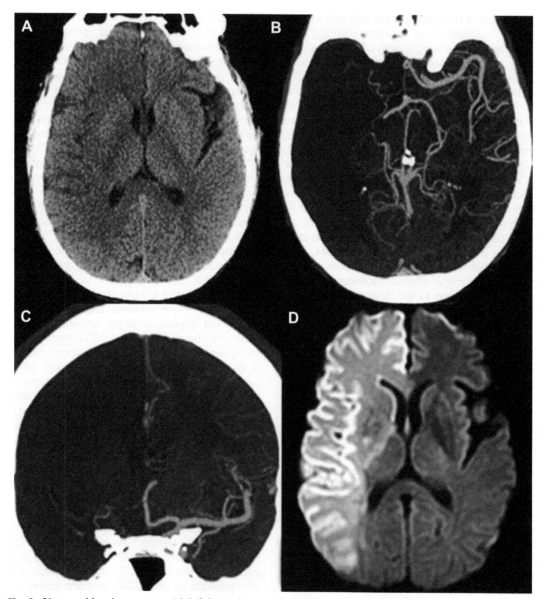

Fig. 6. 61-year-old male presents with left hemiplegia and NIHSS score 23. NCCT (A) shows extensive loss of gray-white matter differentiation in the right hemisphere. CTA collapsed maximum intensity projection images in the axial (B) and coronal (C) planes show a right ICA T occlusion with absence of the right ACA vessels, consistent with an isolated hemisphere. Despite presentation within the IA treatment window, MR imaging at 4.7 hours post ictus shows complete infarction of the right ACA and MCA territories on diffusion MR imaging (D).

A1 segment diminishes the perfusion pressure through the pial collaterals, resulting in greater and more rapid infarct growth in the MCA territory. This finding was reported in 1 study of 49 patients with AIS who underwent MR imaging/MR angiography within 6 hours of stroke onset and before IV tPA treatment.[72] Of the 47 patients with documented vessel occlusions, patients with ICA occlusions (n = 12) had significantly larger mean pretreatment diffusion lesion volumes (84.8 ± 75.2 cm³ vs 32 ± 41.6 cm³) than those with M1 occlusions (n = 19). In addition, patients with ICA occlusions had significantly larger perfusion defects on pretreatment TTP maps (161.2 ± 38.9 cm³ vs 127.5 ± 40.9 cm³). Moreover, it has been shown that relative infarct growth is greater for terminal ICA occlusions than for M1 occlusions after normalizing for the absolute volume of hypoperfusion.[73] Numerous imaging studies have confirmed these findings.[22,54,74,75]

The Importance of the Neurologic Examination

Numerous studies have shown that baseline NIHSS score is a strong predictor of clinical outcome.[76,77] The predictive power of the NIHSS derives from its measurement of both the size and eloquence of the tissue at risk. A recent study has shown the usefulness of NIHSS score thresholds for predicting good and poor functional outcome with high probability.[78] In this study of patients with anterior circulation stroke imaged within 9 hours of onset, all patients with an NIHSS score greater than 20 had poor outcome (90-day mRS score 3–6), and all with an NIHSS score less than 8 had good outcome (90-day mRS score 0–2), regardless of treatment. The lower threshold is supported by another study[79] reporting that patients with AIS with NIHSS score of 8 or greater had a significantly higher rate of subsequent neurologic worsening. Using baseline NIHSS score alone, the most appropriate patients to treat with reperfusion therapy may be those with NIHSS scores of 8 or greater and 20 or less, a range used in the DIAS trial.[37]

The Importance of Absolute Infarct Size

Considerable evidence shows that final infarct size is a critical determinant of clinical outcome (**Box 2**).[80–83] In a substudy of the ASAP (Acute Stroke Accurate Prediction) trial[82] involving 169 patients with median NIHSS score of 6 (mild to moderate severity), infarct growth was an independent predictor of excellent 90-day outcome (mRS score 0–1). In a subgroup analysis of the EPITHET trial,[80] which included 72 patients with median NIHSS score of 12 (moderate to severe strokes), infarct volume had a strong correlation with 90-day NIHSS score (Spearman $\rho = 0.81$; $P<.01$). In a study of 81 patients with IAT with anterior circulation PAO and median NIHSS score of 18,[83] final infarct volume was the best discriminator of good 3-month outcome (mRS score ≤ 2) in receiver operating characteristic analysis (area under the curve = 0.883).

Reperfusion therapy limits the size of the final infarct by salvaging the ischemic penumbra.[80,84–89] Patients with large baseline infarcts have little to no hope of treatment benefit, and should be excluded from the risks of therapy, which include iatrogenic emboli, intracerebral hemorrhage (ICH), and reperfusion edema.[90,91] Therefore, imaging of parenchymal injury at the time of presentation can provide important information for treatment decision making (**Fig. 7**).

Recent evidence suggests that the core infarct volume threshold for poor outcomes may be

---

Box 2
Is the volume of irreversible ischemic injury small (<70–100 cm³)?

Rationale for core infarct imaging:

- Despite the proven benefits of revascularization, most patients treated by IAT within the current time window (6–8 hours post ictus) have poor outcomes.
- Final infarct volume is an important predictor of clinical outcome.
- Studies using various imaging modalities (xenon-enhanced CT, MR imaging DWI, CTA source images, and CT perfusion imaging) have shown that pretreatment core infarct size predicts the clinical response to reperfusion, and that core infarct volume less than 70 to 100 cm³ may be an effective treatment target.

Imaging Approach:

- Diffusion MR imaging provides the most accurate and reliable estimate of the core infarct in the hyperacute setting (within 6 hours of onset).
- Ischemic change on NCCT quantified using the Alberta Stroke Program Early CT Score (ASPECTS) has been shown to influence treatment response. NCCT is limited by low sensitivity and high interrater variability.
- Using postprocessed CT perfusion maps, regions of reduced cerebral blood volume (CBV) are believed to represent irreversible tissue injury. The major limitation to this approach is the questionable reliability of perfusion imaging as a result of nonstandardized acquisition, postprocessing, and analysis methods.
- CTA source image hypoattenuation approximates tissue with CBV depression, under pseudosteady state conditions.

Recommendations:

- Core infarct estimation represents an important step in the evaluation of patients with AIS, and may predict the clinical response to reperfusion.
- Diffusion MR imaging is the test of choice. Advanced CT methods are more widely available, but have potential limitations.

---

even lower than the traditional criterion of one-third of the MCA territory (~100 cm³). Three studies have shown that baseline diffusion lesion volume greater than 70 cm³ is highly specific for poor outcomes with or without therapy.[78,92,93] In

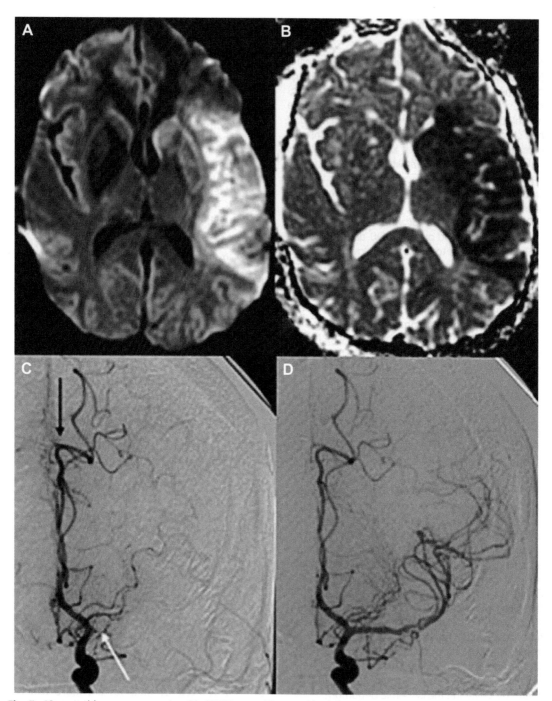

Fig. 7. 48-year-old woman presents with NIHSS score 14 caused by left MCA M1 segment occlusion. MR imaging (A, B) performed at 100 minutes after onset reveals a large baseline infarct (96 cm³ volume). Pretreatment (C) and posttreatment (D) angiograms show successful revascularization of the proximal M1 occlusion (arrow) at 5 hours after onset. She was dependent (mRS score 3) at 3 months.

a retrospective study of 34 patients who underwent pretreatment MR imaging followed by IAT,[74] there were 6 patients with baseline diffusion lesion size greater than 70 cm³ (futile group), all of whom had a poor 3-month outcome (mRS score 3–6) despite reperfusion in 3 patients. Within the study population, the patients in the futile group had the largest infarct growth.

The Complementary Roles of Vessel Imaging, Neurologic Examination, and Parenchymal Evaluation

A recent study has shown the added value of combining knowledge obtained from the neurologic examination with data from vascular and parenchymal imaging.[78] The investigators found that a diffusion lesion greater than 72 cm^3 or an NIHSS score greater than 20 predicted poor outcome with high probability. Similarly, an MTT lesion volume less than 47 cm^3 or NIHSS score less than 8 predicted good outcome with high probability. For practical purposes, the MTT threshold is equivalent to the absence of a PAO. In an analysis of prognostic yield, the NIHSS thresholds alone predicted outcome in 42.6% of cases. The diffusion and perfusion thresholds alone predicted outcome in 53.7%. Using all 3 thresholds together, outcome was predicted in 70.4%. Most outcomes (63.2%) were predicted by either a clinical or imaging threshold alone, suggesting that these parameters are highly complementary, likely because they measure different aspects of acute stroke. The NIHSS measures the neurologic severity of an ischemic insult, whereas diffusion and perfusion imaging reflect the cellular and vascular physiology of acute ischemia, respectively. Using these clinical and imaging thresholds, it follows that patients with a PAO (eg, MTT lesion $\geq$47 cm^3), small infarct size (eg, diffusion lesion $\leq$72 cm^3) and significant neurologic deficit (NIHSS score between 8 and 20) have an indeterminate outcome and seem to be a target population for revascularization therapy.

USING DIFFUSION MR IMAGING TO SELECT PATIENTS FOR IAT

There has been a marked growth in the use of endovascular revascularization therapies in recent years.[94] Proponents of IAT cite the improved revascularization rates of PAOs compared with IV tPA.[4,95–97] However, there remains little evidence for better clinical outcomes with this approach. The only RCT to show such a benefit was the PROACT II (Prolyse in Acute Cerebral Thromboembolism II) study.[4] The MERCI (Mechanical Embolus Removal in Cerebral Ischemia),[98] Multi MERCI,[97] and Penumbra Pivotal[99] trials were prospective, single-arm studies of mechanical devices that used reperfusion, rather than clinical outcome, as their primary end points. Because of this evidence, IAT is still considered by many experts as experimental.[100]

The major criteria for proceeding to IAT include a proximal cerebral artery occlusion and a significant neurologic deficit (NIHSS score >8 or 10), satisfying 2 of the 3 criteria mentioned in the preceding section. However, brain parenchymal evaluation consists of (1) an NCCT scan without an extensive infarct (more than one-third of the MCA territory) or significant mass effect, and (2) presentation within 8 hours of stroke onset. There is increasing criticism of this approach to parenchymal imaging. In response, the Stroke Therapy Academic Industry Roundtable[100] has recommended the use of imaging-based penumbral selection for extended window trials such as for IAT. However, an effective imaging selection criterion in this patient population has yet to be validated.

Can the Perfusion-diffusion Mismatch Identify Favorable Candidates for IAT?

The primary requirement for IAT is the presence of a PAO, such as the ICA or proximal MCA. Given the large parenchymal territory supplied by these vessels, the mismatch approach is a poor discriminator for identifying candidates for IAT with a favorable collateral physiology. One reason is that perfusion imaging methods are highly sensitive for identifying hypoperfused tissue, but not specific for delineating true territory at risk. In a recent analysis of 116 patients with ICA or proximal MCA occlusions, 90 of 93 (96.8%) patients with baseline DWI lesion volume 100 mL or less had at least 100% mismatch.[101] The results were similar when using nonthresholded MTT or TTP with a 4 second delay.

Estimating a Significant Penumbra: The Importance of Pretreatment Core Infarct Volume in Patients with Anterior Circulation PAO

Although the true extent of the penumbra cannot be known with certainty in the clinical setting, it can be reasonably assumed that this territory is large in patients with PAO who present with significant neurologic deficit (eg, NIHSS >10.) On average, the MCA territory and the ICA territory (ACA + MCA) constitute approximately 250 to 300 cm^3 and 400 to 450 cm^3 of brain tissue, respectively (**Box 3**).[102] Therefore, substantial tissue at risk is likely present even when the core infarct exceeds 100 cm^3 (about one-third of the MCA territory).[101] In this setting, the benefit of penumbral salvage is outweighed by the extensive deficit and procedural risk related to the large infarct core. This finding suggests that treatment response in anterior circulation PAO patients may be better predicted by baseline infarct size, rather than the size of the penumbra. This idea is

---

Box 3
Is there a large volume of brain at risk for infarction in the absence of reperfusion?

Rationale for penumbral imaging:

- Reperfusion yields a clinical benefit only if there is salvage of a substantial amount of hypoperfused but viable tissue.
- Studies using penumbral imaging for patient selection have supported a clinical benefit of reperfusion therapy beyond current time windows, confirming physiologic evidence that suggests that collateral physiology may be more important than time for treatment response.

Imaging Approach:

- The most commonly used approach is the MR imaging perfusion/diffusion mismatch, in which the penumbral tissue is defined as tissue with abnormal perfusion but normal diffusion signal. The CT perfusion MTT-CBV mismatch is an analogous model.
- MTT and TTP are the most commonly used parameters for evaluating abnormal perfusion. Some studies have used a quantitative threshold-based approach to exclude regions of benign oligemia.
- However, numerous studies have failed to show a clinical or tissue benefit using the mismatch approach.
- A simpler approach to identifying a significant penumbra is the combination of a PAO, significant clinical deficit (NIHSS score $\geq$10), and small core infarct (<70–100 cm^3).

Recommendations:

- Penumbral assessment is critical for identifying whether reperfusion can lead to tissue salvage and improved outcome.
- Until current perfusion methods are refined and standardized, a simpler approach using vessel status, clinical deficit, and core infarct size seems to be sufficient for patient selection for IAT.

---

supported by a study in which 36 patients with MCA M1 occlusions were evaluated with xenon-enhanced CT within 6 hours of symptom onset.[103] The investigators found that the core infarct volume (% MCA territory with cerebral blood flow [CBF] <8 mL/100 g/min) was an independent predictor of favorable outcome (mRS score 0–1; OR 0.85; 95% CI 0.74–0.98), whereas the penumbral volume (% MCA territory with CBF = 8–20 mL/100 g/min) was not associated with outcome

in univariate or multivariate analysis (P = .5). In this study, the treatments were variable: 26 patients received IV and/or IA therapy, and 10 patients were not treated.

The usefulness of core infarct size for treatment selection in PAO is supported by multiple studies reporting (1) that patients with large pretreatment diffusion lesions do poorly despite successful reperfusion, and (2) that patients with small diffusion lesions do well largely depending on timely reperfusion. Several studies have reported that patients with PAO who have early extensive diffusion imaging lesions have a worse clinical course with a significantly higher risk of malignant brain swelling.[22,104,105] Furthermore, the DEFUSE study showed that patients with acute stroke with early (3–6 hours after onset) and extensive infarcts generally have poor outcomes despite early reperfusion.[39] In this study, only 1 of 6 patients with a malignant profile (diffusion MR imaging lesion $\geq$100 cm^3 and/or perfusion lesion $\geq$100 cm^3 with $\geq$8 seconds of T_{max} delay) had a favorable outcome despite early reperfusion in 3 patients. As mentioned earlier, the core infarct volume threshold for poor outcomes may be as low as 70 cm^3.[78,92,93]

For patients with PAO who do not have extensive infarcts on hyperacute imaging (<6 hours), clinical and tissue outcome is strongly dependent on early reperfusion. A post hoc analysis of DEFUSE[106] showed that patients with PAO with diffusion MR imaging lesion volume less than 25 mL had marked improvement in outcomes if they underwent early reperfusion (OR 12.5; 95% CI 1.8–83.9). Similarly, among patients with anterior circulation PAO treated with IAT,[74] those with a pretreatment diffusion lesion volume less than 70 cm^3 had higher rates of good outcomes (3-month mRS score $\leq$2) with early reperfusion (64%) compared with late (17%) or no (0%) reperfusion (P<.016). Furthermore, there was greater infarct growth in patients who underwent delayed or no reperfusion. Despite differences in the threshold, these studies show the importance of core infarct size in shaping the clinical response to reperfusion, and suggest that patients with PAO with small core infarcts may represent a target population for IAT. Further studies are needed to better define the relationship between core infarct size, early reperfusion, and clinical outcome in this patient population.

The importance of baseline core infarct size in patients treated with IAT has also been shown in studies using CT-based methods for infarct delineation, including NCCT (using ASPECTS classification; **Fig. 8**),[107,108] CTA source images,[109] and CT perfusion CBV maps.[75]

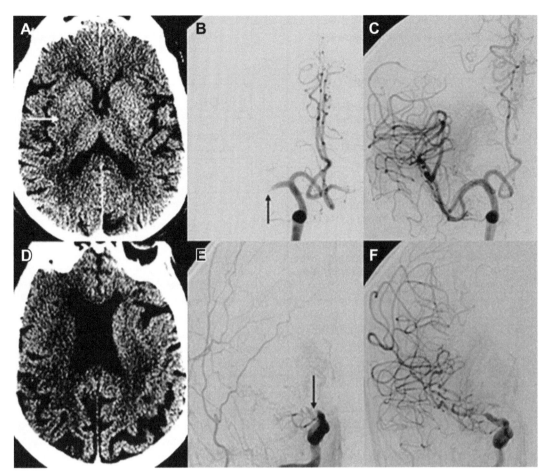

Fig. 8. The patient in (*A*), (*B*), and (*C*) presented with NIHSS score 14 secondary to right M1 occlusion. Baseline NCCT (*A*) performed 2 hours 30 minutes after onset revealed subtle ischemic change in the right putamen (ASPECTS score 9; *white arrow*). Pretreatment (*B*) and posttreatment (*C*) angiograms showed Thrombolysis in Cerebral Infarction (TICI) score 2B revascularization of the M1 occlusion (*black arrow*). The patient was independent (mRS score 2) at 3 months. The patient in (*D*), (*E*), and (*F*) presented with an NIHSS score of 13 caused by right terminal ICA occlusion. Baseline NCCT (*D*) performed 2 hours after onset revealed extensive ischemic change involving the basal ganglia and the frontal and parietal regions (ASPECTS score 2). Pretreatment (*E*) and posttreatment (*F*) angiograms showed TICI 2A reperfusion of the terminal ICA occlusion (*arrow*). The patient subsequently died.

USING DIFFUSION MR IMAGING TO IDENTIFY PATIENTS AT HIGH RISK FOR TREATMENT-RELATED HEMORRHAGE

The benefits of reperfusion therapy must be balanced against its risks, particularly posttreatment ICH (**Box 4**). A clinically significant ICH may be defined based on symptoms or via radiographic criteria.[110] sICH is any hemorrhage that occurs early (24–36 hours) after stroke treatment and is associated with neurologic deterioration, usually an NIHSS increase of 4 or more points or a 1-point deterioration in level of consciousness. From studies of IV and IA therapies, sICH often results in significant morbidity and mortality.[3,4,111]

Alternatively, a clinically significant ICH may be defined as a parenchymal hematoma type 2 (PH2) using the European Cooperative Acute Stroke Study (ECASS) radiographic criteria.[112] PH2 is a dense hematoma involving greater than 30% of the infarct with significant mass effect, and has been shown to have a negative effect on both short-term and long-term clinical outcomes.[111,113,114]

Evidence from both IV and IA studies suggests that pretreatment neuroimaging may be able to identify patients at high risk for hemorrhagic transformation. Early ischemic changes on NCCT (eg, loss of gray-white matter differentiation, effacement of sulci) have been associated with sICH and parenchymal hematomas,[115–117] although

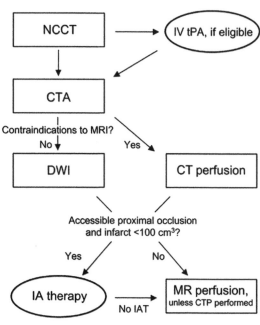

Fig. 9. Massachusetts General Hospital imaging triage algorithm for patients with AIS.

SUMMARY AND RECOMMENDATIONS

Combined imaging and clinical evaluation is a promising approach to improving patient selection for stroke reperfusion therapies. Specifically, vessel status, clinical stroke severity, and core infarct size have been shown to influence outcomes after IV and IA treatment. Noninvasive vessel imaging is best performed with CTA, although MR angiography performs sufficiently well. Concurrent imaging of the neck vessels provides important information for evaluating stroke mechanism and for planning subsequent intervention. Core infarct determination is a key element of the imaging evaluation, and is best performed with diffusion MR imaging. In the setting of anterior circulation stroke, a core infarct size of less than 70 to 100 cm³ seems to identify patients who benefit from revascularization. Therefore, if there is a major vessel occlusion with a significant stroke syndrome (NIHSS score ≥10) and a small core infarct size (volume <70–100 cm³), there is likely a clinically significant penumbra. Core infarct size may be a useful indicator of treatment risk, specifically for significant ICH. Data suggest that a similar core infarct volume threshold of 100 cm³ may identify those patients with a marked risk for symptomatic ICH. Based on the data presented in this review, Massachusetts General Hospital has adopted a new imaging triage protocol for patients with AIS, which is presented in **Fig. 9.**

other studies were not able to confirm these findings.[118,119] MR imaging seems to provide a better assessment of clinically significant hemorrhage risk than NCCT.[31,120] In a retrospective multicenter study of 645 patients with anterior circulation ischemic stroke treated with IV or IA thrombolysis,[121] diffusion MR imaging lesion size was an independent risk factor for sICH (OR 1.080; 95% CI 1.012–1.153 per 10 mL increase). Numerous studies[120,122,123] have confirmed this finding. Moreover, the increased risk in patients with large diffusion lesions seems to be further increased when there is subsequent reperfusion. In a post hoc analysis of the DEFUSE study,[120] only the interaction between diffusion lesion volume and reperfusion status was an independent predictor of sICH when reperfusion was included in the model. Therefore, an acute infarct volume threshold may not only identify patients who respond to reperfusion but may also be used to exclude patients who are at an increased risk of harm from treatment. Evidence suggests that a diffusion MR imaging lesion volume of greater than 100 cm³ is a marker of increased sICH risk, with a 16.1% risk of sICH among patients treated with IV or IA thrombolysis in 1 study.[121]

REFERENCES

1. Lloyd-Jones D, Adams R, Carnethon M, et al. Heart disease and stroke statistics–2009 update: a report from the American Heart Association Statistics Committee and Stroke Statistics Subcommittee. Circulation 2009;119(3):e21–181.

2. Hacke W, Kaste M, Bluhmki E, et al. Thrombolysis with alteplase 3 to 4.5 hours after acute ischemic stroke. N Engl J Med 2008;359(13):1317–29.

3. Tissue plasminogen activator for acute ischemic stroke. The National Institute of Neurological Disorders and Stroke rt-PA Stroke Study Group. N Engl J Med 1995;333(24):1581–7.

4. Furlan A, Higashida R, Wechsler L, et al. Intra-arterial prourokinase for acute ischemic stroke. The PROACT II study: a randomized controlled trial. Prolyse in Acute Cerebral Thromboembolism. JAMA 1999;282(21):2003–11.

5. Rha JH, Saver JL. The impact of recanalization on ischemic stroke outcome: a meta-analysis. Stroke 2007;38(3):967–73.

6. Lo EH, Dalkara T, Moskowitz MA. Mechanisms, challenges and opportunities in stroke. Nat Rev Neurosci 2003;4(5):399–415.

7. Mintorovitch J, Yang GY, Shimizu H, et al. Diffusion-weighted magnetic resonance imaging of acute focal cerebral ischemia: comparison of signal intensity with changes in brain water and Na+, K(+)-AT-Pase activity. J Cereb Blood Flow Metab 1994; 14(2):332–6.

8. Sykova E, Svoboda J, Polak J, et al. Extracellular volume fraction and diffusion characteristics during progressive ischemia and terminal anoxia in the spinal cord of the rat. J Cereb Blood Flow Metab 1994;14(2):301–11.

9. Wick M, Nagatomo Y, Prielmeier F, et al. Alteration of intracellular metabolite diffusion in rat brain in vivo during ischemia and reperfusion. Stroke 1995;26(10):1930–3 [discussion: 1934].

10. Mullins ME, Schaefer PW, Sorensen AG, et al. CT and conventional and diffusion-weighted MR imaging in acute stroke: study in 691 patients at presentation to the emergency department. Radiology 2002;224(2):353–60.

11. Gonzalez RG, Schaefer PW, Buonanno FS, et al. Diffusion-weighted MR imaging: diagnostic accuracy in patients imaged within 6 hours of stroke symptom onset. Radiology 1999;210(1):155–62.

12. Fiebach JB, Schellinger PD, Jansen O, et al. CT and diffusion-weighted MR imaging in randomized order: diffusion-weighted imaging results in higher accuracy and lower interrater variability in the diagnosis of hyperacute ischemic stroke. Stroke 2002; 33(9):2206–10.

13. Heiss WD, Sobesky J, Smekal U, et al. Probability of cortical infarction predicted by flumazenil binding and diffusion-weighted imaging signal intensity: a comparative positron emission tomography/magnetic resonance imaging study in early ischemic stroke. Stroke 2004;35(8):1892–8.

14. Mohr JP, Biller J, Hilal SK, et al. Magnetic resonance versus computed tomographic imaging in acute stroke. Stroke 1995;26(5):807–12.

15. Chalela JA, Kidwell CS, Nentwich LM, et al. Magnetic resonance imaging and computed tomography in emergency assessment of patients with suspected acute stroke: a prospective comparison. Lancet 2007;369(9558):293–8.

16. Fiebach J, Jansen O, Schellinger P, et al. Comparison of CT with diffusion-weighted MRI in patients with hyperacute stroke. Neuroradiology 2001; 43(8):628–32.

17. Grant PE, He J, Halpern EF, et al. Frequency and clinical context of decreased apparent diffusion coefficient reversal in the human brain. Radiology 2001;221(1):43–50.

18. Kidwell CS, Saver JL, Starkman S, et al. Late secondary ischemic injury in patients receiving intraarterial thrombolysis. Ann Neurol 2002;52(6): 698–703.

19. Schaefer PW, Hassankhani A, Putman C, et al. Characterization and evolution of diffusion MR imaging abnormalities in stroke patients undergoing intra-arterial thrombolysis. AJNR Am J Neuroradiol 2004;25(6):951–7.

20. Kidwell CS, Saver JL, Mattiello J, et al. Thrombolytic reversal of acute human cerebral ischemic injury shown by diffusion/perfusion magnetic resonance imaging. Ann Neurol 2000;47(4):462–9.

21. Fiehler J, Knudsen K, Kucinski T, et al. Predictors of apparent diffusion coefficient normalization in stroke patients. Stroke 2004;35(2):514–9.

22. Arenillas JF, Rovira A, Molina CA, et al. Prediction of early neurological deterioration using diffusion- and perfusion-weighted imaging in hyperacute middle cerebral artery ischemic stroke. Stroke 2002;33(9):2197–203.

23. Olivot JM, Mlynash M, Thijs VN, et al. Relationships between cerebral perfusion and reversibility of acute diffusion lesions in DEFUSE: insights from RADAR. Stroke 2009;40(5):1692–7.

24. Chalela JA, Kang DW, Luby M, et al. Early magnetic resonance imaging findings in patients receiving tissue plasminogen activator predict outcome: insights into the pathophysiology of acute stroke in the thrombolysis era. Ann Neurol 2004;55(1):105–12.

25. Latchaw RE, Alberts MJ, Lev MH, et al. Recommendations for imaging of acute ischemic stroke. A scientific statement from the American Heart Association. Stroke 2009;40(11):3646–78.

26. Schellinger PD, Bryan RN, Caplan LR, et al. Evidence-based guideline: the role of diffusion and

perfusion MRI for the diagnosis of acute ischemic stroke: report of the Therapeutics and Technology Assessment Subcommittee of the American Academy of Neurology. Neurology 2010;75(2):177–85.

27. Clark WM, Albers GW, Madden KP, et al. The rtPA (alteplase) 0- to 6-hour acute stroke trial, part A (A0276g): results of a double-blind, placebo-controlled, multicenter study. Thrombolytic therapy in acute ischemic stroke study investigators. Stroke 2000;31(4):811–6.

28. Clark WM, Wissman S, Albers GW, et al. Recombinant tissue-type plasminogen activator (Alteplase) for ischemic stroke 3 to 5 hours after symptom onset. The ATLANTIS Study: a randomized controlled trial. Alteplase Thrombolysis for Acute Noninterventional Therapy in Ischemic Stroke. JAMA 1999;282(21):2019–26.

29. Hacke W, Kaste M, Fieschi C, et al. Intravenous thrombolysis with recombinant tissue plasminogen activator for acute hemispheric stroke. The European Cooperative Acute Stroke Study (ECASS). JAMA 1995;274(13):1017–25.

30. Hacke W, Kaste M, Fieschi C, et al. Randomised double-blind placebo-controlled trial of thrombolytic therapy with intravenous alteplase in acute ischaemic stroke (ECASS II). Second European-Australasian Acute Stroke Study Investigators. Lancet 1998;352(9136):1245–51.

31. Schellinger PD, Thomalla G, Fiehler J, et al. MRI-based and CT-based thrombolytic therapy in acute stroke within and beyond established time windows: an analysis of 1210 patients. Stroke 2007;38(10):2640–5.

32. Thomalla G, Schwark C, Sobesky J, et al. Outcome and symptomatic bleeding complications of intravenous thrombolysis within 6 hours in MRI-selected stroke patients: comparison of a German multicenter study with the pooled data of ATLANTIS, ECASS, and NINDS tPA trials. Stroke 2006;37(3):852–8.

33. Kohrmann M, Juttler E, Fiebach JB, et al. MRI versus CT-based thrombolysis treatment within and beyond the 3 h time window after stroke onset: a cohort study. Lancet Neurol 2006;5(8):661–7.

34. Ribo M, Molina CA, Rovira A, et al. Safety and efficacy of intravenous tissue plasminogen activator stroke treatment in the 3- to 6-hour window using multimodal transcranial Doppler/MRI selection protocol. Stroke 2005;36(3):602–6.

35. Reddrop C, Moldrich RX, Beart PM, et al. Vampire bat salivary plasminogen activator (desmoteplase) inhibits tissue-type plasminogen activator-induced potentiation of excitotoxic injury. Stroke 2005; 36(6):1241–6.

36. Liberatore GT, Samson A, Bladin C, et al. Vampire bat salivary plasminogen activator (desmoteplase): a unique fibrinolytic enzyme that does not promote neurodegeneration. Stroke 2003;34(2):537–43.

37. Hacke W, Albers G, Al-Rawi Y, et al. The Desmoteplase in Acute Ischemic Stroke Trial (DIAS): a phase II MRI-based 9-hour window acute stroke thrombolysis trial with intravenous desmoteplase. Stroke 2005;36(1):66–73.

38. Furlan AJ, Eyding D, Albers GW, et al. Dose Escalation of Desmoteplase for Acute Ischemic Stroke (DEDAS): evidence of safety and efficacy 3 to 9 hours after stroke onset. Stroke 2006;37(5):1227–31.

39. Albers GW, Thijs VN, Wechsler L, et al. Magnetic resonance imaging profiles predict clinical response to early reperfusion: the diffusion and perfusion imaging evaluation for understanding stroke evolution (DEFUSE) study. Ann Neurol 2006;60(5):508–17.

40. Kane I, Sandercock P, Wardlaw J. Magnetic resonance perfusion diffusion mismatch and thrombolysis in acute ischaemic stroke: a systematic review of the evidence to date. J Neurol Neurosurg Psychiatry 2007;78(5):485–91.

41. Schabitz WR. MR mismatch is useful for patient selection for thrombolysis: no. Stroke 2009;40(8):2908–9.

42. Mishra NK, Albers GW, Davis SM, et al. Mismatch-based delayed thrombolysis: a meta-analysis. Stroke 2010;41(1):e25–33.

43. Hacke W, Furlan AJ, Al-Rawi Y, et al. Intravenous desmoteplase in patients with acute ischaemic stroke selected by MRI perfusion-diffusion weighted imaging or perfusion CT (DIAS-2): a prospective, randomised, double-blind, placebo-controlled study. Lancet Neurol 2009;8(2):141–50.

44. Davis SM, Donnan GA, Parsons MW, et al. Effects of alteplase beyond 3 h after stroke in the Echoplanar Imaging Thrombolytic Evaluation Trial (EPITHET): a placebo-controlled randomised trial. Lancet Neurol 2008;7(4):299–309.

45. Rivers CS, Wardlaw JM, Armitage PA, et al. Do acute diffusion- and perfusion-weighted MRI lesions identify final infarct volume in ischemic stroke? Stroke 2006;37(1):98–104.

46. Kane I, Carpenter T, Chappell F, et al. Comparison of 10 different magnetic resonance perfusion imaging processing methods in acute ischemic stroke: effect on lesion size, proportion of patients with diffusion/perfusion mismatch, clinical scores, and radiologic outcomes. Stroke 2007;38(12):3158–64.

47. Davis SM, Donnan GA. MR mismatch and thrombolysis: appealing but validation required. Stroke 2009;40(8):2910.

48. Butcher KS, Parsons M, MacGregor L, et al. Refining the perfusion-diffusion mismatch hypothesis. Stroke 2005;36(6):1153–9.

49. Christensen S, Mouridsen K, Wu O, et al. Comparison of 10 perfusion MRI parameters in 97 sub-6-hour stroke patients using voxel-based receiver operating characteristics analysis. Stroke 2009; 40(6):2055–61.

50. Kakuda W, Lansberg MG, Thijs VN, et al. Optimal definition for PWI/DWI mismatch in acute ischemic stroke patients. J Cereb Blood Flow Metab 2008; 28(5):887–91.

51. Donnan GA, Baron JC, Ma H, et al. Penumbral selection of patients for trials of acute stroke therapy. Lancet Neurol 2009;8(3):261–9.

52. Coutts SB, Simon JE, Tomanek AI, et al. Reliability of assessing percentage of diffusion-perfusion mismatch. Stroke 2003;34(7):1681–3.

53. Toth G, Albers GW. Use of MRI to estimate the therapeutic window in acute stroke: is perfusion-weighted imaging/diffusion-weighted imaging mismatch an EPITHET for salvageable ischemic brain tissue? Stroke 2009;40(1):333–5.

54. Parsons MW, Christensen S, McElduff P, et al. Pretreatment diffusion- and perfusion-MR lesion volumes have a crucial influence on clinical response to stroke thrombolysis. J Cereb Blood Flow Metab 2010;30(6):1214–25.

55. Smith WS, Lev MH, English JD, et al. Significance of large vessel intracranial occlusion causing acute ischemic stroke and TIA. Stroke 2009; 40(12):3834–40.

56. Smith WS, Tsao JW, Billings ME, et al. Prognostic significance of angiographically confirmed large vessel intracranial occlusion in patients presenting with acute brain ischemia. Neurocrit Care 2006; 4(1):14–7.

57. Sims JR, Rordorf G, Smith EE, et al. Arterial occlusion revealed by CT angiography predicts NIH stroke score and acute outcomes after IV tPA treatment. AJNR Am J Neuroradiol 2005;26(2): 246–51.

58. Davis SM, Donnan GA. Basilar artery thrombosis: recanalization is the key. Stroke 2006;37(9):2440.

59. Maas MB, Furie KL, Lev MH, et al. National Institutes of Health Stroke Scale score is poorly predictive of proximal occlusion in acute cerebral ischemia. Stroke 2009;40(9):2988–93.

60. Cipriano LE, Steinberg ML, Gazelle GS, et al. Comparing and predicting the costs and outcomes of patients with major and minor stroke using the Boston Acute Stroke Imaging Scale neuroimaging classification system. AJNR Am J Neuroradiol 2009;30(4):703–9.

61. Staroselskaya IA, Chaves C, Silver B, et al. Relationship between magnetic resonance arterial patency and perfusion-diffusion mismatch in acute ischemic stroke and its potential clinical use. Arch Neurol 2001;58(7):1069–74.

62. Arnold M, Nedeltchev K, Brekenfeld C, et al. Outcome of acute stroke patients without visible occlusion on early arteriography. Stroke 2004; 35(5):1135–8.

63. Arnold M, Nedeltchev K, Mattle HP, et al. Intra-arterial thrombolysis in 24 consecutive patients with internal carotid artery T occlusions. J Neurol Neurosurg Psychiatry 2003;74(6):739–42.

64. Eckert B, Kucinski T, Neumaier-Probst E, et al. Local intra-arterial fibrinolysis in acute hemispheric stroke: effect of occlusion type and fibrinolytic agent on recanalization success and neurological outcome. Cerebrovasc Dis 2003;15(4): 258–63.

65. Barreto AD, Albright KC, Hallevi H, et al. Thrombus burden is associated with clinical outcome after intra-arterial therapy for acute ischemic stroke. Stroke 2008;39(12):3231–5.

66. Tan IY, Demchuk AM, Hopyan J, et al. CT angiography clot burden score and collateral score: correlation with clinical and radiologic outcomes in acute middle cerebral artery infarct. AJNR Am J Neuroradiol 2009;30(3):525–31.

67. Zaidat OO, Suarez JI, Santillan C, et al. Response to intra-arterial and combined intravenous and intra-arterial thrombolytic therapy in patients with distal internal carotid artery occlusion. Stroke 2002;33(7):1821–6.

68. Gupta R, Vora NA, Horowitz MB, et al. Multimodal reperfusion therapy for acute ischemic stroke: factors predicting vessel recanalization. Stroke 2006;37(4):986–90.

69. Fiehler J, Knudsen K, Thomalla G, et al. Vascular occlusion sites determine differences in lesion growth from early apparent diffusion coefficient lesion to final infarct. AJNR Am J Neuroradiol 2005;26(5):1056–61.

70. Nakano S, Iseda T, Kawano H, et al. Correlation of early CT signs in the deep middle cerebral artery territories with angiographically confirmed site of arterial occlusion. AJNR Am J Neuroradiol 2001; 22(4):654–9.

71. Liebeskind DS. Collateral circulation. Stroke 2003; 34(9):2279–84.

72. Derex L, Hermier M, Adeleine P, et al. Influence of the site of arterial occlusion on multiple baseline hemodynamic MRI parameters and post-thrombolytic recanalization in acute stroke. Neuroradiology 2004;46(11):883–7.

73. Kucinski T, Naumann D, Knab R, et al. Tissue at risk is overestimated in perfusion-weighted imaging: MR imaging in acute stroke patients without vessel recanalization. AJNR Am J Neuroradiol 2005;26(4): 815–9.

74. Yoo AJ, Verduzco LA, Schaefer PW, et al. MRI-based selection for intra-arterial stroke therapy: value of pretreatment diffusion-weighted imaging lesion volume in selecting patients with acute stroke who will benefit from early recanalization. Stroke 2009;40(6):2046–54.

75. Gasparotti R, Grassi M, Mardighian D, et al. Perfusion CT in patients with acute ischemic stroke treated with intra-arterial thrombolysis: predictive

value of infarct core size on clinical outcome. AJNR Am J Neuroradiol 2009;30(4):722–7.

76. Baird AE, Dambrosia J, Janket S, et al. A three-item scale for the early prediction of stroke recovery. Lancet 2001;357(9274):2095–9.

77. Sato S, Toyoda K, Uehara T, et al. Baseline NIH stroke scale score predicting outcome in anterior and posterior circulation strokes. Neurology 2008; 70(24 Pt 2):2371–7.

78. Yoo AJ, Barak ER, Copen WA, et al. Combining acute diffusion-weighted imaging and mean transmit time lesion volumes with National Institutes of Health Stroke Scale Score improves the prediction of acute stroke outcome. Stroke 2010;41(8): 1728–35.

79. DeGraba TJ, Hallenbeck JM, Pettigrew KD, et al. Progression in acute stroke: value of the initial NIH stroke scale score on patient stratification in future trials. Stroke 1999;30(6):1208–12.

80. Ebinger M, Christensen S, De Silva DA, et al. Expediting MRI-based proof-of-concept stroke trials using an earlier imaging end point. Stroke 2009; 40(4):1353–8.

81. Warach S, Pettigrew LC, Dashe JF, et al. Effect of citicoline on ischemic lesions as measured by diffusion-weighted magnetic resonance imaging. Citicoline 010 Investigators. Ann Neurol 2000; 48(5):713–22.

82. Barrett KM, Ding YH, Wagner DP, et al. Change in diffusion-weighted imaging infarct volume predicts neurologic outcome at 90 days: results of the Acute Stroke Accurate Prediction (ASAP) trial serial imaging substudy. Stroke 2009;40(7):2422–7.

83. Hakimelahi R, Romero J, Nogueira RG, et al. Final infarct volume is the best predictor of outcome in large vessel occlusion patients treated with IAT. Paper presented at: American Society of Neuroradiology. Vancouver (BC), May 16–21, 2009.

84. Baron JC. Perfusion thresholds in human cerebral ischemia: historical perspective and therapeutic implications. Cerebrovasc Dis 2001;11(Suppl 1): 2–8.

85. Ginsberg MD, Pulsinelli WA. The ischemic penumbra, injury thresholds, and the therapeutic window for acute stroke. Ann Neurol 1994;36(4): 553–4.

86. Hossmann KA. Viability thresholds and the penumbra of focal ischemia. Ann Neurol 1994; 36(4):557–65.

87. Astrup J, Siesjo BK, Symon L. Thresholds in cerebral ischemia–the ischemic penumbra. Stroke 1981;12(6):723–5.

88. Soares BP, Tong E, Hom J, et al. Reperfusion is a more accurate predictor of follow-up infarct volume than recanalization. A proof of concept using CT in acute ischemic stroke patients. Stroke 2010;41(1):e34–40.

89. Hermier M, Nighoghossian N, Adeleine P, et al. Early magnetic resonance imaging prediction of arterial recanalization and late infarct volume in acute carotid artery stroke. J Cereb Blood Flow Metab 2003;23(2):240–8.

90. Caplan LR. Stroke thrombolysis: slow progress. Circulation 2006;114(3):187–90.

91. King S, Khatri P, Carrozzella J, et al. Anterior cerebral artery emboli in combined intravenous and intra-arterial rtPA treatment of acute ischemic stroke in the IMS I and II trials. AJNR Am J Neuroradiol 2007;28(10):1890–4.

92. Arsava E, Ay H, Singhal AB, et al. An infarct volume threshold on early DWI to predict unfavorable clinical outcome. Paper presented at: International Stroke Conference. New Orleans (LA), February 20–22, 2008.

93. Sanak D, Nosal V, Horak D, et al. Impact of diffusion-weighted MRI-measured initial cerebral infarction volume on clinical outcome in acute stroke patients with middle cerebral artery occlusion treated by thrombolysis. Neuroradiology 2006;48(9):632–9.

94. Hirsch J, Yoo AJ, Nogueira RG, et al. Case volumes of intra-arterial and intravenous treatment of ischemic stroke in the USA. J Neurointerv Surg 2009;1(1):27–31.

95. Wolpert SM, Bruckmann H, Greenlee R, et al. Neuroradiologic evaluation of patients with acute stroke treated with recombinant tissue plasminogen activator. The rt-PA Acute Stroke Study Group. AJNR Am J Neuroradiol 1993;14(1):3–13.

96. Lee KY, Han SW, Kim SH, et al. Early recanalization after intravenous administration of recombinant tissue plasminogen activator as assessed by pre- and post-thrombolytic angiography in acute ischemic stroke patients. Stroke 2007;38(1):192–3.

97. Smith WS, Sung G, Saver J, et al. Mechanical thrombectomy for acute ischemic stroke: final results of the Multi MERCI trial. Stroke 2008;39(4):1205–12.

98. Smith WS, Sung G, Starkman S, et al. Safety and efficacy of mechanical embolectomy in acute ischemic stroke: results of the MERCI trial. Stroke 2005;36(7):1432–8.

99. Penumbra Pivotal Stroke Trial Investigators. The penumbra pivotal stroke trial: safety and effectiveness of a new generation of mechanical devices for clot removal in intracranial large vessel occlusive disease. Stroke 2009;40(8):2761–8.

100. Saver JL, Albers GW, Dunn B, et al. Stroke Therapy Academic Industry Roundtable (STAIR) recommendations for extended window acute stroke therapy trials. Stroke 2009;40(7):2594–600.

101. Hakimelahi R, Copen WA, Schaefer PW, et al. A small DWI lesion in the setting of an anterior circulation proximal artery occlusion predicts the presence of a large diffusion-perfusion mismatch.

Paper presented at: American Society of Neuroradiology Annual Meeting. Vancouver (BC), May 16–21, 2009.

102. van der Zwan A, Hillen B, Tulleken CA, et al. A quantitative investigation of the variability of the major cerebral arterial territories. Stroke 1993; 24(12):1951–9.

103. Jovin TG, Yonas H, Gebel JM, et al. The cortical ischemic core and not the consistently present penumbra is a determinant of clinical outcome in acute middle cerebral artery occlusion. Stroke 2003;34(10):2426–33.

104. Thomalla GJ, Kucinski T, Schoder V, et al. Prediction of malignant middle cerebral artery infarction by early perfusion- and diffusion-weighted magnetic resonance imaging. Stroke 2003;34(8):1892–9.

105. Oppenheim C, Samson Y, Manai R, et al. Prediction of malignant middle cerebral artery infarction by diffusion-weighted imaging. Stroke 2000;31(9): 2175–81.

106. Lansberg MG, Thijs VN, Bammer R, et al. The MRA-DWI mismatch identifies patients with stroke who are likely to benefit from reperfusion. Stroke 2008;39(9):2491–6.

107. Hill MD, Rowley HA, Adler F, et al. Selection of acute ischemic stroke patients for intra-arterial thrombolysis with pro-urokinase by using ASPECTS. Stroke 2003;34(8):1925–31.

108. Hill MD, Demchuk AM, Tomsick TA, et al. Using the baseline CT scan to select acute stroke patients for IV-IA therapy. AJNR Am J Neuroradiol 2006;27(8): 1612–6.

109. Lev MH, Segal AZ, Farkas J, et al. Utility of perfusion-weighted CT imaging in acute middle cerebral artery stroke treated with intra-arterial thrombolysis: prediction of final infarct volume and clinical outcome. Stroke 2001;32(9):2021–8.

110. Khatri P, Wechsler LR, Broderick JP. Intracranial hemorrhage associated with revascularization therapies. Stroke 2007;38(2):431–40.

111. Berger C, Fiorelli M, Steiner T, et al. Hemorrhagic transformation of ischemic brain tissue: asymptomatic or symptomatic? Stroke 2001;32(6):1330–5.

112. Trouillas P, von Kummer R. Classification and pathogenesis of cerebral hemorrhages after thrombolysis in ischemic stroke. Stroke 2006;37(2):556–61.

113. Paciaroni M, Agnelli G, Corea F, et al. Early hemorrhagic transformation of brain infarction: rate, predictive factors, and influence on clinical outcome: results of a prospective multicenter study. Stroke 2008;39(8):2249–56.

114. Fiorelli M, Bastianello S, von Kummer R, et al. Hemorrhagic transformation within 36 hours of a cerebral infarct: relationships with early clinical deterioration and 3-month outcome in the European Cooperative Acute Stroke Study I (ECASS I) cohort. Stroke 1999;30(11):2280–4.

115. Brekenfeld C, Remonda L, Nedeltchev K, et al. Symptomatic intracranial haemorrhage after intra-arterial thrombolysis in acute ischaemic stroke: assessment of 294 patients treated with urokinase. J Neurol Neurosurg Psychiatry 2007; 78(3):280–5.

116. Larrue V, von Kummer RR, Muller A, et al. Risk factors for severe hemorrhagic transformation in ischemic stroke patients treated with recombinant tissue plasminogen activator: a secondary analysis of the European-Australasian Acute Stroke Study (ECASS II). Stroke 2001;32(2):438–41.

117. Intracerebral hemorrhage after intravenous t-PA therapy for ischemic stroke. The NINDS t-PA Stroke Study Group. Stroke 1997;28(11):2109–18.

118. Demchuk AM, Hill MD, Barber PA, et al. Importance of early ischemic computed tomography changes using ASPECTS in NINDS rtPA Stroke Study. Stroke 2005;36(10):2110–5.

119. Patel SC, Levine SR, Tilley BC, et al. Lack of clinical significance of early ischemic changes on computed tomography in acute stroke. JAMA 2001;286(22): 2830–8.

120. Lansberg MG, Thijs VN, Bammer R, et al. Risk factors of symptomatic intracerebral hemorrhage after tPA therapy for acute stroke. Stroke 2007; 38(8):2275–8.

121. Singer OC, Humpich MC, Fiehler J, et al. Risk for symptomatic intracerebral hemorrhage after thrombolysis assessed by diffusion-weighted magnetic resonance imaging. Ann Neurol 2008;63(1):52–60.

122. Singer OC, Kurre W, Humpich MC, et al. Risk assessment of symptomatic intracerebral hemorrhage after thrombolysis using DWI-ASPECTS. Stroke 2009;40(8):2743–8.

123. Selim M, Fink JN, Kumar S, et al. Predictors of hemorrhagic transformation after intravenous recombinant tissue plasminogen activator: prognostic value of the initial apparent diffusion coefficient and diffusion-weighted lesion volume. Stroke 2002;33(8):2047–52.

Diffusion Magnetic Resonance Imaging in Multiple Sclerosis

L. Celso Hygino da Cruz Jr, MD[a,b,c,]*,
Raquel Ribeiro Batista, MD[d],
Roberto Cortes Domingues, MD[e],
Frederik Barkhof, MD, PhD[f]

KEYWORDS

- Multiple sclerosis • Diffusion MR imaging
- Central nervous system • Plaques

Multiple sclerosis (MS) is considered the most common inflammatory autoimmune neurologic disorder, involving especially the white matter (WM), the main pathologic features of which include a primary perivascular inflammation, demyelination, gliosis, and axonal injury.[1,2] MS is a chronic disease, estimated to affect 2.5 million people worldwide, and almost 400,000 persons in only the United States. Women are affected twice to 3 times as frequently as men, and it is uncommon in children, accounting for only about 0.3% to 0.4% of all cases. The symptoms begin most frequently during the third and fourth decades. However, MS can develop after age 50 years, accounting for 10% of cases.[2,3] MS is the most frequent cause of nontraumatic neurologic disability in young and middle-age adults.[1] Thus, early diagnosis is required to promptly begin a more effective treatment.

Conventional magnetic resonance (MR) imaging has become a primary tool for the investigation of MS and for clinical diagnosis over the past 3 decades, since its introduction.[4] MR scans offer the most sensitive way to identify MS lesions and their changes, for example disease accumulation and disease activity.[5] Therefore, the use of MR imaging has had a major effect on early and more precise diagnosis as well as on treatment management, predicting the prognosis of patients (**Fig. 1**).[2]

The role of MR imaging in the diagnosis of MS has been strengthened with the introduction of the McDonald criteria,[6] because this modality is able to determine dissemination in both time and space of the demyelinating lesions. The McDonald criteria include the Barkhof-Tintore MR imaging criteria,[7,8] because a spinal cord lesion can substitute for any of the brain lesions.[6] Nevertheless, in the light of subsequent studies, new insights were added and the previous proposed 2001 criteria were revised at the reconvened international panel during 2005.[9] The Barkhof-Tintore MR imaging criteria were kept in the new diagnostic MS criteria. However, the 2 criteria differ in the extent to which a spinal cord lesion can also assist with fulfillment of dissemination in space.[2]

The authors have nothing to disclose.

[a] Clinics CDPI and Multi-Imagem, Rua Saddock de Sá 266, Rio de Janeiro, Brazil
[b] Clinic IRM, Rua Capitao Salomao 44, Rio de Janeiro, Brazil
[c] Department of Radiology, Federal University of Rio de Janeiro, Rio de Janeiro, Brazil
[d] CDPI Clinic, Av. das Américas, 4666, sala 325, Barra da Tijuca, Rio de Janeiro, CEP: 22649-900, Brazil
[e] CDPI and Multi-Imagem Clinics, Av. das Américas, 4666, sala 325, Barra da Tijuca, Rio de Janeiro, CEP: 22649-900, Brazil
[f] Department of Radiology, Vrije University Medical Centre, De Boelelaan 1117, PO Box 7057, Amsterdam 1007 MB, The Netherlands
* Corresponding author. Rua Saddock de Sá 266, Ipanema, Rio de Janeiro, Brazil CEP: 22411-040.
E-mail address: celsohygino@hotmail.com

Neuroimag Clin N Am 21 (2011) 71–88
doi:10.1016/j.nic.2011.02.006

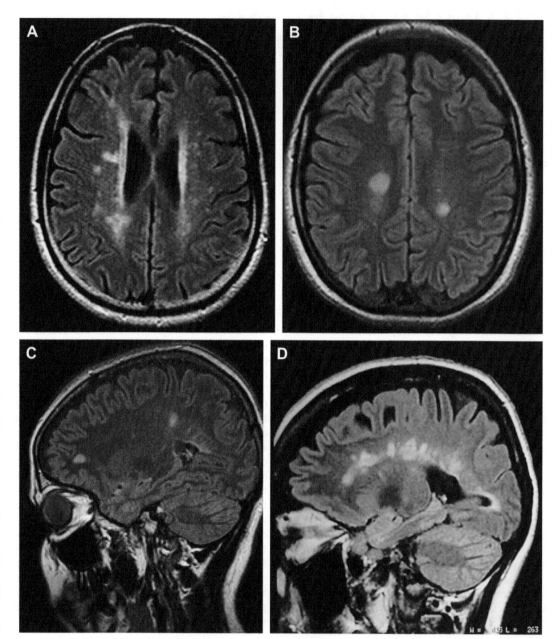

Fig. 1. MS: different imaging features. (*A, B*) Axial fluid-attenuated inversion recovery (FLAIR) shows typical appearance of deep WM plaques like multiple hyperintense lesions in subcortical and cerebral deep WM, mostly ovoid in shape. (*C, D*) Sagittal FLAIR shows demyelinating plaques along the margin of lateral ventricles and the corpus callosum, with the typical radial arrangement, called Dawson fingers.

As mentioned earlier, conventional MR imaging offers the most sensitive way to detect demyelinating plaques and their histopathologic changes over time. It is also useful in helping to determine the diagnosis of clinically defined MS as well as to rule out other conditions that may resemble the disease. Although high sensitivity has been described, the MR specificity is low and these findings may resemble other pathologic conditions, such as those secondary to atherosclerosis. MR imaging contributes decisively to the management of patients with MS, adding useful information regarding conversion to clinically definitive MS, earlier diagnosis, disease prognosis, and treatment response. MR imaging is the most versatile technique for depicting MS lesions. More recently, some investigators have suggested that diffusion tensor imaging (DTI) could play an

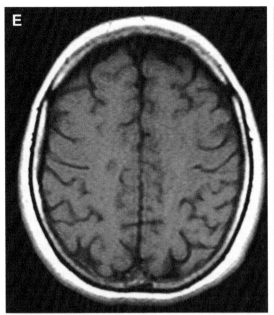

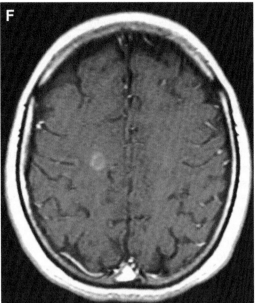

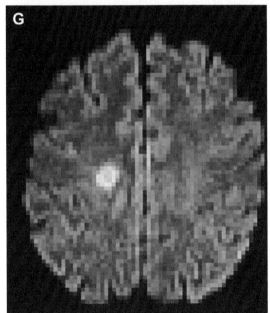

Fig. 1. MS: different imaging features. Axial T1-weighted images before (E) and after (F) gadolinium administration show a single plaque in the right frontal lobe, which shows enhancement after contrast injection, consistent acute inflammatory demyelination. (G) Diffusion-weighted imaging reveals a high signal lesion, which may be related to the acute phase of the disease.

important role in the diagnosis of certain patients, who present with few lesions and more diffuse WM involvement depicted only with fractional anisotropy (FA) measurements.[10]

Nevertheless, predicting the prognosis is not easy, and it depends on several factors. MR imaging could be used to provide certain information relevant for this purpose. Atrophy can be useful, but we also need measures of diffuse damage to the normal-appearing WM (NAWM), and even to the normal-appearing gray matter (NAGM), using DTI for instance.

DIFFUSION MR IMAGING

Diffusion MR imaging (diffusion-weighted imaging [DWI]) has been used in the clinical scenario for the last 2 decades. Since its clinical usefulness in detecting hyperacute infarcts was established,[11] DWI has been studied extensively in the evaluation of other neurologic conditions, such as brain neoplasm,[12] brain abscess,[13] and degenerative diseases.[14]

An increasing improvement in the assessment of MS has been seen in the last few years, leading to a better understanding of its immunopathogenesis, pathologic conditions, and genetics.[2] Because of its ability to detect and quantify disease-related pathologic conditions of the central nervous system, DTI has increasingly been applied to assess patients with MS, not only to investigate plaques but also the NAWM and more recently the gray matter (GM), optic nerve, and spinal cord.[15–17]

PHYSICAL BASIS
Diffusion Sensitization

DWI is based on the random or Brownian motion of water molecules. In the brain, the presence of some tissue structures restricts free water motion. MR imaging makes it possible to estimate the diffusivity of water molecules.[18] Most diffusion measurements are made using a variant of the Stejskal and Tanner sequence, by applying the 2 equal and opposite gradient pulses (compensating for the effects of uniform gross movement like flow), to determine the amount of signal loss, as a function of the magnitude of diffusion.[19] Echo-planar imaging spin-echo (SE) T2-weighted sequences are used, because of their ability to reduce motion artifacts and their rapid acquisition time. The signal intensity on DWI is influenced by both T2 tissue effect and the tissue diffusion characteristics. To exclude the T2 effect and to reflect solely the diffusion effect itself, an apparent diffusion coefficient (ADC) map is generated.[20] Although the results of DWI seem to be promising, it is important to consider the multicenter variability of the method.[21]

DTI

The magnitude of diffusion depends on the direction in which it is measured. A full characterization of diffusion can be obtained in terms of a tensor, a 3 × 3 matrix that accounts for the correlation existing between molecular displacements along orthogonal directions. From the quantitative parameters of DTI it is possible to derive ADC, mean diffusivity (MD), the average of the ADCs measured in the 3 orthogonal directions, as well as an anisotropy measure such as FA. FA is a quantitative measure of deviation from isotropy and reflects the degree of alignment of cellular structures and tissue coherence.[22–24] Because interpreting a tensor representation can be nonintuitive, scalar metrics have been proposed to simplify DTI data. FA

measures the fraction of the total magnitude of diffusion anisotropy, varying from completely isotropic diffusion, denoted as 0, up to complete anisotropic diffusion, denoted as 1.[25,26]

MS Plaques

One can speculate that in the acute phase of the plaque formation, an expanded extracellular volume is caused by astrocyte proliferation, perivascular inflammation, and demyelination, all representing pathologic stigmata of the initial step in plaque formation, whereas in its chronic stage, a more pronounced increase in extracellular space represents axonal loss and tissue destruction.[27]

Although T2-weighted and fluid-attenuated inversion recovery (FLAIR) sequences are highly sensitive for MS lesions, they lack histopathologic specificity (Fig. 2). This finding may be explained because inflammation, edema, demyelination, gliosis, and axonal loss are all represented as areas of high signal intensity on these sequences. Thus, they are not able to differentiate between different plaque subtypes. Mildly T1-weighted SE imaging can be more specific and can determine whether the lesion is acute or chronic. T1-weighted SE imaging seems to be more specific than T2-weighted imaging for identifying clinically relevant lesions.[28] Hypointense lesions on T1-weighted SE, the so-called black holes, represent chronic plaques, which may correlate with disease progression and disability.[29] Contrast-enhanced T1-weighted imaging is routinely used in clinical assessment of patients with MS to depict acute lesions. In the acute inflammatory phase, a disruption of the blood-brain barrier occurs, and an acute lesion appears first as a nodule-enhancing lesion and subsequently progresses to a ring-enhancing lesion.[30] MR imaging can be 5 to 10 times more sensitive in depicting acute plaques, representing disease activity, than the clinical evaluation of relapses, which suggests that most of the enhancing lesions are clinically silent.[31]

Diffusion MR imaging has been used to evaluate MS plaques. Some acute plaques may show restricted diffusion (Fig. 3), mostly at their margin. This pattern of enhancement is not specific for demyelinating disease, but its diagnosis can be suspected, because it is frequently peripheral and discontinuous (Fig. 4). This imaging characteristic may also be useful in the differential diagnosis with other expansive lesions, such as gliomas, which can present restricted diffusion within the solid portion of the lesion, secondary to high cellularity.

Diffusion MR imaging has been used to differentiate acute from chronic MS plaques, using ADC and FA. Although some investigators have used

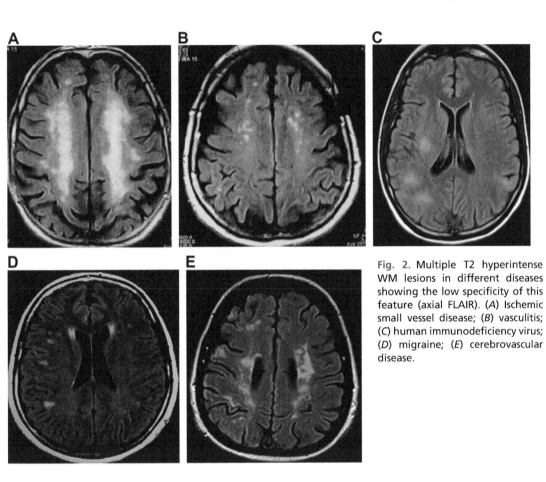

A **B** **C**

D **E**

Fig. 2. Multiple T2 hyperintense WM lesions in different diseases showing the low specificity of this feature (axial FLAIR). (*A*) Ischemic small vessel disease; (*B*) vasculitis; (*C*) human immunodeficiency virus; (*D*) migraine; (*E*) cerebrovascular disease.

DWI and DTI to try to make such a distinction, the results are inconsistent. Initial papers suggested that ADC is increased within MS plaques compared with normal WM.[32] Current evidence indicates that the pathologic substrate of MS lesions is different among MS subgroups and that disease progression may be associated with neuronal and axonal loss.[33] Therefore the increase in diffusivity possibly reflects expanded free water content within the lesion, although the relative contribution from edema, demyelination, and axonal loss is difficult to determine. The highest diffusion values seem to be found in hypointense lesions, the so-called black hole, compared with enhancing lesions and isointense lesions.[34] However, hypointensities on T1-weighted images do not solely represent tissue destruction of the late stages of the disease but may also be associated with acute lesions, resulting in enlargement of the extracellular space as a result of edema and inflammation, a process that is potentially reversible at follow-up.[35] Acute edematous lesions were found to sometimes have even higher ADC values than chronic lesions. Thus, predicting

activity of the disease based on the DWI findings, measured through ADC maps, is unreliable.[34,36]

In general, MS lesions have decreased FA values on DTI when compared with the contralateral NAWM and normal control subjects (**Fig. 5**).[37] The reduction in the FA values within the plaques indicates the disruption of myelin and axonal structures that leads to disorganization and increased extracellular space.[5] Some investigators reported that reduction in FA values observed in enhancing plaques is lower than in nonenhancing plaques, suggesting that DTI can indicate disease activity.[38] FA values can also be found to be reduced in ring-enhancing plaques compared with homogenous enhancing lesions.[36] However, conflicting results have been reported when FA values are used to differentiate acute from chronic plaques. Some reports were not able to depict any statistical difference between these 2 histopathologic MS plaque subtypes.[36,38–40]

In an acute lesion tissue damage can be permanent, related to neurodegeneration, and on the other hand it can be transient, as observed in

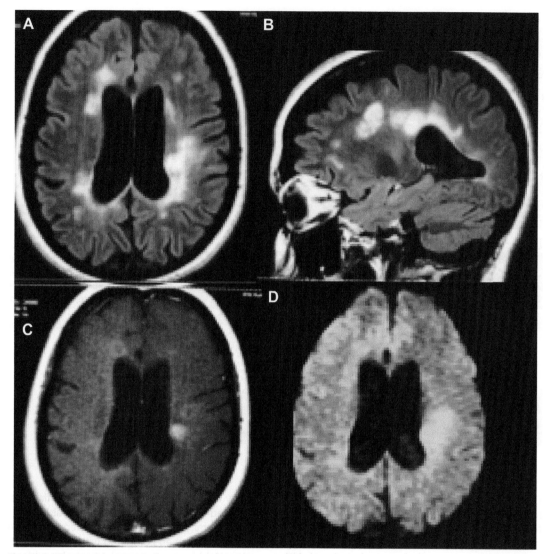

Fig. 3. A 37-year-old woman who presented with a 40-day history of progressive paresthesia, weakness of both legs. (*A, B*) Axial and sagittal FLAIR shows multiple hyperintense lesions along the margin of the body of lateral ventricles and corpus callosum, suggesting demyelination plaques. (*C*) Gadolinium-enhanced axial T1-weighted image shows ring enhancement of the right frontal lesion and homogeneous enhancement of the left parietal lesion, both suggesting acute inflammation. (*D*) DWI shows a high signal in both lesions, which may be related to acute disease.

edema, demyelination, and remyelination.[41] The postprocessing of DTI data may add new information regarding the cytoarchitecture and histopathologic alterations related to MS. The tensor model provides, besides the FA and MD, other measures of the diffusion direction. For each vector, a value known as an eigenvalue is attributed (λ_1, λ_2, and λ_3). Axial diffusivity (eigenvalue λ_1) is defined as the diffusion along the long axis and is higher than across the main fibers. It indicates a rate for the diffusion of water parallel to a bundle of axons or tract. Radial diffusivity is the one observed at

the other 2 perpendicular plans, represented by the average of eigenvalue λ_2 and λ_3, and represents the rate of the diffusion of water perpendicular to the axons.[42,43] Demyelination in general leads to reduction in radial diffusivity values, whereas axonal damage leads to axial diffusivity alterations.[42] Increased radial diffusivity relates to demyelination, and decreased radial diffusivity is seen during remyelination.[44] Based on these findings regarding axial and radial diffusivities alterations related to histopathologic intrinsic characteristics of MS plaques, a recent study

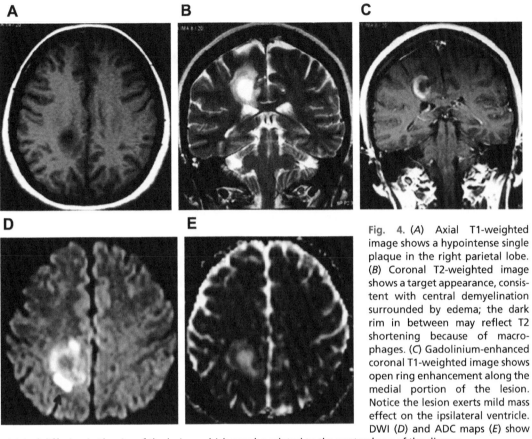

A **B** **C**

D **E**

Fig. 4. (A) Axial T1-weighted image shows a hypointense single plaque in the right parietal lobe. (B) Coronal T2-weighted image shows a target appearance, consistent with central demyelination surrounded by edema; the dark rim in between may reflect T2 shortening because of macrophages. (C) Gadolinium-enhanced coronal T1-weighted image shows open ring enhancement along the medial portion of the lesion. Notice the lesion exerts mild mass effect on the ipsilateral ventricle. DWI (D) and ADC maps (E) show restricted diffusion in the rim of the lesion, which may be related to the acute phase of the disease.

suggests that DTI can determine the plaque subtype: acute, subacute, or chronic.[45] Such a distinction is hard to make using FA values and MD. Although these are preliminary results, the investigators suggest that eigenvalues may be more sensible than FA and MD measurement when the demyelinating process is the most important damage. In the acute plaque, the demyelinating process is predominant, with altered radial diffusivity. A mixed pattern of histopathologic damage is observed in chronic plaques, including demyelination, altering radial diffusivity, and axonal loss, altering axial diffusivity.[45]

Clinical Correlation

Conventional MR imaging findings do not correlate well with clinical manifestations of disease activity.[46] MS lesions on T2-weighted images are spatially and histopathologically nonspecific. Lesion load provides useful information in monitoring the disease and its treatment response. However, lesion load may not adequately account for the patient's functional state.[47] Nonetheless, brain atrophy correlates strongly with clinical deficiency, although the lesion load does not show such a correlation.[48] Thus, destructive process underlying MS-related brain atrophy may not merely depend on the severity of T2 lesion load.[15]

The increased use of MR imaging in the assessment of MS has disclosed that the extent of WM abnormalities measured using conventional MR imaging contributes only partially to the clinical manifestations of the disease, including accumulation of irreversible disability.[49] The advent of new advanced MR imaging sequences may play an important role in the assessment of patients with MS and may therefore contribute to explaining the discordance between conventional MR imaging findings and clinical status, especially analyzing the NAWM and GM. Axonal damage is a key feature in MS lesions, occurring within both acute and chronic plaques, as well as in the NAWM. There is increasing evidence that axonal damage has a strong effect on permanent neurologic deficits.[50] Increased GM disease might be

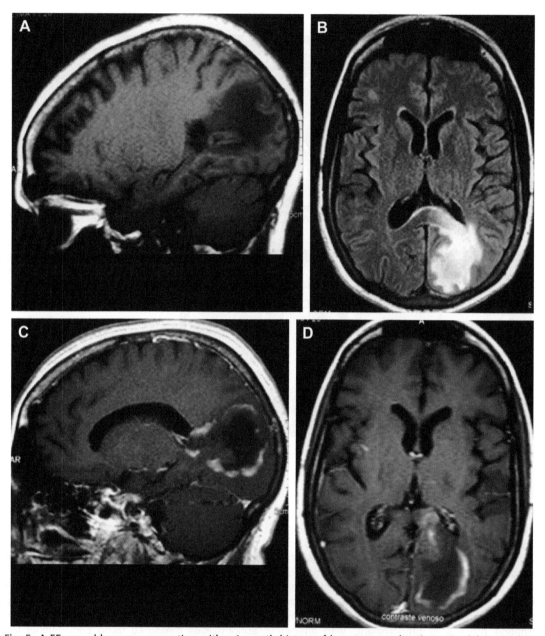

Fig. 5. A 55-year-old woman presenting with a 1-month history of homonymous hemianopsia. (*A*) Sagittal T1-weighted image shows a large hypointense occipital lesion, hyperintense on axial FLAIR (*B*). (*C*) Sagittal T1-weighted image and gadolinium-enhanced axial image (*D*) shows heterogeneous enhancement along the wall of the lesion, suggesting acute disease.

an additional factor contributing to the presence and severity of cognitive impairment in patients with progressive MS.[51] Some investigators have suggested that GM diffusivity changes may be viewed as a hallmark of the more disabling and progressive stages of the disease,[52] because the accumulation of damage in focal lesions and NAWM occurs even during the earliest nondisabling phases of MS.[53] GM diffusivity changes have also been related to neuropsychologic impairment in MS.[54]

Despite disappointing preliminary data, diffusion imaging seems to present a better correlation with clinical disability. The pathologic damage detected by DTI in clinically eloquent NAWM regions is a significant factor contributing to MS disability.[55] Overall, diffusion studies indicate that the severity of damage within T2-visible lesions

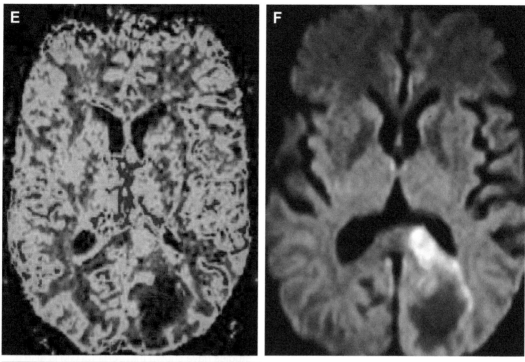

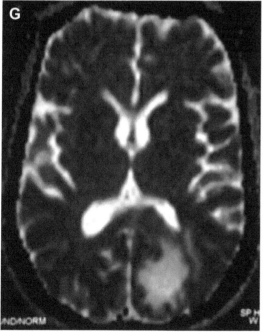

Fig. 5. A 55-year-old woman presenting with a 1-month history of homonymous hemianopsia. (E) Relative cerebral blood volume map does not show a high perfusion. (F) Axial DWI and ADC maps (G) show restricted diffusion along the medial wall of the lesion, suggesting acute phase.

and in the NAGM, as well as in clinically eloquent WM tracts, has a significant effect on neurologic disability.[15] DTI measures may thus contribute to composite MR-based scores, explaining otherwise unexplained variance in MS-related disability.[53,56]

NAWM

Conventional MR imaging has limitations in assessing lesion burden and delineating tissue damage, which are known to occur beyond the visible margins of MS plaques.[15] However, the findings at conventional MR imaging do not correlate well with the specific pathologic or clinical course of MS. Recent evidence from histopathologic studies has shown that the disease processes of MS involve not only the plaques seen on conventional MR images but also the WM regions that seem to be normal.[57] The extension of disease beyond the boundaries of plaques has important ramifications in disease assessment, because the quantification of disease burden is an important surrogate marker for disability progression. An imaging examination that depicts greater disease burden than that seen at conventional MR imaging could provide valuable additional information for both drug trials and patient treatment.[58] With the advent of diffusion MR imaging as a quantitative MR technique, the ability to better detect and characterize the disease burden, including occult microscopic disease changes, has improved greatly.[5] Although these results seem to be promising, it is also important to consider the multicenter variability in DTI measurements, which can be influenced by the type of scanner, the magnetic field strength, and the number of diffusion gradient pulse directions applied.[21]

Several studies have shown diffusion changes in the NAWM in patients with MS, suggesting that the histopathologic abnormalities may be widespread. These diffusion abnormalities can be characterized as an increase in MD and ADC values, as well as a decrease in FA values, which is in agreement with findings from magnetization transfer ratio studies.[37] Such alterations in the NAWM tend to be more severe in perilesional regions[58] and in sites where visible MS plaques are usually located, suggesting subtle microstructural changes.[36,38,39] Local alterations in DTI parameters may herald the future appearance of new focal lesions.[59]

Although most of the studies show increased diffusivity and reduced anisotropy in the NAWM, some studies did not find any significant difference in these analyses.[60] These disagreements can possibly be explained by the different forms of postprocessing of data obtained by DTI. A subsequent study with the same patient cohort using histogram analysis did report subtle abnormalities.[61]

However, NAWM damage is only partially correlated with the extent of focal lesions and the severity of intrinsic damage, suggesting that diffusivity changes in NAWM are not entirely dependent on retrograde degeneration of axons transected in MR conventional visible plaques.[41]

Similar alterations can perhaps already be observed in patients presenting with clinically isolated syndrome (CIS), suggestive of MS, using histogram analysis of segmented diffusion maps of the brain.[62]

Some reports also showed DTI alterations in the normal-appearing corpus callosum, which may precede abnormalities in other NAWM regions, suggesting preferential occult injury to this location.[45,63] The cumulative bridging effects of the corpus callosum resulting in Wallerian degenerative changes from the connecting distal WM plaques may play an important role in the relationship between the corpus callosum diffusion abnormalities and the cerebral lesion load.[64] In agreement with these imaging findings, a postmortem MS study showed quantitative reduction in total number and attenuation of axons passing through the corpus callosum that grossly appeared normal.[65]

GM

Recently, new insights have been added in GM assessment with the advent of modern scanners and advanced MR techniques. Postmortem studies have shown that cerebral GM is also pathologically involved in patients with MS. Cerebral GM lesions occur in many patients with MS.[66] In addition to axonal injury, the presence of cortical plaques has been identified in several different types, according to their topography within the cortex.[67] Microglial activation predominates in the characterization of cortical plaques, instead of infiltrating lymphocytes, which occurs to a lesser extent. Moreover, neuronal apoptosis, loss of dendritic arborization, and transected and demyelinated axons represent the involvement of neuroaxonal structures in the pathophysiology of the cortical plaques.[66,68] The loss of dendrites and axons contributes to reducing the diffusion anisotropy even more.[69] Retrograde degeneration of GM neurons secondary to WM damage is also likely to occur, contributing to the GM damage. The discrepancy regarding patient clinical status and lesion burden assessed by conventional MR sequences can be partially explained by the lack of depicting NAWM abnormalities and GM lesions as well.[49]

Although histopathologic studies show cortical lesions, reliable detection of these lesions with conventional MR sequences is challenging.[70] There is a low sensitivity in the detection of GM lesion because of their small size, partial volume effects with cerebrospinal fluid (CSF) and relaxation characteristics similar to the GM on T2-weighted and FLAIR images.[71] Advanced MR imaging techniques, such as the double inversion recovery (DIR) sequence, are superior to conventional T2-weighted and FLAIR images (Fig. 6),[72] like other sequences (phase-sensitive inversion recovery) that better depict the cortical-WM junction.[73] Both CSF and WM are selectively suppressed. DIR sequence has some limitations

regarding its inherent sensitivity to noise, and flow-related artifacts, which can result in false-positive findings.[72]

Using the DTI sequence to assess cortical lesions, geometric distortions may be observed,

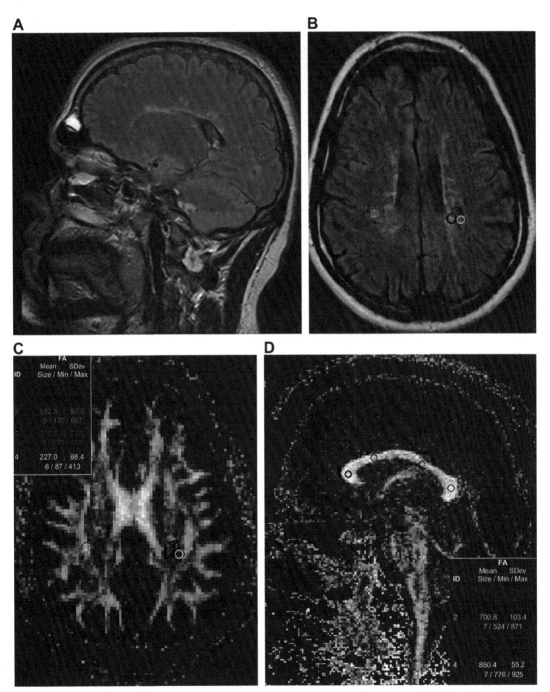

Fig. 6. (A) Sagittal and axial FLAIR (B) shows demyelinating plaques along the margin of the lateral ventricles and the corpus callosum. (C) In the axial FA map, regions of interest were drawn in the plaque, periplaque regions, NAWM. Note that a difference in FA values between lesion, periplaque region, and NAWM can be observed. (D) Midsagittal FA map shows placement of region of interest in the corpus callosum. Note the reduction of FA values in the corpus callosum.

especially if these sequences use echo-planar imaging. To minimize this problem, DTI analysis of cortical lesions requires accurate coregistration of DW images to the images used for lesion detection. Advanced nonlinear image registration methods have the potential to reduce this artifact.[74] DTI has shown GM involvement, which seems to be greater in the progressive form of MS. DTI may reflect the severity of cortical dysfunction, associated with memory and attention deficits in patients with MS, because a correlation between GM MD and cognitive impairment could be shown.[75] Discordant results were reported in the FA value measurement of NAGM. Using bulk histogram analysis, FA values were reduced in NAGM.[76] A more recent report showed an increase in mean FA values in cortical lesions in patients with MS when compared with healthy control subjects.[77] However, results from the same patient cohort using histogram analysis of the entire GM showed a reduction in FA values, in agreement with previous reports, probably because of a widespread microstructural alteration.[77] Conflicting results were described when GM damage in different MS phenotypes was assessed with DTI. Although a significant reduction in GM diffusivity was observed in patients with secondary progressive (SP) MS, no difference was noted in patients with relapsing remitting (RR) MS. These findings may point to a more extensive pathologic abnormality in progressive forms of MS than in patients with RRMS, supporting the concept that in part GM MS lesions are secondary to WM damage.[49] This report is consisted with the more profound cognitive impairment found in patients with SPMS[78] and with accelerating cortical atrophy in progressive MS.[79]

Optic Nerve

Acute demyelinating optic neuritis is often the initial clinical manifestation of MS, and MS is the most common cause of optic neuritis. A clinical challenge arises when predicting which patients presenting with optic neuritis will develop MS.[80] In absence of other clinical manifestations, optic neuritis is referred to as one of the CISs suggestive of MS. Typical findings on conventional MR imaging include a swollen nerve and hyperintensity on T2-weighted and short-tau inversion recovery images, which may enhance on gadolinium-enhanced T1-weighted images. Although these findings are typically related to optic neuritis, they are nonspecific because ischemia and infection can present similarly.[81]

DTI is a surrogate marker of the structural integrity of the optic nerve, with increases in MD and reductions in FA in case of neuritis. DTI can also be applied to further detection of early optic nerve alterations, before abnormalities detected on conventional MR imaging.[81] Despite the potential usefulness of DTI in the clinical scenario in the assessment of the optic nerve, its acquisition is still a technical challenge. This structure is small, mobile, and has a surface area susceptible to volume ratio, leading to increased partial volume contamination to bone and intraconal fat.[15] Applying the gradient pulse in fewer directions, the diffusion sequence can be performed with a shorter acquisition time. Nonetheless, most previous studies concentrated on ADC measurement. ADC is increased in the diseased optic nerve and has a close correlation with visual activity and clinical measures of visual functioning.[82] DTI measures the integrity of the axons in the optic nerve and is related to physiologic findings, like evoked potentials. Special DTI techniques may be required for examination of this structure.[83] Reduction in the connectivity of the optic radiations was also shown in patients with optic neuritis, suggesting a mechanism of transsynaptic degeneration secondary to the damage.[84]

Pediatric MS

MS is an increasingly recognized condition in the pediatric population. Although MS typically affects young adults in the second and third decades, it has been increasingly recognized to occur in children. Clinical symptoms related to MS can occur before the age of 18 years in about 10% of cases.[85,86] Although the underlying pathophysiology of disease does not vary with age, it seems that MS in the pediatric population has a more inflammatory course. Children have accrued physical disability more slowly than adults.[87] Nonetheless, they have significant cognitive dysfunctions.[88]

In a previous report, only a slight increase of ADC in the NAWM was found.[89] In another study, an increased ADC and decreased FA values in the NAWM of pediatric patients with MS compared with healthy controls was reported.[90] A more recent study concluded that more diffuse damage is present in the early stages of pediatric MS, because DTI measures indicate abnormalities in the WM-containing lesions or not in the principal pathways.[91] The absence or mildness of DTI abnormalities in the NAWM may explain a favorable clinical status in the pediatric MS population.[90] Because DTI has an exquisite ability to depict subtle alterations in the NAWM during the early course of the disease, it can contribute to the management of patients and serve as an outcome in clinical trials. Moreover, DTI may also be useful to assess the effect of MS on specific neurologic functions.[91]

Diffusion Tractography

Recently, DTI tractography has been used to better depict more subtle abnormalities related to MS in main fiber tracts. DTI tractography may increase the specificity of MR imaging findings, thereby improving the strength of their relationship with clinical findings.[15] DTI postprocessing techniques, such as tract-based analysis, provide an opportunity for further studies of the connectivity and function of the main fiber tracts.[92] However, streamline algorithms have difficulty in passing through the GM, areas where fibers cross, and through damaged WM, because of uncertainty in the principal diffusion direction within the voxel when FA decreases.[93] Fiber tract disruption caused by the transection of lesions can be directly visualized on fiber tractography.[94] Such lesions may be associated with significantly fewer fiber tracts and lower FA.[95] Fiber tract loss observed in the corticospinal tract according with lesion load supports the concept of Wallerian degeneration and axonal transection[96] and correlates with clinical measures of locomotor disability.[97] Moreover, DTI tractography may show that patients presenting with CIS have increased diffusivity and lesion load in the corticospinal tract.[98] DTI tractography can detect subtle pathologic abnormalities beyond macroscopic lesions in WM main fiber tracts in MS and in addition may also increase the specificity in the assessment of specific neurologic deficits.[46,99] Tract-based DTI analysis uses spatial normalization with subsequent group comparison. Thus, results obtained from this technique should be interpreted conservatively.

High field

High-field MR systems provide a higher signal-to-noise ratio (SNR), allowing the acquisition of thinner and volumetric sections, with higher spatial resolution as well as increasing contrast-to-noise. These findings may contribute to increasing the sensitivity for detection of MS plaques (**Fig. 7**).[100,101] Moreover, the susceptibility effects in high-field strength scanners are boosted, allowing an improvement in the appreciation of microvascularity and its relationship with MS plaques.

These new insights, regarding the assessment of patients with clinically suspected MS, increase the sensitivity for lesion detection, and may allow an earlier definite diagnosis and initiation of appropriate treatment, which may in turn influence clinical management.[100,102] Thus, high-field MR imaging further strengthens the role of MR imaging in the study of MS.

The higher SNR provided by high-field MR systems can achieve higher-quality DTI. Although high-field MR systems have contributed to the evaluation of patients with MS, the susceptibility-induced signal intensity loss and distortion near the skull base and air sinuses is also prominent and should be carefully considered in clinical applications.[5] Nonetheless, the improvement in radiofrequency coils and sequence acquisition has the advantage of performing diffusion imaging at higher field strengths, achieving increased SNR for more detailed compounds that might be obscured in lower field scanners.

Technical Developments

The best acquisition and postprocessing strategies for diffusion MR imaging studies in patients with MS remain a matter of debate. Some drawbacks are associated with DTI in the assessment of multiple fibers crossing within a single voxel. The interscanner variability and issues related to high-field MR system acquisition may also alter the results regarding the analysis of specific areas in the brain. Moreover, DTI tractography still has some technical limitations, which may lead to erroneous fiber tracking and FA analysis.[103] Higher-strength MR scanners and multiple-receiver coils with parallel imaging data acquisition techniques have the potential to improve DTI acquisition because they can provide a better SNR, enhancing spatial resolution.[104] A parallel imaging approach can reduce the distortions seen in echo-planar imaging, but has the disadvantage that the SNR is poorer. Periodically rotated overlapping parallel lines with enhanced reconstruction also allows the acquisition of diffusion imaging at high spatial resolution with minimal distortion.[103]

Diffusion spectrum imaging is a novel approach developed to minimize the adverse effects in the crossing fibers within a single voxel. With this technique, it is possible to more accurately detect variations in diffusion along different directions, measuring the diffusion coefficient at high angular resolution.[105]

There are other approaches that do not require any assumptions about diffusion within a voxel, such as q-space formalism, which measures the displacement profile. It has been used to estimate the three-dimensional displacement distribution of water molecules, allowing the characterization of the slow restricted diffusion component, which is

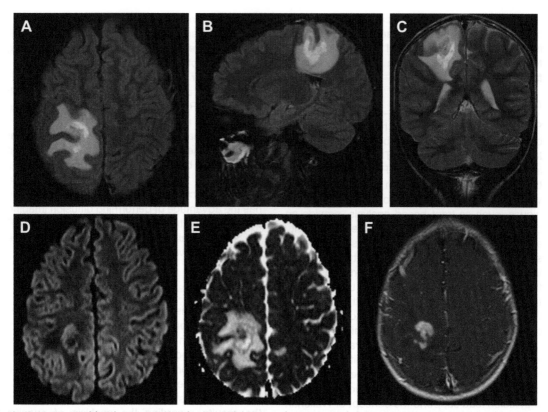

Fig. 7. A 7-year-old girl presenting with a 4-week history of progressive left hemiparesis. (*A–C*) Axial, sagittal, and coronal FLAIR shows a large hyperintense right frontoparietal lesion with lesion-in-a-lesion appearance, suggesting demyelinating plaque. (*D, E*) Axial DWI shows mildly hyperintense signal of the rim part, mildly hypointense on ADC maps, which may show restricted diffusion, observed in acute disease. (*F*) Gadolinium-enhanced axial T1-weighted image shows heterogeneous enhancement of the lesion, mostly peripheral, suggesting acute disease.

probably mainly dependent on axonal membranes and modulated by myelin layers. In principle, this approach improves the ability to differentiate between demyelination, axonal loss, and inflammation in MS.[106]

Other approaches measure the diffusion along different directions with a high angular resolution. The resulting three-dimensional representation of diffusivity can be broken down into a set of orthogonal three-dimensional functions, the so-called spherical harmonics.[107]

The knowledge of the underlying anatomy is a prerequisite to a better analysis of pathologic changes in tissue microstructures, to avoid misinterpretation of the postprocessed DTI data. When comparing DTI data in patients with those in healthy controls, therefore, it is imperative to consider regions that match anatomically. Recently, several methods have been described for handling this uncertainty in a probabilistic fashion. The subjectivity of placing a region-of-interest approach to collect information for

analyzing DTI data can be replaced by histogram analysis of MD and FA maps.[103] A more elegant approach is to perform nonlinear spatial normalization of DTI data in an anatomic reference frame to facilitate the analysis and allow a voxel-based assessment that does not require a priori hypothesis.[108] Registration may also be improved by matching based on the whole of the DTI, rather than just a simple image intensity.[109]

The contribution of such new DTI technical acquisition in the analysis of patients with MS is promising but still needs to be validated.

SUMMARY

New information has been incorporated into the evaluation of patients with MS in recent years. Advances in MR imaging were essential to better understand the pathophysiology and clinical management of patients with MS. Besides the known high sensitivity in identifying demyelinating plaques, new advanced MR imaging techniques, including diffusion imaging, increased the histo-pathologic specificity of these lesions. There has also been an improvement in the characterization of the NAWM and recently a better identification of cortical involvement.

The advent of advanced MR imaging sequences may play an important role in the assessment of patients with MS and may therefore contribute to explaining the discordance between conventional MR imaging findings and clinical status, especially analyzing the NAWM and GM.

Nonetheless, multicenter studies using advanced diffusion MR imaging acquisition and postprocess-ing are still necessary for continuous improvement in technical and postprocessing features to create a better understanding of disease and the useful-ness of MR imaging in clinical practice.

REFERENCES

1. Rodriguez M, Silva A, Ward J, et al. Impairment, disability and handicap in multiple sclerosis: a popu-lation-based study in Olmsted Country, Minnesota. Neurology 1994;44:28–33.

2. Inglese M. Multiple sclerosis: new insights and trends. AJNR Am J Neuroradiol 2006;27:954–7.

3. Nusbaum AO, Rapalino O, Fung K, et al. White matter diseases and inherited metabolic disor-ders. In: Atlas S, editor. Magnetic resonance imaging of the brain and spine. 4th edition. Phil-adelphia: Lippincott Williams & Wilkins; 2009. p. 343–444.

4. Young IR, Hall AS, Pallis CA, et al. Nuclear magnetic resonance imaging of the brain in multiple sclerosis. Lancet 1981;2(8255):1063–6.

5. Ge Y. Multiple sclerosis: the role of MR imaging. AJNR Am J Neuroradiol 2006;27:1165–76.

6. McDonald WI, Compston A, Edan G, et al. Recommended diagnostic criteria for multiple scle-rosis: guidelines from the International Panel on the Diagnosis of Multiple Sclerosis. Ann Neurol 2001; 50:121–7.

7. Barkhof F, Filippi M, Miller DH, et al. Comparison of MRI criteria at first presentation to predict conver-sion to clinically definitive multiple sclerosis. Brain 1997;120:2059–69.

8. Tintore M, Rovira A, Martinez MJ, et al. Isolated demyelinating syndromes: comparison of different MR imaging criteria to predict conversion to clini-cally definitive multiple sclerosis. AJNR Am J Neu-roradiol 2000;21:702–6.

9. Polman CH, Reingold SC, Edan G, et al. Diagnostic criteria for multiple sclerosis: 2005 revisions to the "McDonald Criteria". Ann Neurol 2005;58:840–6.

10. Zwemmer JN, Bot JC, Jelles B, et al. At the heart of primary progressive multiple sclerosis: three cases with diffuse MRI abnormalities only. Mult Scler 2008;14:428–30.

11. Warach S, Chien D, Li W, et al. Fast magnetic reso-nance diffusion-weighted imaging of acute human stroke. Neurology 1992;42:1717–23.

12. Cruz LC Jr, Souensen AG. Diffusion tensor magnetic resonance imaging of brain tumors. Neu-rosurg Clin N Am 2005;16:115–34.

13. Guo AC, Provenzale JM, Cruz LC Jr, et al. Cerebral abscesses: investigation using apparent diffusion coefficient maps. Neuroradiology 2001;43:370–4.

14. Parente DB, Gasparetto EL, Cruz LC Jr, et al. Potential role of diffusion tensor MRI in the differen-tial diagnosis of mild cognitive impairment and Alzheimer's disease. AJR Am J Roentgenol 2008; 190:1369–74.

15. Rovaris M, Gass A, Bammer R, et al. Diffusion MRI in multiple sclerosis. Neurology 2005;65:1526–32.

16. Cruz LC Jr, Domingues RC, Gasparetto EL. Diffu-sion tensor imaging of the cervical spinal cord of patients with relapsing-remising multiple sclerosis: a study of 41 cases. Arq Neuropsiquiatr 2009;67: 391–5.

17. Rueda F, Cruz LC Jr, Domingues RC, et al. Diffu-sion tensor MR imaging evaluation of the corpus callosum of patients with multiple sclerosis. Arq Neuropsiquiatr 2008;66:449–53.

18. Holodny AI, Ollenschlager M. Diffusion imaging in brain tumor. Neuroimaging Clin N Am 2002;12:107–24.

19. Stejskal E, Tanner J. Spin diffusion measurements: spin echoes in the presence of time-dependent field gradient. J Chem Phys 1965;42:288–92.

20. Romero JM, Schaefer PW, Grant PE, et al. Diffusion MR imaging of acute ischemic stroke. Neuroimag-ing Clin N Am 2002;12:35–53.

21. Pagani E, Hirsch JG, Pouwels PJ, et al. Intercenter differences in diffusion tensor MRI acquisition. J Magn Reson Imaging 2010;31:1458–68.

22. Le Bihan D, Mangin JF, Poupon C, et al. Diffusion tensor imaging: concepts and applications. J Magn Reson Imaging 2001;13:534–46.

23. Pierpaoli C, Jezzard P, Baser PJ, et al. Diffusion tensor MR imaging of the human brain. Radiology 1996;201:637–48.

24. Basser PJ, Pierpaoli C. Microstructural and physio-logical features of tissues elucidated by quantita-tive-diffusion-tensor-MRI. J Magn Reson B 1996; 111:209–19.

25. Melhem ER, Mori S, Mukundan G, et al. Diffusion tensor MR imaging of the brain and the white matter tractography. AJR Am J Roentgenol 2002; 178(1):3–16.

26. Ito R, Mori S, Melhem ER. Diffusion tensor MR imaging and tractography. Neuroimaging Clin N Am 2002;12(1):1–19.

27. Castriota-Scanderbeg A, Tomaiuolo F, Sabatini U, et al. Demyelinating plaques in relapsing-remitting

and secondary-progressive multiple sclerosis: assessment with diffusion MR imaging. AJNR Am J Neuroradiol 2000;21:862–8.

28. van Walderveen MA, Barkhof F, Hommes OR, et al. Correlating MRI and clinical disease activity in multiple sclerosis: relevance of hypointense lesions on short-TR/short-TE (T1-weighted) spin-echo images. Neurology 1995;45:1684–90.

29. Truyen L, van Waesberghe JH, van Walderveen MA, et al. Accumulation of hypointense lesions ("black holes") on T1 spin-echo MRI correlates with disease progression in multiple sclerosis. Neurology 1996; 47:1469–76.

30. Grossman RI, Braffman BH, Brorson JR, et al. Multiple sclerosis: serial study of gadolinium-enhanced MR imaging. Radiology 1998;169:117–22.

31. Barkhof F, Scheltens P, Frequin ST, et al. Relapsing-remitting multiple sclerosis: sequential enhanced MR imaging vs clinical findings in determining disease activity. AJR Am J Roentgenol 1992;159: 1041–7.

32. Horsfield MA, Larsson HB, Jones DK, et al. Diffusion magnetic resonance imaging in multiple sclerosis. J Neurol Neurosurg Psychiatry 1998; 64(Suppl 1):S80–4.

33. Barnes D, Munro PM, Youl BD, et al. The long-standing multiple sclerosis lesion: a quantitative MRI and electron microscopic study. Brain 1991; 114:1271–80.

34. Roychowdhury S, Maldjian JA, Grossman RI. Multiple sclerosis: comparison of trace apparent diffusion coefficients with MR enhancement pattern of lesions. AJNR Am J Neuroradiol 2000;21:869–74.

35. van Waesberghe JH, van Walderveen MA, Castelijns JA, et al. Patterns of lesion development in multiple sclerosis: longitudinal observations with T1-weighted spin-echo and magnetization transfer MR. AJNR Am J Neuroradiol 1998;19:675–83.

36. Bammer R, Augustin M, Strasser-Fuchs S, et al. Magnetic resonance diffusion tensor imaging for characterizing diffuse and focal white matter abnormalities in multiple sclerosis. Magn Reson Med 2000;44:583–91.

37. Filippi M, Inglese M. Overview of diffusion-weighted magnetic resonance studies in multiple sclerosis. J Neurol Sci 2001;186(Suppl 1):S37–43.

38. Filippi M, Cercignani M, Inglese M, et al. Diffusion tensor magnetic resonance imaging in multiple sclerosis. Neurology 2001;56:304–11.

39. Filippi M, Iannucci G, Cercignani M, et al. A quantification study of water diffusion in multiple sclerosis lesions and normal-appearing white matter using echo-planar imaging. Arch Neurol 2000;57:1017–21.

40. Castriota-Scanderbeg A, Sabatini U, Fasano F, et al. Diffusion of water in large demyelinating lesions: a follow-up study. Neuroradiology 2002;44:764–7.

41. Rovaris M, Agosta F, Pagani E, et al. Diffusion tensor MR imaging. Neuroimaging Clin N Am 2009;19:37–43.

42. Song SK, Sun SW, Ramsbottom MJ, et al. Dysmyelination revealed through MRI as increased radial (but unchanged axial) diffusion of water. Neuroimage 2002;17:1429–36.

43. DeBoy CA, Zhang J, Dike S, et al. High resolution diffusion tensor imaging of axonal damage in focal inflammatory and demyelinating lesions in rat spinal cord. Brain 2007;130:2199–210.

44. Song SK, Yoshino J, Le TQ, et al. Demyelination increases radial diffusivity in corpus callosum of mouse brain. Neuroimage 2005;26:132–40.

45. Gasparetto E, Rueda F, Cruz Jr LC, et al. Acute and chronic demyelinating plaques in patients with multiple sclerosis: a diffusion tensor magnetic resonance imaging study. Paper presented at: RSNA Scientific Assembly and Annual Meeting. Chicago, November 30 to December 3, 2008.

46. Kealey SM, Kim Y, Whiting WL, et al. Determination of multiple sclerosis plaque size with diffusion-tensor MR imaging: comparison study with healthy volunteers. Radiology 2005;236(2):615–20.

47. Filippi M, Horsfield MA, Hajnal JV, et al. Quantitative assessment of magnetic resonance imaging lesion load in multiple sclerosis. J Neurol Neurosurg Psychiatry 1998;64(Suppl 1):S88–93.

48. Kalkers NF, Bergers E, Castelijns JA, et al. Optimizing the association between disability and biological markers in MS. Neurology 2001;57:1253–8.

49. Bozzali M, Cercignani M, Sormani MP, et al. Quantification of brain gray matter damage in different MS phenotypes by use of diffusion tensor MR imaging. AJNR Am J Neuroradiol 2002;23:985–8.

50. Trapp BD, Ransohoff R, Rudick R. Axonal pathology in multiple sclerosis: relationship to neurologic disability. Curr Opin Neurol 1999;12:295–302.

51. Camp SJ, Stevenson VL, Thompson AJ, et al. Cognitive function in primary progressive and transitional progressive multiple sclerosis: a controlled study with MRI correlates. Brain 1999; 122:1341–8.

52. Rovaris M, Judica E, Ceccarelli A, et al. A 3-year diffusion tensor MRI study of grey matter damage progression during earliest clinical stage of MS. J Neurol 2008;255:1209–14.

53. Pulizzi A, Rovaris M, Judica E, et al. Determinants of disability in multiple sclerosis at various disease stages: a multiparametric magnetic resonance study. Arch Neurol 2007;64:1163–8.

54. Rovaris M, Riccitelli G, Judica E, et al. Cognitive impairment and structural brain damage in benign multiple sclerosis. Neurology 2008;71:1521–6.

55. Ciccarelli O, Werring DJ, Wheeler-Kingshott CA, et al. Investigation of MS normal-appearing brain using diffusion tensor MRI with clinical correlations. Neurology 2001;56:926–33.

56. Mainero C, De Stefano N, Iannucci G, et al. Correlates of MS disability assessed in vivo using aggregates of MR quantities. Neurology 2001;56: 1331–4.

57. Lucchinetti CF, Bruck W, Rodriguez M, et al. Distinct patterns of multiple sclerosis pathology indicates heterogeneity in pathogenesis. Brain Pathol 1996;6:259–74.

58. Guo AC, MacFall JR, Provenzale JM. Multiple sclerosis: diffusion tensor MR imaging for evaluation of normal-appearing white matter. Radiology 2002; 222:729–36.

59. Rocca MA, Cercignani M, Iannucci G, et al. Weekly diffusion-weighted imaging of normal-appearing white matter in MS. Neurology 2000; 55:882–4.

60. Griffin CM, Chard DT, Ciccarelli O, et al. Diffusion tensor imaging in early relapsing-remitting multiple sclerosis. Mult Scler 2001;7:290–7.

61. Rachid W, Hadjiprocopis A, Griffin CM, et al. Diffusion tensor imaging of early relapsing-remitting multiple sclerosis with histogram analysis using automated segmentation and brain volume correction. Mult Scler 2004;10:9–15.

62. Gallo A, Rovaris M, Riva R, et al. Diffusion tensor MRI detects normal-appearing white matter damage unrelated to short-term disease activity in patients at the earlier stage of multiple sclerosis. Arch Neurol 2005;62:803–8.

63. Ge Y, Law M, Johnson G, et al. Preferential occult corpus callosum in multiple sclerosis measured by diffusion tensor imaging. J Magn Reson Imaging 2004;20:1–7.

64. Ciccarelli O, Werring DJ, Barker GJ, et al. A study of the mechanisms of normal-appearing white matter damage in multiple sclerosis using diffusion tensor imaging: evidence of Wallerian degeneration. J Neurol 2003;250:287–92.

65. Evangelou N, Esiri MM, Smith S, et al. Quantitative pathological evidence for axonal loss in normal appearing white matter in multiple sclerosis. Ann Neurol 2000;47:391–5.

66. Peterson JW, Bo L, Morks S, et al. Transected neuritis, apoptotic neurons, and reduced inflammation in cortical multiple sclerosis lesions. Ann Neurol 2001;50:389–400.

67. Kidd D, Barkhof F, McConnell R, et al. Cortical lesions in multiple sclerosis. Brain 1999;122:17–26.

68. Bo L, Vedeler CA, Nyland H, et al. Intracortical multiple sclerosis lesions are not associated with increased lymphocyte infiltration. Mult Scler 2003; 9:323–31.

69. McKinstry RC, Mathur A, Miller JH, et al. Radial organization of developing preterm human cerebral cortex revealed by non-invasive water diffusion anisotropy MRI. Cereb Cortex 2002;12: 1237–43.

70. Wegner C, Esiri MM, Chance SA, et al. Neocortical neuronal, synaptic, and glial loss in multiple sclerosis. Neurology 2006;67:960–7.

71. Cercignani M, Bozzali M, Iannucci G, et al. Magnetization transfer and mean diffusivity of normal appearing white and grey matter from patients with multiple sclerosis. J Neurol Neurosurg Psychiatry 2001;70:311–7.

72. Pouwels PJ, Kuijer JP, Mugler JP 3rd, et al. Human gray matter: feasibility of single-slab 3D double inversion-recovery high-spatial-resolution MR imaging. Radiology 2006;241:873–9.

73. Hou P, Hasan KM, Sitton CW, et al. Phase-sensitive T1 inversion recovery imaging: a time-efficient interleaved technique for improved tissue contrast in neuroimaging. AJNR Am J Neuroradiol 2005; 26:1432–8.

74. Jezzard P, Barnett AS, Pierpaoli C. Characterization of and correction for eddy current artifacts in echo planar diffusion imaging. Magn Reson Med 1998;39:801–12.

75. Rovaris M, Iannucci G, Falautano M, et al. Cognitive dysfunction in patients with mildly disabling relapsing-remitting multiple sclerosis: an exploratory study with diffusion tensor MR imaging. J Neurol Sci 2002;195:103–9.

76. Vreken H, Pouwels PJ, Geurts JJ, et al. Altered diffusion tensor in multiple sclerosis normal-appearing brain tissue: cortical diffusion changes seem related to clinical deterioration. J Magn Reson Imaging 2006;23:628–36.

77. Poonawalla AH, Hasan KM, Gupta RK, et al. Diffusion-tensor MR imaging of cortical lesions in multiple sclerosis: initial findings. Radiology 2008; 246(3):880–6.

78. Heaton RH, Nelson LM, Thompson DS, et al. Neuropsychological findings in relapsing remitting and chronic progressive multiple sclerosis. J Consult Clin Psychol 1985;53:103–10.

79. Fisher E, Lee JC, Nakamura K, et al. Gray matter atrophy in multiple sclerosis: a longitudinal study. Ann Neurol 2008;64:255–65.

80. Arnold AC. Evolving management of optic neuritis and multiple sclerosis. Am J Ophthalmol 2005; 139:1101–8.

81. Glisson CC, Galetta SL. Nonconventional optic nerve imaging in multiple sclerosis. Neuroimaging Clin N Am 2009;19:71–9.

82. Hickman SJ, Wheeler-Kingshott CA, Jones SJ, et al. Optic nerve diffusion measurement from diffusion weighted imaging in optic neuritis. AJNR Am J Neuroradiol 2005;26:951–6.

83. Anand Trip S, Wheeler-Kingshott CA, Jones SJ, et al. Optic nerve diffusion tensor imaging in optic neuritis. Neuroimage 2006;30:498–505.

84. Ciccarelli O, Toosy AT, Hickman SJ, et al. Optic radiation changes after optic neuritis detected by

tractography-based group mapping. Hum Brain Mapp 2005;25:308–16.

85. Chitnis T. Pediatric multiple sclerosis. Neurologist 2006;12:299–310.

86. Chitnis T, Glanz B, Jaffin S, et al. Demographics of pediatric-onset multiple sclerosis in a MS center population from the Northeastern United States. Mult Scler 2009;15:627–31.

87. Simone IL, Carrara D, Tortorella C, et al. Course and prognosis in early-onset MS: comparison with adult-onset forms. Neurology 2002;59:1922–8.

88. Gorman MP, Healy BC, Polgar-Turcsanyi M, et al. Increased relapse rate in pediatric-onset compared with adult-onset multiple sclerosis. Arch Neurol 2009;66:54–9.

89. Mezzapesa DM, Rocca MA, Falini A, et al. A preliminary diffusion tensor and magnetization transfer magnetic resonance imaging study of early-onset multiple sclerosis. Arch Neurol 2004;61:366–8.

90. Tortorella C, Rocca MA, Mezzapesa D, et al. MRI quantification of gray and white matter damage in patients with early-onset multiple sclerosis. J Neurol 2006;253:903–7.

91. Vishwas MS, Chitnis T, Pienaar R, et al. Tract-based analysis of callosal, projection, and association pathways in pediatric patients with multiple sclerosis: a preliminary study. AJNR Am J Neuroradiol 2010;31:121–8.

92. Basser PJ, Pajevic S, Pierpaoli C, et al. In vivo fiber tractography using DT-MRI data. Magn Reson Med 2000;44:625–32.

93. Jones DK. Determining and visualizing uncertainty in estimates of fiber orientation from diffusion tensor MRI. Magn Reson Med 2003;49:7–12.

94. Ge Y, Tuvia K, Law M, et al. Corticospinal tract degeneration in brainstem in patients with multiple sclerosis: evaluation with diffusion tensor tractography. Int Soc Magn Reson Med 2005;394.

95. Soohoo S, Ge Y, Law M, et al. Lesional fractional anisotropy, diffusivity and fiber tractography in patient with multiple sclerosis with DTI at 3 Tesla. In: Proceedings of the 43rd Annual Meeting of the American Society of Neuroradiology. Toronto; 2005. p. 108.

96. Trapp BD, Peterson J, Ransohoff RM, et al. Axonal transection in the lesions of multiple sclerosis. N Engl J Med 1998;338:278–85.

97. Wilson M, Tench CR, Morgan PS, et al. Pyramidal tract mapping by diffusion tensor magnetic resonance imaging in multiple sclerosis: improving correlations with disability. J Neurol Neurosurg Psychiatry 2003;74:203–7.

98. Pagani E, Filippi M, Rocca MA, et al. A method for obtaining tract-specific diffusion tensor MRI measurements in the presence of disease: application to patient with clinically isolated syndromes suggestive of multiple sclerosis. Neuroimage 2005;26:258–65.

99. Lin F, Yu C, Jiang T, et al. Diffusion tensor tractography-based group mapping of pyramidal tract in relapsing-remitting multiple sclerosis patients. AJNR Am J Neuroradiol 2007;28:278–82.

100. Kollia K, Maderwald S, Putzki N, et al. First clinical study on ultra-high-field MR imaging in patients with multiple sclerosis: comparison of 1.5T and 7T. AJNR Am J Neuroradiol 2009;30:699–702.

101. Keiper MD, Grossman RI, Hirsch JA, et al. MR identification of white matter abnormalities in multiple sclerosis: a comparison between 1.5T and 4T. AJNR Am J Neuroradiol 1998;19:1489–93.

102. Tan IL, van Shijndel RA, Pouwels PJ, et al. MR venography of multiple sclerosis. AJNR Am J Neuroradiol 2000;21:1039–42.

103. Pagani E, Bammer R, Horsfield MA, et al. Diffusion MRI in multiple sclerosis: technical aspects and challenges. AJNR Am J Neuroradiol 2007;28: 411–20.

104. Bammer R, Auer M, Keeling SL, et al. Diffusion tensor imaging using single-shot SENSE-EPI. Magn Reson Med 2002;48:128–36.

105. Frank LR. Anisotropy in high angular resolution diffusion-weighted MRI. Magn Reson Med 2001; 45:935–9.

106. Assaf Y, Ben-Bashat D, Chapman J, et al. High b-value q-space analyzed diffusion-weighted MRI: application to multiple sclerosis. Magn Reson Med 2002;47:115–26.

107. Frank LR. Characterization of anisotropy in high angular resolution diffusion-weighted MRI. Magn Reson Med 2002;47:1083–99.

108. Alexander DC, Pierpaoli C, Basser PJ, et al. Spatial transformation of diffusion tensor magnetic resonance images. IEEE Trans Med Imaging 2001;20: 1131–9.

109. Park HJ, Kubicki M, Shenton ME, et al. Spatial normalization of diffusion tensor MRI using multiple channels. Neuroimage 2003;20:1995–2009.

Diffusion Imaging in Brain Infections

Emerson L. Gasparetto, MD, PhD[a,b,*], Rafael F. Cabral, MD[a,b],
L. Celso Hygino da Cruz Jr, MD[a,c,d],
Romeu C. Domingues, MD[a,b]

KEYWORDS
- Diffusion imaging • Brain infection
- Diffusion-weighted MR imaging

Infections of the central nervous system (CNS) continue to be a worldwide health problem, mainly in poor and developing countries. Because treatment options are available for most causes of CNS infection, the correct differential diagnosis must be obtained as early as possible. Clinical presentation and laboratory data are useful for differential diagnosis, but medical imaging is also important.

Magnetic resonance (MR) imaging is the method of choice for patients with CNS infections because it provides high anatomic resolution and tissue contrast, multiplanar acquisition, and high sensitivity to contrast enhancement. In addition, advanced MR imaging techniques, such as MR spectroscopy, diffusion-weighted imaging (DWI), diffusion tensor imaging (DTI), and dynamic-susceptibility contrast-enhanced perfusion MR imaging, provide metabolic and functional information about lesions, improving the diagnostic assessment. Of these advanced techniques, the DWI provides potentially unique information on brain tissue viability because its image contrast is dependent on the molecular motion of water, which may be substantially altered by infectious diseases.[1] The aim of this review is to discuss the main clinical applications of DWI in the differential diagnosis of CNS infections, assessing the most common DWI findings in each type of infection.

VIRAL INFECTION
Herpetic Encephalitis

Herpes simplex virus type 1 (HSV-1) is the major causative agent of herpetic encephalitis and fatal sporadic encephalitis, with a high mortality rate. Laboratory findings are nonspecific, and isolation of HSV-1 from the cerebrospinal fluid is rare.[2] MR imaging demonstrates early edematous changes in herpes encephalitis, with an increased signal in the temporal and inferior frontal lobes on T2-weighted imaging (T2-WI). This hyperintense signal involves both the cortex and white matter, and may be seen as early as 48 hours after the onset of symptoms.[3] Herpes encephalitis typically shows heterogeneously restricted diffusion in the early stages of disease, when the inflammatory reaction is more severe. In some cases, DWI shows parenchymal alterations characterized by hyperintensity on DWI, even before abnormalities are noted on conventional MR imaging sequences, such as T2-weighted and fluid attenuation inversion recovery (FLAIR) images. The decrease in water diffusion is caused by cytotoxic edema, and is usually associated with irreversible neuronal damage undergoing necrosis, and poor outcome (Fig. 1). DWI may also reveal large extensions and a higher number of lesions than T2-WI, and is the method of choice for monitoring treatment response.[4] Facilitated diffusion with high apparent diffusion coefficient (ADC) values is seen later, in parallel with the development of vasogenic edema and encephalomalacia (Fig. 2).[5]

Human Immunodeficiency Virus

CNS involvement is an early feature of human immunodeficiency virus (HIV) infection. Although MR imaging is a sensitive technique for visualizing

[a] Department of Radiology, University Federal of Rio de Janeiro, Rio de Janeiro, Brazil
[b] CDPI - Clinica De Diagnostico por Imagem, Rio De Janeiro, Brazil
[c] Clinics CDPI and Multi-Imagem, Rua Saddock de Sá 266, Rio de Janeiro, Brazil
[d] Clinic IRM, Rua Capitao Salomao 44, Rio de Janeiro, Brazil
* Corresponding author. Estrada Da Barra Da Tijuca 1006 Ap 1106, 22641-003 Rio De Janeiro, Brazil.
E-mail address: egasparetto@gmail.com

Neuroimag Clin N Am 21 (2011) 89–113
doi:10.1016/j.nic.2011.01.011
1052-5149/11/$ – see front matter © 2011 Published by Elsevier Inc.

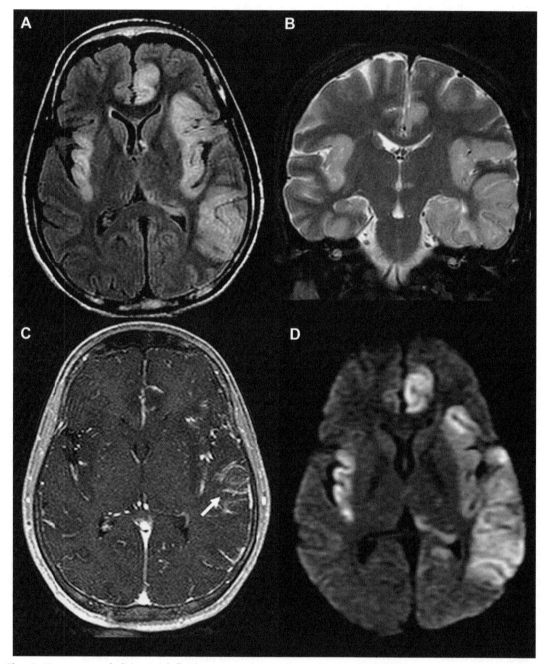

Fig. 1. Herpes encephalitis. Axial fluid-attenuated inversion recovery (FLAIR) (*A*) and coronal T2-weighted imaging (T2-WI) (*B*) show characteristic hyperintense signal in bilateral insular, left frontal, and temporal cortices, with mild patchy enhancement (*arrow* in *C*; T1-WI after gadolinium administration). Heterogeneous high signal intensity (reduced diffusion) is seen in the same areas on diffusion-weighted imaging (*D*).

the effects of HIV in the brain, it cannot show early pathologic involvement. MR imaging features of brain HIV infection include bilateral symmetric increased T2-WI signal intensity in the white matter, and cerebral atrophy.[6] At this stage, DWI may be normal or show "T2 shine-through" effects (**Fig. 3**). HIV-positive patients in more advanced stages may develop dementia, also known as AIDS dementia complex, or HIV-associated dementia (HAD). HAD occurs in 20% to 30% of untreated adult patients.[7] The clinical symptoms of HAD include disabling cognitive impairment accompanied by motor dysfunction, a change in behavior, or both.[8]

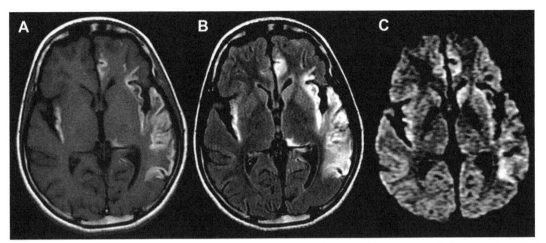

Fig. 2. Herpes encephalitis. The follow-up MR imaging of the same case of herpes encephalitis reveals cortical high signal in the bilateral insular and left frontal, parietal, and periatrial region (laminar cortical necrosis) on axial T1-WI without contrast (*A*). FLAIR (*B*) and DWI (*C*) show reduction of cytotoxic edema in the lesions.

Data from recent studies suggest that DTI might be sensitive for detecting early CNS involvement in HIV infection. Abnormal fractional anisotropy (FA) in the frontal white matter and internal capsules of HIV-positive patients has been demonstrated.[9] In another study, a decrease in FA in the corpus callosum and an increase in mean diffusivity in the subcortical white matter were associated with high viral loads and low CD4 counts.[8] However, the findings of brain areas with abnormal DWI and DTI findings, and the relationship between those variables and the clinical and laboratorial data, are discordant with other studies.[9,10]

Progressive Multifocal Leukoencephalopathy

Progressive multifocal leukoencephalopathy (PML) is a serious subacute demyelinating disease of the CNS caused by JC polyoma virus infection of oligodendrocytes.[11] JC virus infects approximately 70% of the human population and typically remains latent until reactivation by an immunodeficient state (common in AIDS patients). MR imaging findings suggestive of PML include the presence of bilateral asymmetric white matter lesions that are hyperintense on T2-WI and hypo-intense on T1-weighted imaging (T1-WI), and involve the subcortical "U" fibers with "scalloped" appearance, usually without mass effect. PML lesions usually have no significant mass effect and no contrast enhancement.[12]

Recently, studies have used DWI to evaluate patients with PML, and suggested that DWI may detect areas of active disease more effectively than other sequences. Thus, DWI may be the method of choice for monitoring disease activity and eventual response to treatment.[13] When evaluated by DWI, many PML lesions are characterized by a central core of low signal intensity surrounded by a rim of high signal intensity (area of disease activity) (Fig. 4). The peripheral hyperintense rim progressively loses its signal intensity over time, while sustaining high signal intensity on conventional T2-WI.[14] Recent studies also suggest that DWI may be useful for documenting the response of PML to highly active antiretroviral therapy. Usiskin and colleagues[15] obtained serial ADC measurements using a b value of 3000 s/mm², finding a marked reduction in lesional ADC, and a reconstitution of anisotropy in the affected areas that correlated with treatment response.

Other Infections

Herpes simplex virus type 2 is a major cause of neonatal encephalitis, and CNS is involved in approximately 30% of infected infants.[3,16] Infection can result in microcephaly, seizures, microphthalmia, multicystic encephalomalacia, and death. Early findings, seen on MR imaging, include a reduction of distinction at the gray-white matter interface, and the associated edema may be difficult to distinguish from surrounding unmyelinated immature white matter, because both have an increased signal on T2-WI. Recent data proved that DWI is useful for early herpes encephalitis diagnosis.[17] Lesions of herpes simplex encephalitis is seen on DWI as reduced (cytotoxic edema) or increased (vasogenic edema) movement of water molecules.[18,19]

Cytomegalovirus, a virus in the herpes family, infects most infants by the end of their first year and, although rare in adults, is commonly seen in immunocompromised patients. Characteristic

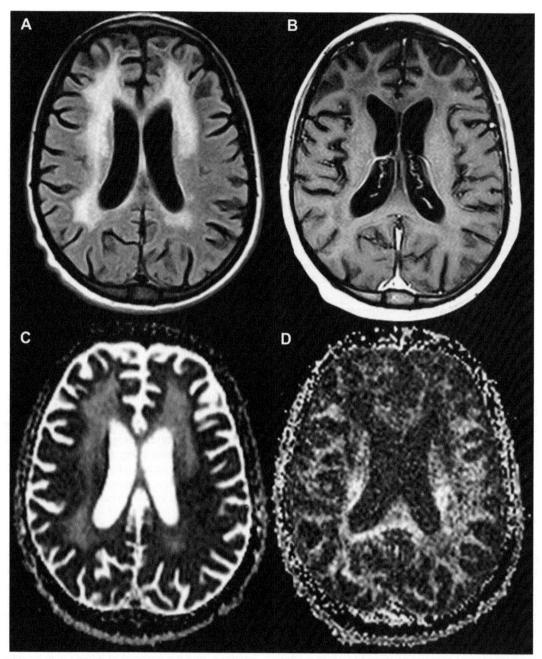

Fig. 3. HIV encephalitis. Axial FLAIR (*A*) reveals asymmetric areas of increased signal intensity without mass effect involving the periventricular white matter, as well as mild brain atrophy. There is no enhancement in postcontrast T1-weighted image (*B*). Apparent diffusion coefficient (ADC) map (*C*) shows increased water diffusibility in the same lesions. Axial fractional anisotropy (FA) map (*D*) shows reduction in the FA in the white matter, which presumably reflects a disruption of the fiber integrity secondary to HIV damage.

lesions are encephalopathy, subependymal spread, and more rarely, nodular focal lesions.[20] Encephalopathy may occur as a rare acute form or, more frequently, a subacute/chronic form, resulting in a condition described as ventriculoencephalitis. MR imaging reveals focal encephalopathy with increased signal on T2-WI and often low signal on T1-WI, with no contrast enhancement. Subependymal spread is usually revealed only after contrast administration, and appears as a thin line of enhancement along the ventricular walls.[21] Subependymal lesions may show reduced

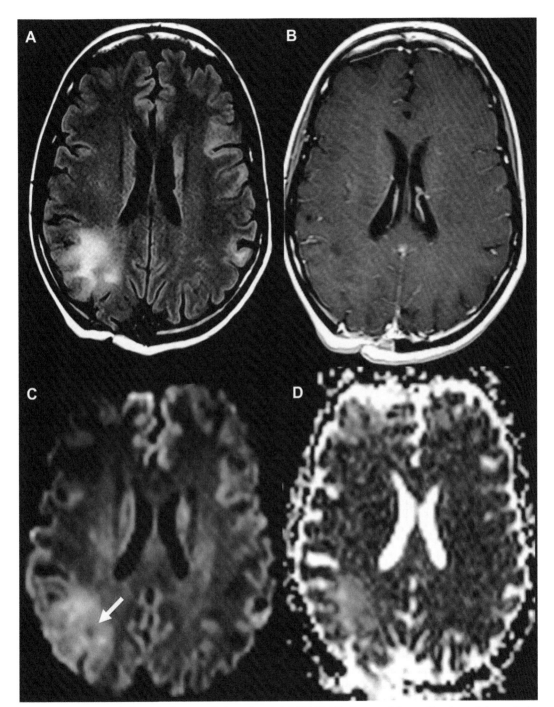

Fig. 4. Progressive multifocal leukoencephalopathy. Axial FLAIR (*A*) shows white matter hyperintense lesions without mass effect in the parietal lobes, larger on the right. Axial postgadolinium T1-WI (*B*) reveals hypointense lesion with no enhancement. Axial DWI (*C*) and ADC map (*D*) show a central core of facilitated diffusibility (*arrow*) surrounded by high signal intensity on DWI and ADC, corresponding to "T2 shine-through" effect (vasogenic edema).

diffusion because of inflammation and cytotoxic edema (Fig. 5).

Influenza virus is associated with various CNS lesions, many of them showing poor prognosis (acute necrotizing encephalopathy, Reye syndrome, and other types of influenza-associated encephalitis/encephalopathy).[22] In acute influenza-associated encephalopathy/encephalitis, MR imaging shows

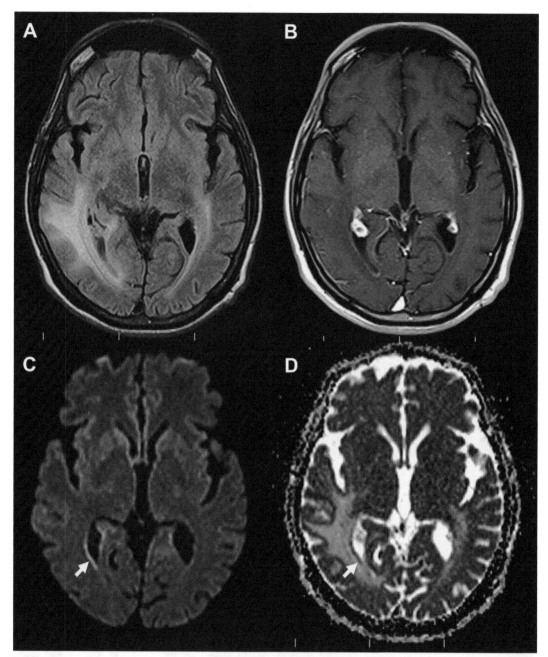

Fig. 5. Cytomegalovirus infection. Axial FLAIR (*A*) demonstrate hyperintense lesion in the white matter adjacent to the posterior horn of the lateral ventricles, better seen on the right side. Axial postcontrast T1-WI (*B*) demonstrates mild subependymal enhancement. DWI (*C*) and the corresponding ADC map (*D*) reveals reduced diffusion in the enhancing lesion (*arrows*).

lesions with diffuse or focal involvement of the cerebral cortex, the entire brain, or the bilateral thalamus.[23,24] Recently, acute encephalopathy syndrome characterized by biphasic seizures and late reduced diffusion was reported.[25] MR imaging shows no acute abnormality during the first 2 days after clinical onset, but reveals reduced diffusion in

the frontal or frontoparietal subcortical white matter, with sparing of the peri-rolandic region, from days 3 to 9. The diffusion abnormality disappears between days 9 and 25, finally resulting in cerebral atrophy.[26]

Subacute sclerosing panencephalitis (SSPE) is a slow progressive neurodegenerative infection by *Morbillivirus* genus viruses, characterized by fatal inflammation and sclerosis of the brain.[27] Clinical manifestations, presence of elevated titers of measles antibodies in the cerebrospinal fluid (CSF) and serum, and abnormal complexes on electroencephalogram establish the diagnosis. There is little correlation between imaging findings and clinical stage.[28] Early findings include a T2-WI signal increase in the frontal, temporal, and occipital white matter; less frequently, pial and parenchymal contrast enhancement, local mass effect, and edema are observed.[29] Focal well-circumscribed areas of hyperintensity on T2-WI can be seen in the basal ganglia, especially the putamen. Atrophy may be the only finding in very slowly progressing cases of subacute sclerosing panencephalitis. For DWI findings, Kanemura and Aihara[30] showed that the regional ADC of the frontal lobe decreased significantly with clinical stage progression, and increased to normal range during clinical improvement. Oguz and colleagues[29] demonstrated increased diffusion of the periventricular white matter and centrum semiovale and reduced diffusion of the arcuate fibers. Finally, Trivedi and colleagues[31] showed that FA values were significantly lower in the periventricular white matter in patients with SSPE and normal findings on conventional imaging, compared with the periventricular white matter of the controls in all cerebral lobes.

BACTERIAL INFECTION
Cerebritis and Pyogenic Abscess

Cerebritis is the earliest manifestation of a cerebral pyogenic infection that may progress to a brain abscess.[32,33] The histopathologic findings are characterized by a localized but poorly demarcated area of parenchymal softening with scattered necrosis, edema, vascular congestion, petechial hemorrhage, and perivascular inflammatory infiltrates at pathology studies.[34] T1-WI MR imaging shows an ill-defined area of isointensity or hypointensity and subtle mass effect, with minimal or absent contrast enhancement. On FLAIR and T2-WI, the infected tissue is hyperintense.[35] Cerebritis can appear as slightly reduced diffusion on DWI, probably related to hypercellularity, brain ischemia, or cytotoxic edema.[32,33]

Pyogenic brain abscesses account for only 2% of intracranial mass lesions, commonly viewed as circumscribed, enlarging, focal infections. Brain abscesses may occur from hematogenic dissemination of extracranial foci, from the extension of meningeal or nasosinusal infections, or after trauma and surgical procedures. MR imaging of a typical abscess with a central liquefactive necrosis shows that the center of the cavity is slightly hyperintense

to CSF, while the surrounding edematous brain is slightly hypointense to the normal brain parenchyma on T1-WI. On T2-WI the signal intensities are variable, depending on the protein composition and viscosity of the material in the central cavity. Usually an isointense-to-slightly hyperintense rim appears on T1-WI, and is hypointense on T2-WI. Ring enhancement after gadolinium administration is frequently seen, with a smooth and thin-walled ring that is often thinner along the medial margin.[36]

DWI usually shows reduced diffusion in the center of pyogenic brain abscesses (**Fig. 6**).[37] This appearance might be related to the high viscosity and cellularity of pus, which restricts water proton mobility.[38] However, care is needed when interpreting DWI and ADC maps of pyogenic abscesses, because small lesions may have normal ADC values.[39] In addition, in the early stages of a pyogenic abscess, during capsule formation, reduced diffusion may be restricted to the wall of the lesion, making differential diagnosis from another infectious causes of brain abscesses and necrotic tumors difficult (**Fig. 7**). ADC values may vary with the age of an abscess and the course of therapy. Ketelslegers and colleagues[40] reported a case of a pyogenic abscess in which the ADC values increased from 0.63 by 0.79 $\times$ 10^{-3} mm^2, to 1.10 by 1.29 $\times$ 10^{-3} mm^2 over 3 weeks of treatment. Another potential factor that may influence ADC values in an abscess is host immune status. In many studies, absolute ADC values are used rather than ADC ratios. Absolute values may be more susceptible to errors in measurement.[41]

DWI is also used to distinguish brain abscesses from necrotic or cystic neoplasms.[41–43] Fertikh and colleagues[41] assessed DWI findings for a series of 53 patients with ring-enhancing masses in the brain (26 abscesses and 23 neoplasms). The mean ADC ratios were significantly higher in neoplasms than in abscesses (2.45 vs 1.12). The accuracy of ADC ratios in discriminating abscesses from neoplasms, determined by the area under the receiver operating characteristic curve, was high, 0.91 $\pm$ 0.04 (mean $\pm$ standard error of the mean). ADC ratios were significantly higher in neoplasms than in pyogenic abscesses, but no difference was seen in ADC ratios between neoplasms and nonbacterial abscesses. In addition, the efficiency of the DWI increased from 87% to 94.3% when information about the presence of a T2 hypointense rim was added. The investigators concluded that ADC measurements significantly helped in distinguishing brain abscesses from necrotic or cystic neoplasms, and that ADC measurements were more reliable in cases of bacterial abscesses than in nonbacterial cases. This finding is important because

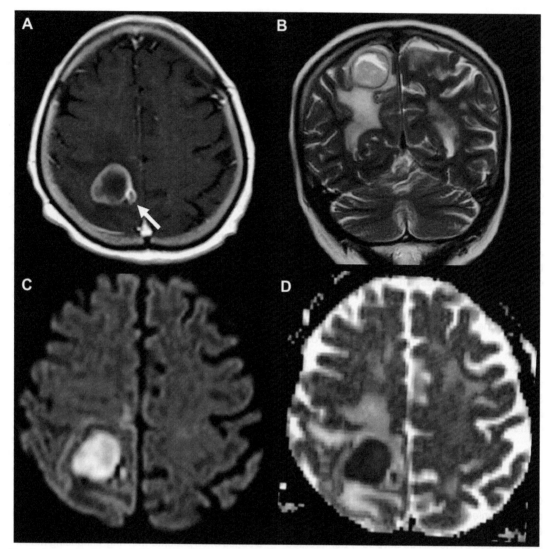

Fig. 6. Pyogenic abscess. Axial postgadolinium T1-WI (*A*) shows a ring-enhancing lesion surrounded by vasogenic edema with mass effect in the right parietal lobe, as well as a daughter lesion (*arrow*) in the medial aspect of the lesion. Coronal T2-WI (*B*) demonstrates a hypointense rim in the lesion, corresponding to both hemorrhage and free radical formation in the abscess capsule. DWI (*C*) and the ADC map (*D*) reveal the characteristic reduced diffusion of the abscess content (pus).

cerebral abscesses can be stereotactically aspirated, avoiding a formal craniotomy in tumor treatment (**Fig. 8**).[41]

Tuberculosis

Meningitis is the most common intracranial manifestation of tuberculosis (TB). It is usually more prominent in the basilar cisterns, especially around the circle of Willis. However, tuberculomas, tuberculous abscess, and cerebral ischemia and infarction are not uncommon findings. The most common imaging findings associated with CNS TB include enhancement of the basal cisterns,

granulomata, calcifications, hydrocephalus, meningeal enhancement, and infarction, most often of the basal ganglia.[44] Coexistent pulmonary TB is seen in 25% to 83% of cases of CNS TB.[45] Tuberculous leptomeningitis from CNS TB may directly involve intracranial arteries through the inflammatory infiltrate, or indirectly through reactive endarteritis obliterans, resulting in thrombosis and infarction.[46] Infarctions are even more common in children.[47] The middle cerebral artery and its branches are most often affected, especially the small perforating branches supplying the basal ganglia. In these patients, DWI is essential for differentiating between direct extension of the infection

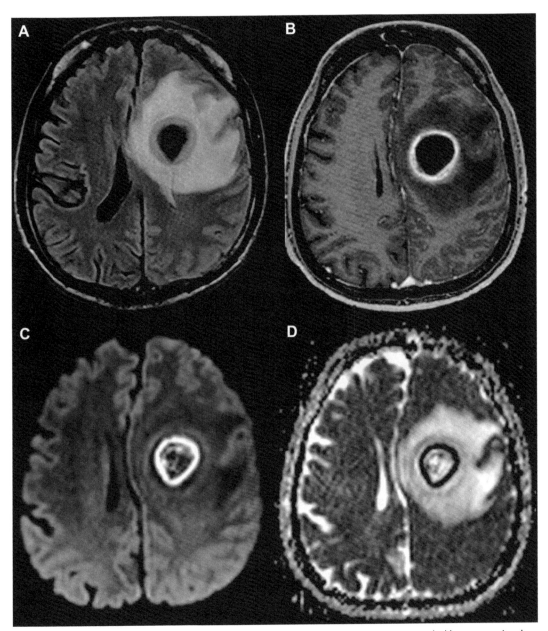

Fig. 7. Pyogenic abscess. Axial FLAIR (*A*) demonstrates a round hypointense mass surrounded by vasogenic edema in the left frontal lobe. Postgadolinium T1-WI (*B*) shows the lesion with ring enhancement. DWI (*C*) and the ADC map (*D*) reveal reduced diffusion in abscess capsule and facilitated diffusion in the core of the lesion. The histologic evaluation defined the diagnosis of early-stage *Streptococcus viridans* abscess.

to the brain parenchyma, and infarction. Reduced diffusion is usually seen in the infarction, while direct extension of the infection results in more heterogeneous signal intensity on DWI and ADC maps.[48–50]

Tuberculomas are granulomas that usually develop from either hematogenous spread or extension from CSF via cortical veins or small penetrating arteries. On T2-WI, they are usually

hypointense and show nodular enhancement in the early stages. During this phase, the tuberculomas may present with heterogeneous signal intensity on DWI and ADC maps, showing reduced or increased diffusion (**Figs. 9** and **10**).[51] As they mature, they develop a T2-WI hypointense center surrounded by an isointense capsule corresponding to solid caseation necrosis, and have ring enhancement. Tuberculous abscesses are more

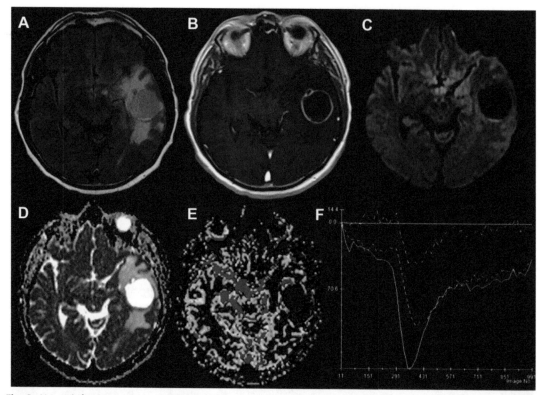

Fig. 8. Necrotic brain tumor (metastasis of lung cancer). FLAIR image (*A*) shows a left temporal cystic-appearing mass with surrounding vasogenic edema. Postgadolinium T1-WI (*B*) demonstrates ring enhancement of the lesion and a daughter lesion. DWI (*C*) and ADC map (*D*) show facilitated diffusion in the lesion. The relative cerebral blood volume map (perfusion imaging) (*E*) and the mean curve (*F*) demonstrate high perfusion in the wall of the lesion, suggesting the diagnosis of tumor instead of abscess.

common in HIV-infected patients. These abscesses range from 3 to 20 cm³ and are hypointense on T1-WI and hyperintense on T2-WI, showing well-defined rim enhancement on postcontrast images.[44] Although tuberculous abscesses may show reduced diffusion in the walls and increased diffusion in the center of the lesion, comparative analysis of ADC values from the walls of the pyogenic, tuberculous, and fungal abscesses have shown no significant differences.[52]

Syphilis

Neurosyphilis is a sexually transmitted disease caused by *Treponema pallidum*.[53] Symptomatic cases can be divided into 4 types, based on the predominant clinical features: meningeal, vascular, general paresis, and tabes dorsalis. The most common forms of neurosyphilis are meningeal and vascular.[44] Pathologically the meningeal form has acute inflammatory meningeal infiltrate, with neuritis and gumma formation. The vascular form is characterized by vascular endarteritis, causing irregular stenosis of medium or large vessels; and

syphilitic gummas may occur in the parenchyma or may be extra-axial, and are characterized by areas of granulated tissue surrounded by mononuclear cells and epithelial fibroblasts.[54]

Neurosyphilis has a wide range of imaging findings, such as atrophy, white matter lesions, infarctions, gummas, meningeal enhancement, and arteritis.[55] Evidence of infarctions of various ages may be seen, and meningovascular syphilis should always be considered when evaluating an HIV-infected patient who presents with cerebral infarction. The infarcts are typically located in the perforating artery territory of the basal ganglia and brainstem (**Fig. 11**). DWI is important for these patients, because it shows acute infarctions as reduced diffusion.[44] For cerebral gummas, MR imaging shows hypointense to isointense lesions on T1-WI, and hyperintense lesions associated with central nodular enhancement and surrounding edema on T2-WI.[56] Reduced diffusion of water molecules can also be seen in these lesions. The exact mechanism for restricted diffusion in the gumma is unclear, but may be due to cytotoxic edema of inflammatory cells.[57]

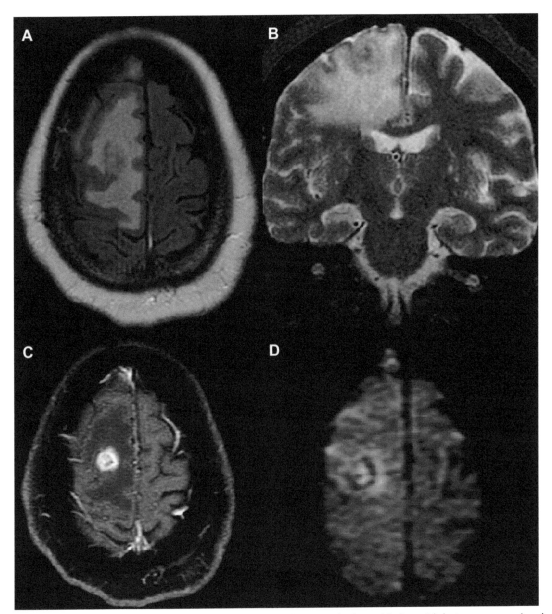

Fig. 9. Tuberculosis. Axial FLAIR (*A*) and coronal T2-WI (*B*) show a right frontal lesion with heterogeneous signal intensity and extensive perilesional vasogenic edema. There is significant enhancement on postcontrast T1-WI (*C*). The DWI (*D*) demonstrates high signal intensity in the center of the lesion, representing reduced diffusion (ADC map not shown).

Others

Septic emboli

Cerebrovascular occlusions by septic embolism usually occur in patients with bacterial endocarditis, history of intravenous drug abuse, or cyanotic heart disease. MR imaging findings may vary from major arterial branch infarction to multiple small abscesses located at the gray-white matter junction, depending on the size of the emboli.[34] As in other abscesses, DWI shows restricted diffusion within the lesions because of the pus content. In cases of very small lesions, reduced diffusion may not be seen.[39]

Meningitis

Meningitis, an acute or chronic inflammatory process of the pia-arachnoid, is potentially serious in childhood because of the possibility of developing cerebral infarcts.[58] DWI is a simple method for assessing the vascular and neurologic

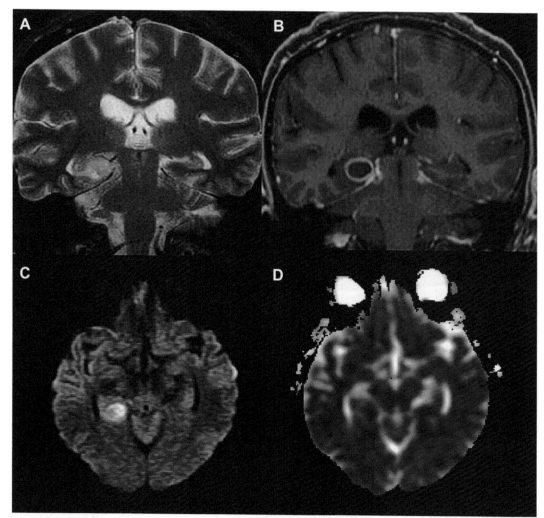

Fig. 10. Tuberculosis. Coronal T2-WI (*A*) and postcontrast T1-WI (*B*) show a heterogeneous lesion with predominant high signal intensity on T2-WI and ring enhancement, located on the right hippocampus. Not also the meningeal enhancement on the tentorium bilaterally. The DWI (*C*) and ADC map (*D*) demonstrate reduced diffusion on the center of the lesion.

complications of bacterial meningitis. Infarcts, which are frequent, may be related to septic vasculitis, and the frontal lobes are most commonly involved. The size, location, and multiplicity of the infarcts correlate with outcome. Infratentorial lesions are associated with a poor outcome, whereas patients with a favorable outcome develop only a few small scattered lesions.[59]

Empyema

Subdural and epidural empyemas account for about 30% of intracranial infections.[60] Empyemas usually develop as a complication of sinusitis, otitis media, meningitis, trauma, or craniotomy. Both subdural and epidural empyemas appear as extracerebral collections of fluid showing intense enhancement of the surrounding membrane.[61] On extra-axial collections, patients with subdural empyemas show a high signal on DWI, which is confirmed on ADC maps as restricted diffusion. However, epidural empyemas may also appear as areas of low signal, or a mixture of high and low signals on DWI (**Fig. 12**).[62] Therefore, the high signal on DWI and markedly diminished ADC distinguishes extra-axial empyemas from reactive effusions.[58]

Pyogenic intraventricular empyema (PIE) is characterized by the presence of pus in the ventricles. Rupture of a brain abscess is the most common cause, but extension of meningitis into the ventricles and a neurosurgical procedure or

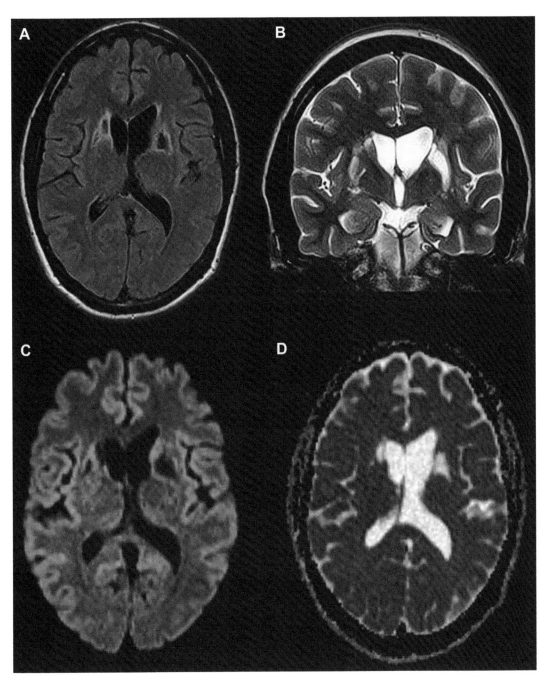

Fig. 11. Meningovascular syphilis. Axial FLAIR (*A*) and coronal T2-WI (*B*) demonstrate basal ganglia lesions that are isointense to cerebrospinal fluid, compatible with previous infarction (encephalomalacia). Axial DWI (*C*) shows hypointense signal intensity, and corresponding ADC map (*D*) reveals hyperintense signal in these lesions indicating facilitated diffusibility.

device are also described.[63] DWI is the most sensitive MR sequence for PIE diagnosis,[64] and it is characterized by high signal intensity in the dependent portion of the ventricles and low signal intensity on ADC maps.

FUNGAL INFECTION
Cryptococcosis

The cryptococcosis is caused by *Cryptococcus neoformans* and is the most common CNS fungal infection in patients with AIDS. The main forms of

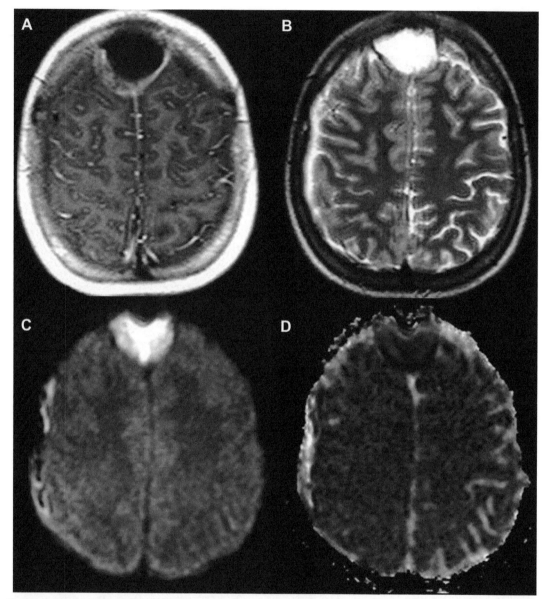

Fig. 12. Empyema. Postcontrast T1-WI (A) and T2-WI (B) show an extra-axial midline frontal lesion with high signal intensity on T2-WI and peripheral enhancement. The DWI (C) and ADC map (D) demonstrate reduced diffusion in the lesion. In addition, a small right frontoparietal subdural fluid collection with mixed areas of reduced and facilitated diffusion is apparent.

cryptococcal infection are meningitis, pseudocysts, and cryptococcomas. The meningitis is seen histopathologically as thickening and opacification of the leptomeninges, with mild inflammatory infiltrate. The pseudocysts have a "soap bubble" appearance and are more commonly seen in the basal ganglia. Histologically cryptococcomas can present as either a chronic granulomatous reaction with fewer cryptococci, or as lesions that contain numerous cryptococci that are associated with mild inflammation.[44]

Although MR imaging may appear normal in patients with cryptococcal meningitis, mild meningeal enhancement can be seen as well as areas of high signal intensity on T2-WI in the white matter, which represents vasogenic edema. Pseudocysts in the basal ganglia have a signal intensity that is similar to the CSF, and the DWI and ADC maps may show facilitated water diffusion as T2 shine-through (Fig. 13). Cryptococcomas are rare, and usually present on MR imaging T1 and T2 prolongation with ring or nodular enhancement,

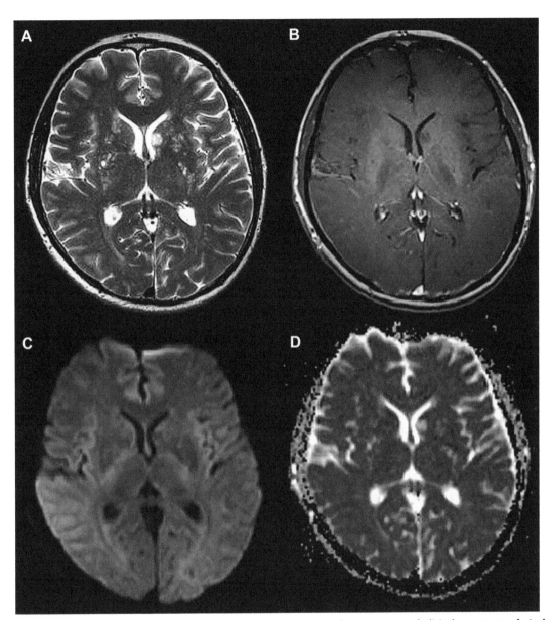

Fig. 13. Cryptococcosis. Axial T2-WI (*A*) of a patient with cryptococcal meningoencephalitis demonstrates foci of increased signal in the basal ganglia bilaterally, mainly in the left caudate. These lesions did not enhance on post-contrast T1-WI (*B*). Axial DWI (*C*) shows hypointense signal, and corresponding ADC map (*D*) reveals hyperintense signal in these lesions indicating facilitated water diffusion.

with surrounding vasogenic edema. Although only a few reports have described DWI findings for cryptococcal lesions, usually cryptococcomas do not show reduced diffusion, a finding that may help distinguish them from pyogenic abscesses.[65–67] Lesions with ring enhancement and viable organisms are reported to have facilitated diffusion in the center from necrosis.[66] However, lesions with a chronic granulomatous reaction may present with heterogeneous signal

intensity on DWI and ADC maps, and occasionally contain areas of restricted diffusion.[65]

Aspergillosis

Aspergillosis can affect the CNS through direct extension from the nasosinusal infection or, more commonly, from hematogenous dissemination of *Aspergillus fumigatus*. In addition to abscess formation, cerebral aspergillosis presents as meningitis, vascular invasion with thrombosis and infarction, hemorrhage, or aneurysm formation. Vascular involvement is common in these patients, and vessel wall invasion results from not only infectious lesions but also from ischemic and hemorrhagic infarcts. Histologic evaluation shows lesions with central area of coagulative necrosis, neutrophils, perivascular hemorrhage, and thrombosis of vessels from the periphery of the lesion. The brain parenchyma around the lesions may present with vasogenic edema, perivascular neutrophilic infiltrates, or mild gliosis.[68]

The imaging patterns that have been described in patients with CNS aspergillosis are multiple cortical and subcortical regions with T2 hyperintensity, multiple ring-enhancing lesions, and dural enhancement adjacent to enhancing lesions of the paranasal sinuses or calvaria. In brain abscesses, MR imaging shows low signal intensity on T1-WI, with occasional high signal foci from hemorrhaging or iron/manganese deposits. T2-WI shows high signal intensity lesions with peripheral low signal intensity from hemorrhaging, which is more clear on T2*-gradient echo sequence images (Fig. 14). Perilesional edema may be present, and contrast enhancement is absent or mild and ring-like.[44]

DWI findings for CNS aspergillosis have been variable.[52,69] Luthra and colleagues[52] found reduced diffusion in the projections and wall of a fungal abscess, while the abscess core did not exhibit reduced diffusion, a pattern unlike that seen for pyogenic and tuberculous abscesses. However, homogeneous[69] and heterogeneous[68,70] areas of high signal intensity on DWI have been seen in aspergillosis. Caution is necessary when interpreting DWI alone, because both early hemorrhage and infarction, commonly seen in CNS aspergillosis, can lead to reduced diffusion.[71]

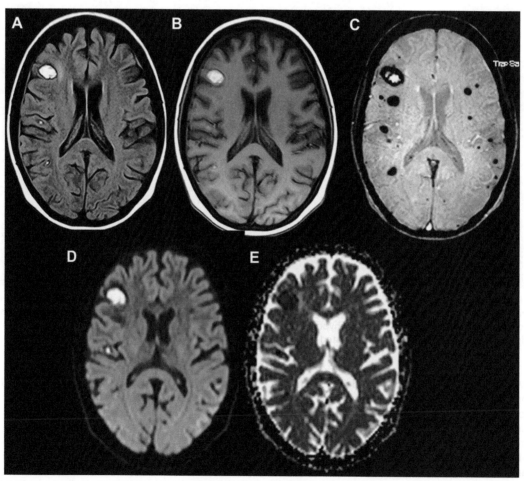

Fig. 14. Aspergillosis. FLAIR (*A*) and T1-WI (*B*) show multiple hyperintense lesions in the corticomedullary junction. Susceptibility weighted imaging (*C*) demonstrates multiple lesions with blood deposits, some of them with restricted diffusion on DWI (*D*) and ADC map (*E*).

Others

DWI findings have also been reported for less common CNS fungal infections, such as mucormycosis, candidiasis, histoplasmosis, and coccidioidomycosis. Tung and Rogg[33] demonstrated reduced diffusion in a case of cerebritis secondary to fronto-ethmoidal mucormycosis sinusitis. Like aspergillosis, candidiasis can present as small lesions with reduced diffusion or large lesions with heterogeneous signal intensity on DWI, due to hemorrhage, infarction, and infection.[72] Histoplasmomas are rare CNS lesions[73] that show no reduced diffusion, making them difficult to distinguish from tumors.[74] In a case of CNS coccidioidomycosis, reduced diffusion was seen in the wall and intracavitary projections of the abscess.[75]

PARASITIC INFECTIONS
Toxoplasmosis

Toxoplasmosis is caused by the obligate intracellular protozoan *Toxoplasma gondii*. Neurologic manifestations are usually related to the reactivation of a latent infection, and are more common in immunosuppressed individuals such as AIDS patients. Histologic evaluation may show 3 different forms of focal lesion: necrotizing abscess, abscess in organization, and chronic abscess. Parenchymal lesions have 3 distinct zones: a central avascular zone with a few microorganisms and coagulative necrosis; an intermediate zone engorged by blood vessels, and containing numerous intracellular and extracellular

tachyzoites; and a peripheral zone with fewer vascular abnormalities, encysted organisms (bradyzoites), and a few tachyzoites. The inflammatory reaction is more intense in the intermediate zone, and usually capsule formation is absent.

MR imaging shows lesions more frequently in the basal ganglia, thalamus, and corticomedullary junction. On T2-weighted sequences, toxoplasmosis lesions are hypointense to isointense and are surrounded by high signal-intensity vasogenic edema. Hemorrhage may occasionally be seen, and postcontrast T1-WI reveals multiple nodular lesions or ring-enhancing lesions. In some cases, a small eccentric nodule rests alongside an enhancing ring. This "target sign" is highly suggestive of toxoplasmosis, but is seen in fewer than 30% of cases. Lesions from toxoplasmosis are usually multiple, and are solitary in fewer than 15% of cases.[44]

Advanced MR imaging techniques such as DWI, MR spectroscopy, and dynamic contrast-enhanced perfusion have improved the diagnostic accuracy of MR imaging for evaluating patients with CNS toxoplasmosis. The presence of high lipid/lactate and nearly normal choline/N-acetyl aspartate ratios by MR spectroscopy, as well as low relative cerebral blood volume (hypoperfusion) suggest a diagnosis of toxoplasmosis instead of lymphoma. In addition, lymphoma can present as reduced diffusion from high cellularity, and an increased nuclear/cytoplasmic ratio.[76] DWI findings for toxoplasmosis lesions are more variable. The center of the abscess is usually isointense or slightly hypointense on DWI compared with normal

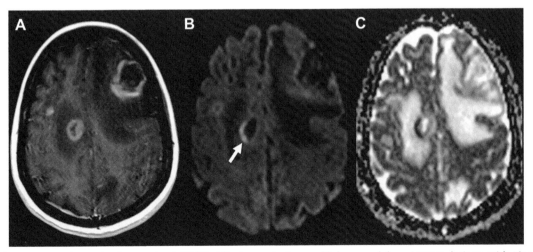

Fig. 15. Toxoplasmosis. Postcontrast T1-WI (*A*) demonstrates multiple round hypointense lesions with ring enhancement. DWI (*B*) shows the heterogeneity of these lesions on diffusion imaging (*B*, DWI and *C*, ADC map), with areas of reduced diffusion (*arrow*) and T2 shine-through effect on the wall, and facilitated diffusion on the center of the lesion.

contralateral white matter. Moreover, the wall is isointense or relatively hyperintense compared with the abscess center. On ADC map images, the abscess center may have a signal intensity that is similar to or higher than the unaffected white matter, while the abscess wall is slightly hypointense (**Figs. 15** and **16**).[77] Thus, areas of reduced diffusion can be seen in the walls of toxoplasmosis lesions but not in the necrotic centers, because pus is absent. This finding helps in differential diagnosis between toxoplasmosis and pyogenic abscesses.[43]

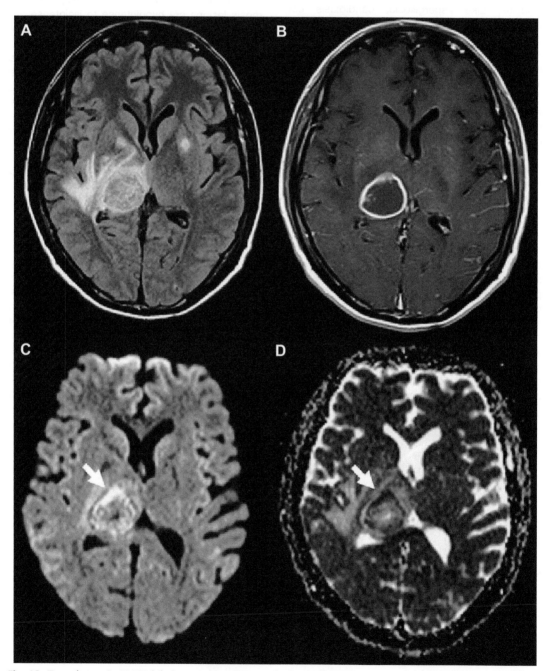

Fig. 16. Toxoplasmosis. FLAIR (*A*) shows a hyperintense lesion in the right thalamus with vasogenic edema and ring-enhancement on postcontrast T1-WI (*B*). A small lesion is also seen on the left lentiform nucleus. DWI (*C*) and ADC map (*D*) show areas of restricted diffusion on the periphery of the lesion (*arrows*) and T2 shine-through effect on the center of the lesion.

Cysticercosis

Neurocysticercosis is caused by encysted larvae of *Taenia solium* and is one of the most common CNS parasitic infections. Humans can be an intermediate or a definitive host. As definitive hosts, humans eat undercooked pork that is infected with viable larvae (cysticerci). On reaching the brain or any other part of the body, the larvae begin a regular life cycle from vesicular cysticercosis until involution, passing through 4 pathologic forms: vesicular, colloidal, granular nodular, and calcified.[78]

Imaging findings in each stage of cysticercosis reflect underlying changes in the disease process and host response. The vesicular stage has multiple cystic-appearing lesions (5–20 mm) with thin walls, and mild or no contrast enhancement. A 2- to 4-mm scolex is identified within the cyst. On DWI, the cysts show facilitated diffusion and the scoleces may show reduced diffusion, presenting as low signal intensity on ADC maps (**Fig. 17**). The cysts are preferentially located in the gray-white matter junction, but can also be seen in the basal ganglia, cerebellum, and brainstem. In the colloidal stage, the larvae begin to degenerate and an inflammatory reaction occurs, resulting in a thicker capsule and perilesional vasogenic edema. These lesions give a low signal on T1-WI and high signal on T2-WI, with ring enhancement and a surrounding halo of high signal on T2-WI. Depending on the severity of the inflammatory response, some lesions in the colloidal stage may have reduced diffusion. In the granular nodular stage, the cysts retract and form granulomatous nodules that may have ring or nodular enhancement, with or without vasogenic edema. In the calcified stage, lesions shrink and completely calcify. These lesions are better seen by computed tomography (CT) scan and T2*-gradient echo or susceptibility weighted imaging sequences. DWI is not useful during the granular nodular and calcified stages.[78–80]

Amebiasis and Echinococcosis

DWI findings are rarely reported for other uncommon CNS parasitic infections, such as amebiasis and echinococcosis. Several amebic organisms may be found in the CNS, such as *Entamoeba histolytica*, *Naegleria fowleri*, and *Acanthamoeba* species. These infections are rare, and the different etiologic agents cause different histopathological patterns. *E histolytica* is the etiologic agent in cerebral amebiasis, which affects patients between 20 and 40 years, and is more common in men. *N fowleri* is the pathogen that causes meningoencephalitis, which is a rare but fatal infection. Finally, *Acanthamoeba* species infection results in granulomatous encephalitis in immunocompromised individuals. In patients with cerebral amebiasis, MR imaging demonstrates single or multiple ring-enhancing lesions with vasogenic edema.[81,82] Although the center of the lesion may show facilitated diffusion, vascular invasion may be seen, resulting in areas of reduced diffusion in the periphery.[83] Echinococcosis affects the CNS in fewer than 1% of cases, and is more commonly diagnosed in childhood. Hydatid disease is most frequently located in the brain hemispheres,

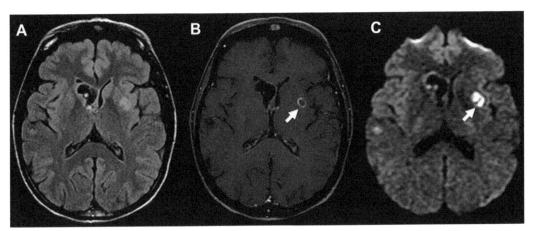

Fig. 17. Cysticercosis. FLAIR (*A*), postcontrast T1-WI (*B*), and DWI (*C*) show cysticercosis in different phases. A cystic-appearing lesion with a mural nodule (scolex) that has high signal on DWI is seen in the right caudate (vesicular stage). Also, a lesion at the colloidal stage is seen on the left lentiform nucleus. This lesion has high signal intensity on FLAIR and ring enhancement (*arrow*), as well as demonstrating reduced diffusion on DWI (*arrow*). Another small lesion with high signal intensity on DWI is seen on the right temporal lobe.

particularly in the territory of the middle cerebral artery. MR imaging shows well-defined, cystic-appearing masses with a signal intensity similar to the CSF and no contrast enhancement.[84,85] Although no previous studies have provided DWI findings for patients with brain hydatid disease, the signal intensity of these lesions on DWI and ADC maps is probably similar to the signal intensity of CSF.

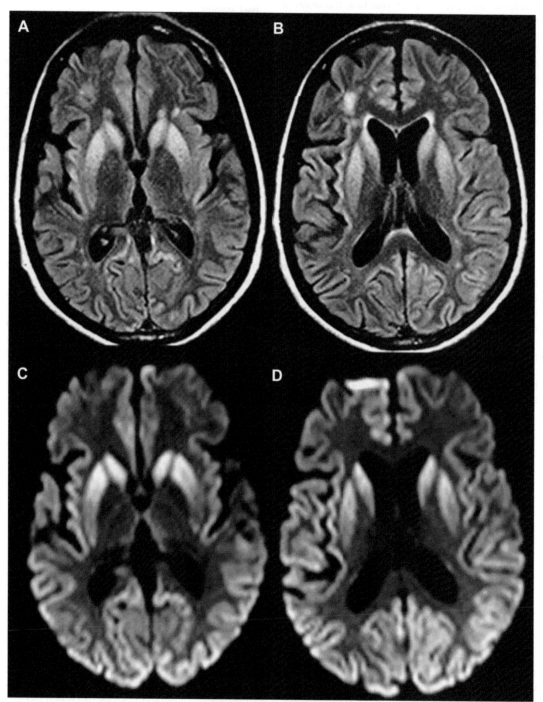

Fig. 18. Creutzfeldt-Jakob disease. FLAIR (*A, B*) shows hyperintense signal in the striatum and in the cortex bilaterally. DWI (*C, D*) reveals reduced diffusion in the same regions.

PRION DISEASES

The prion diseases, also known as transmissible spongiform encephalopathies, are progressive neurodegenerative diseases, with Creutzfeldt-Jakob disease (CJD) the most common. CJD has 4 forms: genetic, iatrogenic, new variant, and sporadic. The most frequent type is sporadic CJD, corresponding to 85% of cases, followed by the genetic form (10%–15%), with the iatrogenic and new variant forms the most rare.

Histopathological features of CJD include spongiform changes, neuronal loss, astrocytosis, and amyloid plaque formation. Although CJD is classically characterized by progressive dementia, myoclonic jerks, and periodic sharp-wave electroencephalographic activity, these features are frequently absent. As a result, most CJD cases cannot be clinically distinguished from other dementing illnesses. In addition, although progressive brain atrophy and areas of high signal intensity in the cerebral cortex and basal ganglia

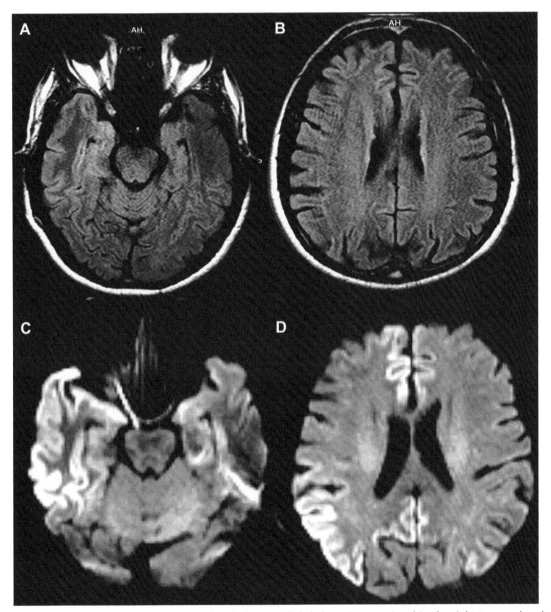

Fig. 19. Creutzfeldt-Jakob disease. FLAIR (*A, B*) shows a slightly hyperintense signal in the right temporal and frontal cortices, as well as in the parietal and occipital cortices bilaterally. These lesions have reduced diffusion on DWI (*C, D*).

can be seen on T2-WI, conventional MR imaging may be normal in as many as 20% of patients.[1]

DWI has emerged as the most sensitive sequence for the diagnosis of human prion diseases, particularly for sporadic CJD, in which increased sensitivity for signal intensity changes in the cortex is observed. The combined use of DWI and FLAIR sequences increases the diagnostic sensitivity and specificity for sporadic CJD to up to 90%.[86] DWI abnormalities reported for CJD include regions of reduced diffusion (high signal intensity on DWI and low signal intensity on ADC map) in the cortex, caudate nucleus, putamen, and thalamus, with a distribution pattern that does not correspond to arterial circulation (**Fig. 18**). In early-stage CJD, abnormalities are most frequently observed in the cortex, and may be unilateral or bilateral, diffuse or focal, and symmetric or asymmetric (**Fig. 19**). Abnormalities of the basal ganglia may also be unilateral or bilateral, and the caudate nucleus is most often involved.[87] The exact mechanisms for the DWI abnormalities in CJD are not known, but could be related to the abnormal prion deposits and vacuolization of the neuropil.

SUMMARY

DWI is a valuable technique that provides information on the physiologic state of the brain. DWI sequences are useful for evaluating CNS infections, and help in obtaining early and accurate diagnoses. Because treatment options are available for most of the CNS infections, correct and early differential diagnosis is important. Differentiating CNS infections from other causes of brain masses, such as malignant tumors, is essential in avoiding invasive procedures and incorrect treatments. In brief, DWI is a fast imaging sequence that provides valuable information for assessment and differential diagnosis of CNS infections.

REFERENCES

1. Schaefer PW, Grant PE, Gonzalez RG. Diffusion-weighted MR imaging of the brain. Radiology 2000;217:331–45.
2. Weiner LP, Fleming JO. Viral infections of the nervous system. J Neurosurg 1984;61:207–24.
3. Tien RD, Feldberg GJ, Osumi AK. Herpes virus infections of the CNS: MR findings. AJR Am J Roentgenol 1993;161:167–76.
4. Sener RN. Herpes simplex encephalitis: diffusion MR imaging findings. Comput Med Imaging Graph 2001;25(5):391–7.
5. Bulakbasi N, Kocaoglu M. Central nervous system infections of herpesvirus family. Neuroimaging Clin N Am 2008;18:53–84.
6. Olsen WL, Longo FM, Mills CM, et al. White matter disease in AIDS: findings at MR imaging. Radiology 1988;169:445–8.
7. Albright AV, Soldan SS, Gonzalez-Scarano F. Pathogenesis of human immunodeficiency virus-induced neurological disease. J Neurovirol 2003; 9(2):222–7.
8. Thurnher MM, Castillo M, Stadler A, et al. Diffusion-tensor MR imaging of the brain in human immunodeficiency virus-positive patients. AJNR Am J Neuroradiol 2005;26:2275–81.
9. Filippi CG, Ulug AM, Ryan E, et al. Diffusion tensor imaging of patients with HIV and normal-appearing white matter on MR images of the brain. AJNR Am J Neuroradiol 2001;22:277–83.
10. Ragin AB, Storey P, Cohen BA, et al. Disease burden in HIV-associated cognitive impairment: a study of whole-brain imaging measures. Neurology 2004; 63:2293–7.
11. Berger JR, Concha M. Progressive multifocal leukoencephalopathy: the evolution of a disease once considered rare. J Neurovirol 1995;1:5–18.
12. Cosottini M, Tavarelli C, Del Bono L. Diffusion-weighted imaging in patients with progressive multifocal leukoencephalopathy. Eur Radiol 2008;18: 1024–30.
13. Mader I, Herrlinger U, Klose U, et al. Progressive multifocal leukoencephalopathy: analysis of lesion development with diffusion-weighted MRI. Neuroradiology 2003;45(10):717–21.
14. Ohta K, Obara K, Sakauchi M, et al. Lesion extension detected by diffusion-weighted magnetic resonance imaging in progressive multifocal leukoencephalopathy. J Neurol 2001;248(9):809–11.
15. Usiskin SI, Bainbridge A, Miller RF, et al. Progressive multifocal leukoencephalopathy: serial high-b-value diffusion-weighted MR imaging and apparent diffusion coefficient measurements to assess response to highly active antiretroviral therapy. AJNR Am J Neuroradiol 2007;28(2):285–6.
16. Osborn RE, Byrd SE. Congenital infections of the brain. Neuroimaging Clin N Am 1991;1:105–18.
17. Kuker W, Nagele T, Schmidt F, et al. Diffusion-weighted MRI in herpes simplex encephalitis: a report of three cases. Neuroradiology 2004;46:122–5.
18. Teixeira J, Zimmerman RA, Haselgrove JC, et al. Diffusion imaging in pediatric central nervous system infections. Neuroradiology 2001;43:1031–9.
19. Kubota T, Ito M, Maruyama K, et al. Serial diffusion-weighted imaging of neonatal herpes encephalitis: a case report. Brain Dev 2007;29:171–3.
20. Kalayjian RC, Cohen ML, Bonomo RA, et al. Cytomegalovirus clinical and pathologic features. Medicine 1993;72:67–77.

21. Andreula C. Cranial viral infections in the adult. Eur Radiol 2004;14:E132–44.
22. Yoshikawa H, Yamazaki S, Watanabe T, et al. Study of influenza-associated encephalitis/encephalopathy in children during the 1997 to 2001 influenza seasons. J Child Neurol 2001;16:885–90.
23. Yoshikawa H, Watanabe T, Oda Y. Selective, reversible thalamic involvement with influenza A infection. Pediatrics 1998;102:1494–5.
24. Tokunaga Y, Kira R, Takemoto M, et al. Diagnostic usefulness of diffusion-weighted magnetic resonance imaging in influenza-associated acute encephalopathy or encephalitis. Brain Dev 2000;22:451–3.
25. Takanashi J, Oba H, Barkovich AJ, et al. Diffusion MRI abnormalities after prolonged febrile seizures with encephalopathy. Neurology 2006;66:1304–9.
26. Takanashi J, Tsuji M, Amemiya K, et al. Mild influenza encephalopathy with biphasic seizures and late reduced diffusion. J Neurol Sci 2007;256:86–9.
27. Tsuchiya K, Yamauchi T, Furui S, et al. MR imaging vs CT in subacute sclerosing panencephalitis. AJNR Am J Neuroradiol 1988;9:943–6.
28. Anlar B, Saatci I, Kose G, et al. MRI findings in subacute sclerosing panencephalitis. Neurology 1996;47:1278–83.
29. Oguz KK, Celebi A, Anlar B. MR imaging, diffusion-weighted imaging and MR spectroscopy findings in acute rapidly progressive subacute sclerosing panencephalitis. Brain Dev 2007;29:306–11.
30. Kanemura H, Aihara M. Serial diffusion-weighted imaging in subacute sclerosing panencephalitis. Pediatr Neurol 2008;38:430–4.
31. Trivedi R, Gupta RK, Agarawal A. Assessment of white matter damage in subacute sclerosing panencephalitis using quantitative diffusion tensor MR imaging. AJNR Am J Neuroradiol 2006;27:1712–6.
32. Flaris N, Hickey W. Development and characterization of an experimental model of brain abscess in the rat. Am J Pathol 1992;141:1299–307.
33. Tung GA, Rogg JM. Diffusion-weighted imaging of cerebritis. AJNR Am J Neuroradiol 2003;24(6):1110–3.
34. Parker JC Jr, Dyer MC. Neurologic infections due to bacteria fungi, and parasites. In: Doris RL, Robertson DM, editors. Textbook of neuropathology. Baltimore (MD): Williams & Wilkins; 1985. p. 632–703.
35. Falcone S, Post M. Encephalitis, cerebritis, and brain abscess: pathophysiology and imaging findings. Neuroimaging Clin N Am 2000;10:333–53.
36. Haimes AB, Zimmerman RD, Morgello S, et al. MR imaging of brain abscesses. AJR Am J Roentgenol 1989;152:1073–85.
37. Ebisu T, Tanaka C, Umeda M, et al. Discrimination of brain abscess from necrotic or cystic tumors by diffusion-weighted echo planar imaging. Magn Reson Imaging 1996;14:1113–6.
38. Desprechin B, Stadnik T, Koerts G, et al. Use of diffusion-weighted MR imaging in differential diagnosis between intracerebral necrotic tumors and cerebral abscesses. AJNR Am J Neuroradiol 1999;20:1252–7.
39. Guo AC, Provenzale JM, Cruz LC Jr, et al. Cerebral abscesses: investigation using apparent diffusion coefficient maps. Neuroradiology 2001;43:370–4.
40. Ketelslegers E, Duprez T, Ghariani S, et al. Time dependence of serial diffusion-weighted imaging features in a case of pyogenic brain abscess. J Comput Assist Tomogr 2000;24:478–81.
41. Fertikh D, Krejza J, Cunqueiro A, et al. Discrimination of capsular stage brain abscesses from necrotic or cystic neoplasms using diffusion-weighted magnetic resonance imaging. J Neurosurg 2007;106:76–81.
42. Nadal Desbarats L, Herlidou S, de Marco G, et al. Differential MRI diagnosis between brain abscesses and necrotic or cystic brain tumors using the apparent diffusion coefficient and normalized diffusion-weighted images. Magn Reson Imaging 2003;21(6):645–50.
43. Chang SC, Lai PH, Chen WL, et al. Diffusion-weighted MRI features of brain abscess and cystic or necrotic brain tumors: comparison with conventional MRI. Clin Imaging 2002;26(4):227–36.
44. Smith AB, Smirniotopoulos JG, Rushing EJ. Central nervous system infections associated with human immunodeficiency virus infection: radiologic-pathologic correlation. Radiographics 2008;28:2033–58.
45. Bagga A, Kalra V, Ghai OP. Intracranial tuberculoma. Clin Pediatr 1988;27:487–90.
46. Leiguarda R, Berthier M, Starkstein S, et al. Ischemic infarction in 25 children with tuberculous meningitis. Stroke 1988;19:200–4.
47. Schoeman J, Hewlett R, Donald P. MR of childhood tuberculous meningitis. Neuroradiology 1988;30:473–7.
48. Whiteman M, Espinoza L, Post MJ, et al. Central nervous system tuberculosis in HIV-infected patients: clinical and radiographic findings. AJNR Am J Neuroradiol 1995;16(6):1319–27.
49. Sheller JR, Des Prez RM. CNS tuberculosis. Neurol Clin 1986;4(1):143–58.
50. van der Merwe DJ, Andronikou S, Van Toorn R, et al. Brainstem ischemic lesions on MRI in children with tuberculous meningitis: with diffusion weighted confirmation. Childs Nerv Syst 2009;25:949–54.
51. Gasparetto EL, Tazoniero P, de Carvalho Neto A. Disseminated tuberculosis in a pregnant woman presenting with numerous brain tuberculomas: case report. Arq Neuropsiquiatr 2003;61(3B):855–8.
52. Luthra G, Parihar A, Nath K, et al. Comparative evaluation of fungal, tubercular, and pyogenic brain

abscesses with conventional and diffusion MR imaging and proton MR spectroscopy. AJNR Am J Neuroradiol 2007;28:1332–8.

53. Bash S, Hathout GM, Cohen S. Mesiotemporal T2-weighted hyperintensity: neurosyphilis mimicking herpes encephalitis. AJNR Am J Neuroradiol 2001; 22(2):314–6.

54. Berger JR, Waskin H, Pall L, et al. Syphilitic cerebral gumma with HIV infection. Neurology 1992;42(7): 1282–7.

55. Brightbill TC, Ihmeidan IH, Post MJ, et al. Neurosyphilis in HIV-positive and HIV-negative patients: neuroimaging findings. AJNR Am J Neuroradiol 1995; 16(4):703–11.

56. Fadil H, Gonzalez-Toledo E, Kelley BJ, et al. Neuroimaging findings in neurosyphilis. J Neuroimaging 2006;16:286–9.

57. Soares-Fernandes JP, Ribeiro M, Maré M, et al. Diffusion-weighted magnetic resonance imaging findings in a patient with cerebral syphilitic gumma. J Comput Assist Tomogr 2007;31:592–4.

58. Friede RL. Cerebral infarcts complicating neonatal leptomeningitis. Acta Neuropathol 1973;23:245–53.

59. Jan W, Zimmerman RA, Bilaniuk LT, et al. Diffusion-weighted imaging in acute bacterial meningitis in infancy. Neuroradiology 2003;45:634–9.

60. Danzinger A, Price H, Schechter MM. An analysis of 113 intracranial infections. Neuroradiology 1980;19:31–4.

61. Tsuchiya K, Makita K, Furui S, et al. Contrast-enhanced magnetic resonance imaging of sub- and epidural empyemas. Neuroradiology 1992;34: 494–6.

62. Tsuchiya K, Osawa A, Katase S, et al. Diffusion-weighted MRI of subdural and epidural empyemas. Neuroradiology 2003;45:220–3.

63. Pezzullo JA, Tung GA, Mudigonda S, et al. Diffusion-weighted MR imaging of pyogenic ventriculitis. AJR Am J Roentgenol 2003;180:71–5.

64. Han K, Choi DS, Ryoo JW, et al. Diffusion-weighted MR imaging of pyogenic intraventricular empyema. Neuroradiology 2007;49:813–8.

65. Kamezawa T, Shimozuru T, Niiro M, et al. MRI demonstration of intracerebral cryptococcal granuloma. Neuroradiology 2000;42(1):30–3.

66. Ho TL, Lee HJ, Lee KW, et al. Diffusion-weighted and conventional magnetic resonance imaging in cerebral cryptococcoma. Acta Radiol 2005;46(4): 411–4.

67. Patro SN, Kesavadas C, Thomas B, et al. Uncommon presentation of intracranial cryptococcal infection mimicking tuberculous infection in two immunocompetent patients. Singapore Med J 2009;50(4):e133–7.

68. Mueller-Mang C, Castillo M, Mang TG, et al. Fungal versus bacterial brain abscesses: is diffusion-weighted MR imaging a useful tool in the differential diagnosis? Neuroradiology 2007;49(8):651–7.

69. Oner AY, Celik H, Akpek S, et al. Central nervous system aspergillosis: magnetic resonance imaging, diffusion-weighted imaging, and magnetic resonance spectroscopy features. Acta Radiol 2006; 47(4):408–12.

70. Charlot M, Pialat JB, Obadia N, et al. Diffusion-weighted imaging in brain aspergillosis. Eur J Neurol 2007;14(8):912–6.

71. Gabelmann A, Klein S, Kern W, et al. Relevant imaging findings of cerebral aspergillosis on MRI: a retrospective case-based study in immunocompromised patients. Eur J Neurol 2007; 14(5):548–55.

72. Jain KK, Mittal SK, Kumar S, et al. Imaging features of central nervous system fungal infections. Neurol India 2007;55:241–50.

73. Gasparetto EL, Carvalho Neto A, Alberton J, et al. Histoplasmoma as isolated central nervous system lesion in an immunocompetent patient. Arq Neuropsiquiatr 2005;63:689–92.

74. Smith JS, Quiñones-Hinojosa A, Phillips JJ, et al. Limitations of diffusion-weighted imaging in distinguishing between a brain tumor and a central nervous system histoplasmoma. J Neurooncol 2006;79:217–8.

75. Castro S, Bernardes I. Coccidioidal cerebral abscess with peripheral restricted diffusion. J Neuroradiol 2009;36:162–4.

76. Camacho DL, Smith JK, Castillo M. Differentiation of toxoplasmosis and lymphoma in AIDS patients by using apparent diffusion coefficients. AJNR Am J Neuroradiol 2003;24(4):633–7.

77. Chong-Han CH, Cortez SC, Tung GA. Diffusion-weighted MRI of cerebral toxoplasma abscess. AJR Am J Roentgenol 2003;181(6):1711–4.

78. Noujaim SE, Rossi MD, Rao SK, et al. CT and MR imaging of neurocysticercosis. AJR Am J Roentgenol 1999;173(6):1485–90.

79. Gupta RK, Prakash M, Mishra AM, et al. Role of diffusion weighted imaging in differentiation of intracranial tuberculoma and tuberculous abscess from cysticercus granulomas-a report of more than 100 lesions. Eur J Radiol 2005;55(3):384–92.

80. Raffin LS, Bacheschi LA, Machado LR, et al. Diffusion-weighted MR imaging of cystic lesions of neurocysticercosis: a preliminary study. Arq Neuropsiquiatr 2001;59(4):839–42.

81. Kidney DD, Kim SH. CNS infections with free-living amebas: neuroimaging findings. AJR Am J Roentgenol 1998;171:809–12.

82. Schumacher DJ, Tien RD, Lane K. Neuroimaging findings in rare amebic infections of the central nervous system. AJNR Am J Neuroradiol 1995;16: 930–5.

83. McKellar MS, Mehta LR, Greenlee JE, et al. Fatal granulomatous Acanthamoeba encephalitis mimicking a stroke, diagnosed by correlation of results of

sequential magnetic resonance imaging, biopsy, in vitro culture, immunofluorescence analysis, and molecular analysis. J Clin Microbiol 2006;44:4265–9.

84. Pedrosa I, Saíz A, Arrazola J, et al. Hydatid disease: radiologic and pathologic features and complications. Radiographics 2000;20:795–817.

85. Per H, Kumandaş S, Gümüş H, et al. Primary soliter and multiple intracranial cyst hydatid disease: report of five cases. Brain Dev 2009;31:228–33.

86. Hyare H, Thornton J, Stevens J, et al. High-b-value diffusion MR imaging and basal nuclei apparent diffusion coefficient measurements in variant and sporadic Creutzfeldt-Jakob disease. AJNR Am J Neuroradiol 2010;31(3):521–6.

87. Ukisu R, Kushihashi T, Tanaka E, et al. Diffusion-weighted MR imaging of early-stage Creutzfeldt-Jakob disease: typical and atypical manifestations. Radiographics 2006;26:S191–204.

Diffusion Imaging in Traumatic Brain Injury

Emerson L. Gasparetto, MD, PhD[a,b,*],
Fernanda C. Rueda Lopes, MD[a,b],
Roberto C. Domingues, MD[a,c],
Romeu C. Domingues, MD[a,c]

KEYWORDS

- Diffusion imaging • Traumatic brain injury
- Magnetic resonance imaging • Computed tomography

Traumatic brain injury (TBI) is a common and devastating condition that exacts a heavy toll on the affected individuals, their families, and society in general. Worldwide, 10 million deaths and/or hospitalizations annually are directly attributable to TBI.[1] It is reported that 1.4 million people incur TBI in the United States every year, but this statistic does not reflect the true incidence, because many individuals never seek medical attention.[2] The most common causes of TBI are falls, motor vehicle accidents, sports-related injuries, and assaults.

Neuroimaging plays an important role in the evaluation of patients with TBI. Cranial computed tomography (CT) is the modality of choice for the initial assessment of moderate to severe TBI because it is fast, widely available, and highly accurate for the detection of skull fractures and intracranial lesions, which may necessitate immediate surgical intervention.[3] Magnetic resonance (MR) imaging is the method of choice in patients with acute TBI when neurologic findings cannot be explained by CT. MR imaging is also recommended for the evaluation of TBI-related symptoms in the subacute or chronic phases of the injury. After the patient has been stabilized, imaging is directed at providing a clearer picture of the extent of injury and information regarding prognosis. The use of MR imaging is helpful to the physician, because it has a greater spatial resolution than CT, as well as an increased sensitivity to lesions within the brainstem, posterior fossa, and in regions adjacent to bone. Conventional MR imaging sequences usually provide valuable information related to the severity of the TBI, and are informative as to prognosis and the likelihood of long-term disabilities.[3,4]

Advanced MR imaging techniques, such as diffusion-weighted imaging (DWI) and diffusion tensor imaging (DTI), have emerged as powerful noninvasive methods in neuroimaging, but the application of these techniques to TBI is recent.[3,4] DWI describes an MR imaging sequence that is sensitive to the diffusion of water molecules within tissues. Restricted diffusion is expressed as a reduction in the apparent diffusion coefficient (ADC) and results in hyperintense signal intensities on DWI. Reduced diffusion is often interpreted as indicating cytotoxic edema, and is most frequently seen in ischemic stroke.[5] DTI measures both the direction and magnitude of the water-associated proton diffusion. Diffusion in white matter is nonrandom, being primarily constrained to an axis parallel to axons, a property referred to as anisotropy. Changes in fractional anisotropy (FA) are interpreted as alterations in white matter ultrastructure.[6] Both DWI and DTI can show abnormalities in the white matter in the acute and chronic phases after TBI. These findings are sometimes beneath the resolution of standard neuroimaging techniques, such as CT and conventional MR imaging. These measures are often directly applicable to the prognosis of the patient, predicting both the

[a] CDPI – Clínica de Diagnóstico por Imagem, Rio de Janeiro, Brazil
[b] Department of Radiology, University of Rio de Janeiro, Rio de Janeiro, Brazil
[c] Clinic Multi-Imagem, Rio de Janeiro, Brazil
* Corresponding author. Estrada da Barra da Tijuca 1006 ap 1106, 22641-003 Rio de Janeiro, Brazil.
E-mail address: egasparetto@gmail.com

Neuroimag Clin N Am 21 (2011) 115–125
doi:10.1016/j.nic.2011.02.003

duration of coma and outcome in patients with severe TBI.[7]

This article discusses both the current and potential clinical applications of DWI and DTI in patients with TBI.

ACUTE STAGE IMAGING
Acute Hematomas

Intracranial bleeding (intra-axial and extra-axial) are common acute findings after TBI. CT scans and conventional MR imaging sequences are the gold standard imaging techniques for the evaluation of these patients. However, DWI may help in some cases, because in the acute phase, a blood clot may appear with high signal intensity on DWI and low signal intensity on ADC, representing reduced diffusion. In the days after injury, a T2 shine-through effect can be seen and, within weeks, hematomas show facilitated diffusion (**Fig. 1**). In addition, DWI may facilitate detection of small acute and subacute intraventricular hemorrhage, with accuracy equal to that of CT.[8,9]

Diffuse Cerebral Swelling

Severe brain trauma (Glasgow Coma Scale ≤8) triggers a cascade of molecular and cellular events, culminating in a loss of ionic gradients in the brain. Water influx to the intracellular compartment leads to restricted water diffusion. This intracellular edema is cytotoxic, and is similar to that

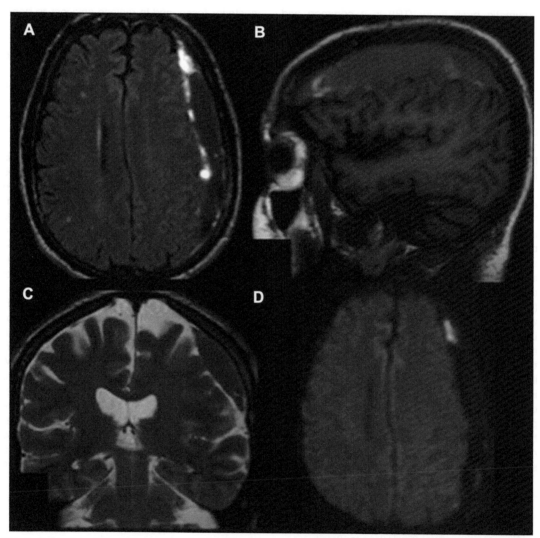

Fig. 1. Subacute subdural hematoma. Axial FLAIR (A), sagittal T1-WI (B), coronal T2-WI (C), and DWI (D) show a right frontoparietal subdural hematoma 3 weeks after the TBI. The signal is heterogeneous in all the sequences, predominantly hypointense on FLAIR, T2-WI, and DWI, and isointense on T1-WI. The DWI shows an area of restricted diffusion in the anterior portion of the hematoma.

seen in ischemia.[10,11] Head injury may also cause damage to the blood-brain barrier, usually around parenchymal lesions, increasing the extracellular water content and resulting in vasogenic edema. Edema itself constitutes a secondary insult resulting from trauma,[8,9] which leads to intracranial hypertension and decreased cerebral perfusion, the main cause of morbidity and mortality after trauma. Intracranial hypertension also leads to increased edema, and can result in ischemic lesions. Thus, diffuse cerebral swelling is represented by an increase in tissue fluid and a combination of cytotoxic and vasogenic edema.[8]

Areas of both cytotoxic and vasogenic edema have high signal intensities on T2-weighted images (T2-WI), and DWI plays a role in differentiating between these injury types.[8,11,12] Cytotoxic edema presents with low ADC values (low signal intensity on ADC maps) and high signal intensities on DWI, reflecting restricted diffusion (Fig. 2).[3,11,12] These changes can be observed as

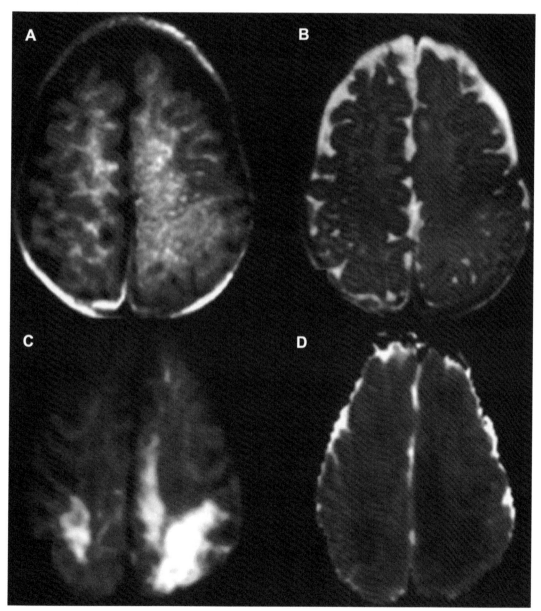

Fig. 2. Cytotoxic edema. Axial T1-WI (A), T2-WI (B), DWI (C), and ADC map (D) show bilateral frontoparietal cytotoxic edema in a 3-month-old child after TBI. Mild signal abnormalities are seen on T1-WI and T2-WI, but the DWI and ADC map show extensive areas of restricted diffusion, indicating cytotoxic edema.

soon as 8 hours after the injury, and are mainly related to diffuse axonal injury (DAI). Within the first 2 weeks after injury, in most cases the edema increases in severity, as the ADC decreases, and normalizes around the 10th day, similar to the pseudonormalization that occurs in ischemia.[11] Animal models are consistent with these observations, showing that ADC values progressively decline after acute head injury, reaching the lowest values 1 to 2 weeks after injury.[13,14] As seen in ischemic lesions, a penumbral area can be observed around the parenchymal traumatic lesion. The penumbra is represented by low ADC values that surround a region with even lower ADC values, and may represent an extension of the lesion.[11] The similarities observed between ischemic and post-TBI lesions lend support to the idea that ischemia and edema are usually associated,[10,12,15,16] as has been shown in animal models.[15] Cytotoxic edema and ischemia are intrinsically correlated to such a high degree that an ischemic injury should be excluded with additional MR imaging sequences if the lesions with restricted diffusion are not located at the predilection sites of DAI.[16]

Cytotoxic edema that occurs without ischemia may be designated as neurotoxic edema.[12] Neurotoxic edema may be instigated by a direct trauma mechanism. Trauma leads to a lesion of the axonal membrane, resulting in the leakage of glutamate into the extracellular space and excitotoxicity injury. High extracellular glutamate induces aberrant calcium and sodium influx into neural cells, resulting in the induction of apoptosis, gliosis, delayed neuronal death, and infarction. Excitotoxicity may be the underlying damage mechanism in the penumbral area surrounding a lesion after head injury.[12,17]

Glial cells such as astrocytes and oligodendrocytes also express glutamate receptors. Alternatively, the intracellular edema may occur in these cells, thus protecting axons from increased glutamate uptake. Intramyelin and neurotoxic edema represent slower forms of cellular swelling and may be responsible for the extended time over which decreased ADC values are observed after TBI.[12]

Vasogenic edema presents with different findings in MR imaging, displaying high signal intensities on the ADC maps and DWI (T2 shine-through effect) or, less commonly, high signals on ADC and low signals on DWI (facilitated diffusion).[11,12] These changes in signal intensities are usually located around a focal parenchymal lesion, such as a hematoma, because the blood clot exerts an osmotic effect on the surrounding brain parenchyma. The clot is usually present after the injury

and stable over the following weeks.[11] These findings suggest that intracellular edema should be more relevant to the clinicians, because it increases over time,[11] and is considered the major contributor to posttraumatic brain swelling in closed-head trauma.[17]

DTI parameters may also be affected by brain swelling. FA reduction may occur as early as 24 hours after trauma, and last for at least 7 days.[18] The entire white matter may show reductions in the FA during this acute phase, based on increased radial diffusivity values with no disturbance in the axial diffusivity.[19] If the ADC values are also increased, vasogenic edema is indicated; this is a reversible and treatable damage mechanism.[19]

Ischemia and Infarction

Hypoxic-ischemic injury is usually seen after TBI and it is related to poor clinical outcome.[20] In most cases, this type of injury is caused by either local or systemic effects.[12,20] Local factors can include cerebral edema with increased intracranial hypertension, as well as intracranial hematomas. These factors can lead to compression of intracranial blood vessels, thereby causing hypoperfusion and ischemia, which can involve a whole hemisphere. Vasospasms induced by subarachnoid hemorrhage may also play a role in cerebral infarction.[9] Systemic factors like hypotension and hypoxia caused by the trauma,[9,12,20] and distal embolization secondary to the vascular dissection or fat embolism, may be involved as well.[9] Acute ischemic areas are easily observed using DWI, because they have reduced diffusion that presents with high signal intensities on DWI and low signal intensities on ADC maps.[9]

SUBACUTE STAGE IMAGING
DAI

DAI results from rotational acceleration and deceleration forces that produce diffuse shear-strain deformations of brain tissue.[16,17] DAI usually takes place at the junction of the gray and white matter, particularly in the corpus callosum (CC), and at the dorsolateral aspect of the upper brain stem,[9,17,21] because the border between these areas and the adjacent tissue differs in density and rigidity.[22] As a result, disruptions in ionic homeostasis and altered permeabilities of the axolemma occur.[12] Initially, damage manifests as the development of axonal bulbs, or retraction balls, with subsequent progression to microglial clusters and long-tract degeneration.[17,21] Axonal disconnection may happen 30 to 60 hours after trauma, leaving both axonal segments with independent myelin sheaths.[21] Axonal injury occurring at acute time points is followed by demyelination and edema at subacute time points.[23] The force of impact causing the brain injury also determines the amount of fiber misalignment and/or disruption.[24]

DWI is a sophisticated tool for the evaluation of DAI lesions, because it is more sensitive than T2-WI and fluid-attenuated inversion recovery (FLAIR) in the acute phase of injury after trauma.[15,25] In addition, the lesion volume depicted with DWI has a stronger correlation with clinical outcome than that obtained from other conventional sequences.[15] The high signal intensity lesions observed with DWI may have high or low ADC values, and this additional information allows the classification of the injury in terms of severity.[25] ADC values significantly decrease in typical DAI lesions observed with conventional MR imaging,[15,17,25] as early as 1 day after the head injury, and decreases persist up to 18 days (Fig. 3).[17] This finding is likely related to cytotoxic

edema,[17] which has previously been associated with DAI.[11] Thus, lesions with low ADC indicate severe head injury and might be predictive of the patient's long-term prognosis.[12,25,26] DAI may also be represented as hemorrhagic lesions, which are better identified with T2*-WI. DWI may miss some of these lesions,[25] because the effect of blood products on ADC is uncertain. Blood clots typically reduce the motion of water molecules. In addition, cytotoxic edema is usually present with such lesions. Hemorrhagic DAI may therefore present with low ADC values.[17]

DAI lesions may be observed using DTI within the first few hours after head trauma.[21,27,28] DTI is susceptible to changes in parenchymal structure that are caused by misalignment of fibers, edema, axonal degeneration, fiber disruption, and demyelination.[24] Experiments with an animal model show that the initial days after trauma are characterized by axonal injury and resultant decreases in axial diffusion. After a week, axonal injury is followed by demyelination, and radial

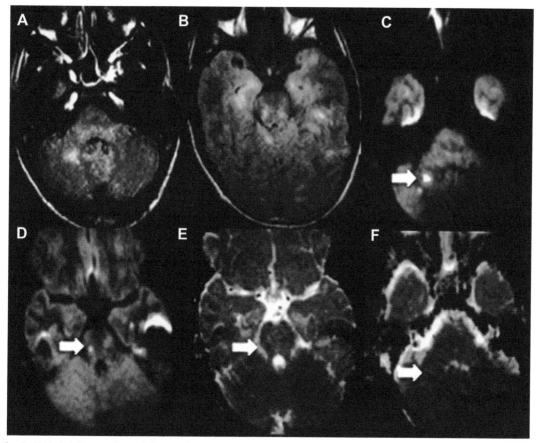

Fig. 3. DAI. Axial FLAIR (*A* and *B*), DWI (*C* and *D*), and ADC map (*E* and *F*) show lesions related to DAI in a 13-year-old boy after TBI. Multiple foci of high signal intensity on FLAIR are seen in the brain stem and cerebellar white matter, some of them showing restricted diffusion (*arrows*).

diffusion is then increased. Thus, the combination of reductions in axial diffusion values from axonal and cytoskeleton misalignment and increasing radial diffusion from demyelination, which favors diffusion in planes perpendicular to axons, leads to decreased FA values.[20,21]

FA measurements may be assessed in normal-appearing white matter (NAWM) on T2-WI to detect DAI.[21] The NAWM of trauma patients has been studied with DTI 1 year after the injury. In these patients, FA values were lower than the controls in the NAWM of the CC, the internal capsule, and the centrum semiovale, and were correlated with clinical outcome (**Fig. 4**).[29] The ADC values in the NAWM of the hemispheres and CC were higher in trauma patients than in controls,[21,30,31] because of the loss of myelinated axon fibers secondary to the trauma.[31,32]

The CC is more susceptible to DAI, because it is a less mobile structure connecting 2 mobile structures, the cerebral hemispheres.[22] This characteristic is more important in the posterior portion of the CC, as indicated by a pathologic-anatomic study.[9,24] The genu of the CC may be affected[9,24] even in mild head trauma. FA decreases and ADC increases in the CC can be observed within the first 3 months after trauma, likely as a result of vasogenic edema, because these changes disappear after 3 months after injury. However, in moderate and severe head trauma, FA decreases in the splenium of the CC are not accompanied by ADC variations within the first 3 months.[24] This finding suggests that lesions in the posterior part of the CC have diffusion patterns distinct from those in the genu, which may reflect more irreversible lesions.[24] Lesions with low ADC, as a result of cytotoxic edema, are also frequently present in the CC during the acute phase of severe TBI (**Fig. 5**).[22,33]

Following the description of all possible TBI lesion patterns on the DWI/ADC maps, a lesion

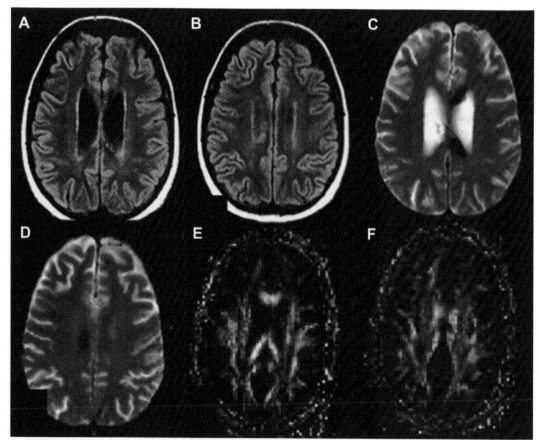

Fig. 4. DAI. Axial FLAIR (*A* and *B*), T2*-WI (*C* and *D*), and FA map (*E* and *F*) show bilateral frontal white matter lesions in a 26-year-old woman 8 months after the TBI. The FLAIR images show almost no significant signal abnormalities on the white matter. There is mild ventricular dilatation and areas of low signal intensity on T2*-WI in the CC and subcortical white matter related to DAI. The FA maps show significant reduction of the FA values on the frontal white matter, mainly at the left side.

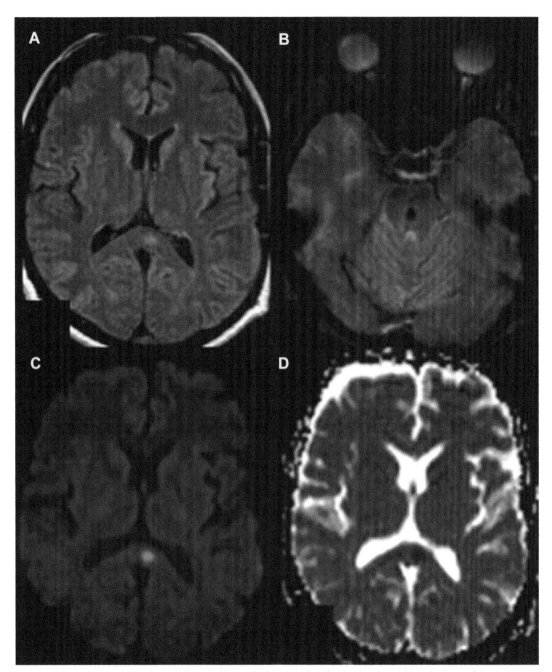

Fig. 5. DAI. Axial FLAIR (*A*), T2*-WI (*B*), DWI (*C*), and ADC map (*D*) show a lesion in the splenium of the CC in a 21-year-old man after TBI. The lesion in the CC has mildly increased signal intensity on FLAIR and restricted water diffusion on DWI and ADC map. Also, there is a focus of low signal intensity on T2*-WI on the brain stem (blood deposits), related to DAI.

classification scheme was developed based on this advanced MR imaging sequence.[12] Type I consists of lesions that are hyperintense on DWI with increased ADC, representing vasogenic edema. Type II lesions are hyperintense with DWI, but with reduced ADC, indicating cytotoxic edema. Type III represents a central hemorrhagic lesion surrounded by an area of hyperintensity on DWI and increased ADC. Lesions were also classified based on size and extent as follows: (A) focal injury, (B) regional/confluent lesion, and (C) extensive/diffuse injury.[9,12]

Fiber tractography is another DTI-based technique for evaluation of the white matter tracts. With the use of a fiber-tracking algorithm, it is possible to distinguish a reduction in the number of fibers in a specific white matter tract.[34–39] This finding may be useful after the third month after the trauma, when axonal loss and secondary degeneration are more common. In acute phases, the presence of edema may disguise the real number of fibers within certain tracts passing through a specific brain region.[34,35] Tractography delineates the point of axonal disruption in brain regions commonly involved in DAI, such as the CC, the brain stem, and the cortical-spinal tract.[27]

Cortical Contusion

Cortical contusions represent a primary injury that occurs at the time of the TBI.[9] This injury is caused by a direct contact of the skull within the brain parenchyma, often at the most anterior portions of the temporal and frontal poles.[17] The impact often results in punctuate hemorrhages in the brain parenchyma,[9] which affect the gray matter but mostly spare the underlying white matter,[8] and may be associated with diffuse subarachnoid hemorrhage.[9] Coup injury occurs at the site of primary impact, and is usually associated with scalp lesions or skull fractures. However, hemorrhagic cerebral cortical contusions are more common and larger in the contracoup area of injury, located at the opposite site of the primary injury. These lesions often contain blood clots, which present small dots of signal hyperintensity on DWI, constituting a pattern of reduced diffusion.[9]

CHRONIC STAGE IMAGING
Hydrocephalus

In severe cases of axonal damage, atrophy of the gray and white matter causes the ventricles to enlarge.[19,32] This widespread brain atrophy may progress over months, or even years, after an injury.[3,32] Atrophy progresses most rapidly in the first year after a trauma,[32] most likely because of Wallerian degeneration of disrupted white matter tracts.[12] However, apoptosis, excitotoxicity, inflammation, and prolonged hypoperfusion may also play significant roles in this type of damage.[12]

Traumatic hydrocephalus may occur secondary to impaired cerebral spinal fluid (CSF) reabsorption at the level of the arachnoid villi (communicating hydrocephalus), which is usually associated with previous subarachnoid hemorrhage. Hydrocephalus can also be secondary to an obstruction of the cerebral aqueduct and fourth-ventricular outflow (noncommunicating hydrocephalus), related

to mass effects from brain herniation or hematoma, mostly during acute phases.[8] DWI does not offer additional information to the conventional MR imaging sequence in patients with posttraumatic hydrocephalus.

Encephalomalacia

Encephalomalacia can develop months or years after a head injury, and is best observed on FLAIR images,[9] usually in the inferior and anterior portions of the frontal and temporal lobes.[8,9] With conventional MR imaging, as well as on DWI and ADC maps,[8] encephalomalacia has a pattern of signal intensities similar to CSF.

Leptomeningeal Cysts

Leptomeningeal cysts may be caused by tears in the dura mater. This dural defect allows expansion of the arachnoid mater at the site of a bone defect, often a suture, presumably as a result of CSF pulsation. The slow widening of the skull defect or suture may be observed.[8] The cyst, which contains primarily CSF, has the same MR imaging characteristics as CSF on the conventional sequences. On DWI, signs of T2 shine-through or facilitated diffusion are seen, making the differential diagnosis with empyema more straightforward.

Chronic Cortical and White Matter Abnormalities

White matter damage is the most prominent feature in patients with TBI, and is associated with low FA values. The FA may behave differently depending on the severity of the head trauma as well as on the interval between trauma and imaging evaluation. Clinically, it is generally believed that acute injury is followed by chronic progressive damage, which leads to long-term cognitive decline. In support of this idea, MR imaging follow-ups in patients 2 years after moderate and severe trauma show FA values progressively lower in the frontal and temporal lobes when compared with MR imaging performed 4 months after the trauma.[23] Decreased FA values may also be seen after a subacute period (3–5 months) after moderate/severe trauma not only with DAI lesions[27] but also in many areas of NAWM, such as the cingulum, the CC, lobar white matter,[24] the posterior limb of the internal capsule, and the cerebral peduncle (**Fig. 6**).[20] This FA reduction is related to increasing radial diffusion and decreasing axial diffusion, with unchanged mean diffusion values.[20]

DTI may also be useful for the evaluation of chronic TBI, resulting from the cumulative effects

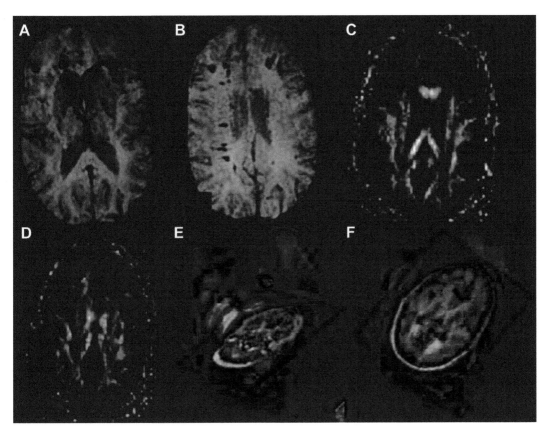

Fig. 6. Chronic cortical and white matter abnormalities. Axial susceptibility-weighted MR phase imaging (SWI) (*A* and *B*), FA map (*C* and *D*), and tractography (*E* and *F*) show severe cortical and white matter lesions related to DAI in a 26-year-old man 8 months after the TBI. Multiple chronic hemorrhagic lesions are seen on SWI, predominating on the left frontal lobe. The FA maps show significant reduction of the FA values (*darker*) on the white matter of the frontal lobes, mainly at the left side. The tractography shows the genu and splenium on the CC and shows significant reduction of the white matter fibers on the genu of the CC, which is more severe on the left.

of repeated blows to the head. Professional boxers evaluated in several studies had many normal-appearing brain areas with low FA and high ADC values, including the CC and the internal capsule.[40,41]

The main goal of evaluating the imaging results of patients with TBI with DWI, and especially DTI, is to find reliable imaging predictors of a patient's outcome.[4,18,20,25] Decreased FA has been reported in patients with poor outcome (Glasgow Outcome Score [GOS] 1–3), when compared with patients with good outcome (GOS 4 and 5).[20,25] Lower FA values in the cerebral peduncle might also predict poor outcome 1 year after the trauma.[20] Low FA values in the splenium of the CC and in the posterior limb of the internal capsule have also been related with poor outcome.[25,41] Evaluation of FA using tract-based statistical analysis was performed and confirmed these findings. This study added the inferior longitudinal fasciculus to the list of affected areas, and highlighted

the importance of lesions in the right side of the brain.[40] As a result, FA may be considered an additional tool for outcome prediction.[18,41]

SUMMARY

Despite advances in MR technology in recent years, CT is still the modality of choice for evaluation of acute TBI. MR imaging is reserved for patients with acute TBI when neurologic findings are incompatible with CT findings. In the subacute and chronic phases after TBI, MR imaging has usefulness in patient evaluation. Advanced MR imaging techniques, such as DWI and DTI, can be useful in improving the neuroimaging evaluation of TBI and enhancing our understanding of the pathophysiologic manifestations of brain trauma. Both DWI and DTI can detect white matter abnormalities that are beneath the resolution of CT and conventional MR imaging. In addition, DWI and DTI findings are instructive to the prognosis in patients with TBI, predicting not only coma duration but also long-term motor and cognitive deficits. Thus, diffusion MR imaging offers additional information over conventional MR imaging alone in patients with TBI, and should be included in MR imaging protocols used for the evaluation of brain trauma. Further studies correlating the findings of diffusion MR imaging with the prognosis of TBI patients will better clarify the role of this technique as a prognostic tool in brain trauma.

REFERENCES

1. Langlois JA, Rutland-Brown W, Wald MM. The epidemiology and impact of traumatic brain injury: a brief overview. J Head Trauma Rehabil 2006;21:375–8.
2. Langlois JA, Marr A, Mitchko J, et al. Tracking the silent epidemic and educating the public: CDC's traumatic brain injury-associated activities under the TBI Act of 1996 and the Children's Health Act of 2000. J Head Trauma Rehabil 2005;20:196–204.
3. Duckworth JL, Stevens RD. Imaging brain trauma. Curr Opin Crit Care 2010. [Epub ahead of print].
4. Gallagher CN, Hutchinson PJ, Pickard JD. Neuroimaging in trauma. Curr Opin Neurol 2007;20:403–9.
5. Schaefer PW, Grant PE, Gonzalez RG. Diffusion-weighted MR imaging of the brain. Radiology 2000;217:331–45.
6. Nucifora PG, Verma R, Lee SK, et al. Diffusion-tensor MR imaging and tractography: exploring brain microstructure and connectivity. Radiology 2007; 245:367–84.
7. Bazarian JJ, Zhong J, Blyth B, et al. Diffusion tensor imaging detects clinically important axonal damage after mild traumatic brain injury: a pilot study. J Neurotrauma 2007;24:1447–59.
8. Le TH, Gean AD. Neuroimaging of traumatic brain injury. Mt Sinai J Med 2009;7(6):145–62.
9. Parizel PM, Van Goethem JW, Özsarlak O, et al. New developments in the neuroradiological diagnosis of craniocerebral trauma. Eur Radiol 2005;15:569–81.
10. Karaarslan E, Arslan A. Diffusion weighted MR imaging in non-infarct lesions of the brain. Eur J Radiol 2008;65:402–16.
11. Pasco A, Ter Minassian A, Chapon C, et al. Dynamics of cerebral edema and apparent diffusion coefficient of water changes in patients with severe traumatic brain injury. A prospective MRI study. Eur Radiol 2006;16:1501–8.
12. Muccio CF, Simone MD, Esposito G, et al. Reversible post-traumatic bilateral extensive restricted diffusion of the brain. A case study and review of the literature. Brain Inj 2009;23:466–72.
13. Albensi BC, Knoblach SM, Chew BG, et al. Diffusion and high resolution MRI of traumatic brain injury in rats: time course and correlation with histology. Exp Neurol 2000;162:61–72.
14. Lescot T, Fulla-Oller L, Po C, et al. Temporal and regional changes after focal traumatic brain injury. J Neurotrauma 2010;27:85–94.
15. Schaefer PW, Huisman TA, Sorensen AG, et al. Diffusion-weighted MR imaging in closed head injury: high correlation with initial glasgow coma scale score and score on modified Rankin scale at discharge. Radiology 2004;233:58–66.
16. Huisman TA. Diffusion-weighted imaging: basic concepts and application in cerebral stroke and head trauma. Eur Radiol 2003;13:2283–97.
17. Liu AY, Maldjian JA, Bagley LJ, et al. Traumatic brain injury: diffusion-weighted imaging findings. AJNR Am J Neuroradiol 1999;20:1636–41.
18. Tollard E, Galanaud D, Perlbarg V, et al. Experience of diffusion tensor imaging and H1 spectroscopy for outcome prediction in severe traumatic brain injury: preliminary results. Crit Care Med 2009;37: 1448–55.
19. Newcombe VF, Williams GB, Nortje J, et al. Analysis of acute traumatic axonal injury using diffusion tensor imaging. Br J Neurosurg 2007;21:340–8.
20. Sidaros A, Engberg AW, Sidaros K, et al. Diffusion tensor imaging during recovery from severe traumatic brain injury and relation to clinical outcome: a longitudinal study. Brain 2008;131:559–72.
21. Arfanakis K, Haughton VM, Carew JD, et al. Diffusion tensor MR imaging in diffuse axonal injury. AJNR Am J Neuroradiol 2002;23:794–802.
22. Chan JH, Tsui EY, Peh WC, et al. Diffuse axonal injury: detection of changes in anisotropy of water diffusion by diffusion-weighted imaging. Neuroradiology 2003;45:34–8.
23. Greenberg G, Mikulis DJ, Ng K, et al. Use of diffusion tensor imaging to examine subacute white matter injury progression in moderate to severe traumatic brain injury. Arch Phys Med Rehabil 2008;89: S45–50.
24. Rutgers DR, Fillard P, Paradot G, et al. Diffusion tensor imaging characteristics of the corpus callosum in mild, moderate and severe traumatic brain injury. AJNR Am J Neuroradiol 2008;29: 1730–5.
25. Huisman TA, Sorensen G, Hergan K, et al. Diffusion-weighted imaging for the evaluation of diffuse axonal injury in closed head injury. J Comput Assist Tomogr 2003;27:5–11.
26. Schaefer PW. Applications of DWI in clinical neurology. J Neurol Sci 2001;186:S25–35.
27. Ahn YH, Kim SH, Han BS, et al. Focal lesions of the corticospinal tract demonstrated by diffusion tensor imaging in patients with diffuse axonal injury. NeuroRehabilitation 2006;21:239–43.
28. Bosnell R, Giorgio A, Johansen-Berg H. Imaging white matter diffusion changes with development and recovery from brain injury. Dev Neurorehabil 2008;11:174–86.

29. Ptak T, Sheridan R, Rhea J, et al. Cerebral fractional anisotropy score in trauma patients: a new indicator of white matter injury after trauma. AJR Am J Roentgenol 2003;181:1401–7.
30. Hou DJ, Tong KA, Ashwal S, et al. Diffusion-weighted magnetic resonance imaging improves outcome prediction in adult traumatic brain injury. J Neurotrauma 2007;24:1558–69.
31. Rugg-Gunn FJ, Symms MR, Barker GJ, et al. Diffusion imaging shows abnormalities after blunt head trauma when conventional magnetic resonance imaging is normal. J Neurol Neurosurg Psychiatry 2001;70:530–3.
32. Mamere AE, Saraiva LA, Matos AL, et al. Evaluation of delayed neuronal and axonal damage secondary to moderate and severe traumatic brain injury using quantitative MR imaging techniques. AJNR Am J Neuroradiol 2009;30:947–52.
33. Takayama H, Kobayashi M, Sugishita M, et al. Diffusion-weighted imaging demonstrates transient cytotoxic edema involving the corpus callosum in a patient with diffuse brain injury. Clin Neurol Neurosurg 2000;102:135–9.
34. Rutgers DR, Toulgoat F, Cazejust J, et al. White matter abnormalities in mild traumatic brain injury: a diffusion tensor imaging study. AJNR Am J Neuroradiol 2008;29:514–9.
35. Wang JY, Bakhadirov K, Devous MD, et al. Diffusion tensor tractography of traumatic diffuse axonal injury. Arch Neurol 2008;65:619–26.
36. Naganawa S, Sato C, Ishihra S, et al. Serial evaluation of diffusion tensor brain fiber tracking in a patient with severe diffuse axonal injury. AJNR Am J Neuroradiol 2004;25:1553–6.
37. Jang SH, Kim DS, Son SM, et al. Clinical application of diffusion tensor tractography for elucidation of the causes of motor weakness in patients with traumatic brain injury. NeuroRehabilitation 2009;24:273–8.
38. Perlbarg V, Puybasset L, Tollard E, et al. Relation between brain lesion location and clinical outcome in patients with severe traumatic brain injury: a diffusion tensor imaging study using voxel-based approaches. Hum Brain Mapp 2009;30:3924–33.
39. Huisman TA, Schwamm LH, Schaefer PW, et al. Diffusion tensor imaging as potential biomarker of white matter injury in diffuse axonal injury. AJNR Am J Neuroradiol 2004;25:370–6.
40. Chappell M, Ulug AM, Zhang L, et al. Distribution of microstructural damage in the brains of professional boxers: a diffusion MRI study. J Magn Reson Imaging 2006;24:537–42.
41. Zhang L, Heier LA, Zimmerman RD, et al. Diffusion anisotropy changes in the brains of professional boxers. AJNR Am J Neuroradiol 2006;27:2000–4.

Diffusion-Weighted Imaging in Neonates

Katyucia Rodrigues, MD[a,*], P. Ellen Grant, MD[b,c,d,e]

KEYWORDS

- Neonatal imaging • Diffusion-weighted imaging
- Pediatric neuroradiology • Hypoxic-ischemic
- Venous injury • Inborn errors of metabolism

Diffusion-weighted imaging (DWI) has become an important tool in pediatric neuroradiology, helping in the evaluation of the encephalopathic and seizing neonate, and adding conspicuity, specificity, and prognostic value to the conventional magnetic resonance (MR) imaging data. DWI also facilitates understanding the pathophysiology and natural time course of ischemic and nonischemic disorders.

As myelination is incomplete in neonates, the detection of edema and the estimate of edema extent on T2-weighted imaging (T2-WI) is difficult. In addition, Fluid-attenuated inversion recovery (FLAIR) is insensitive to acute edema in the newborn brain, due to lack of myelination. DWI with corresponding apparent diffusion coefficient (ADC) maps provide the ability to differentiate edema associated with increased extracellular space and edema associated with metabolic compromise or evolving necrosis. The quantitative nature of ADC maps also provides the potential to detect regions of increased or decreased diffusivity if performed at b values where normal data are available.

Although transport of the acutely ill neonate to the MR imaging scanner can be challenging, it should be performed as soon as clinically possible to search for the presence, pattern, severity, and extent of injury. MR-compatible incubators with built-in coils have provided a means to reduce transport time and minimize transport risk. Incorporation of DWI into the standard MR imaging protocol adds only minutes, yet provides the potential for early detection of the presence and type of perinatal brain injury. This information is valuable to the clinical team as they attempt to determine if acute brain injury is the cause of the clinical symptoms and what type of injury has occurred. Although in most centers providing therapeutic hypothermia MR imaging is typically not performed until the neonate is stable on cooling to maximize therapeutic effectiveness, MR imaging as soon as stable for transport is still preferred. In these cases MR imaging with DWI provides valuable information about the presence of contraindications for therapeutic hypothermia, such as significant hemorrhage or venous thrombosis.

At pediatric centers axial DWI images are typically acquired with maximum b values ranging from 700 to 1000 s/mm². The authors prefer a b value of at least 1000 to 1500 s/mm² because of the improved contrast to noise for regions with decreased ADC.[1,2] Higher b values (~3000 s/mm²) may be useful for improved conspicuity of regions with decreased ADC, but myelinating regions have also become more conspicuous, so detection of very subtle injury requires knowledge of normal

[a] Multi-Imagem/CDPI Clinics, R. Alm. Saddock de Sá, 266-Ipanema, Rio de Janeiro 22411-040, Brazil
[b] Fetal-Neonatal Neuroimaging and Developmental Science Center, Children's Hospital Boston, 1 Autumn Street, 6th Floor, Room AU654, Boston, MA 02115, USA
[c] Division of Newborn Medicine, Department of Medicine, Children's Hospital Boston, 300 Longwood Avenue, Boston, MA, USA
[d] Division of Neuroradiology, Department of Radiology, Children's Hospital Boston, 300 Longwood Avenue, Boston, MA, USA
[e] Harvard Medical School, 25 Shattuck Street, Boston, MA, USA
* Corresponding author.
E-mail address: katy.macedo@gmail.com

Neuroimag Clin N Am 21 (2011) 127–151
doi:10.1016/j.nic.2011.01.012

appearance. Moreover, as signal to noise decreases with increasing b value, these higher b values are most helpful on 3T systems with 32 channel coils.

As with all studies in which DWI is performed, ADC maps must be obtained and used in conjunction with DWI for optimal interpretation. This guideline holds particularly true for the immature brain, where there are normally large variations in ADC values caused by large regional differences in tissue water content. The ADC map is a direct reflection of the rate of water diffusion and is therefore not complicated by T2 contrast. Regions of low T2 due to early myelination can mask otherwise bright regions of decreased ADC on DWI, and regions of high T2 due to extracellular edema can appear bright on DWI, falsely appearing like regions of decreased ADC. Therefore both DWI and ADC maps must be used when evaluating the newborn brain.

ARTERIAL HYPOXIC-ISCHEMIC INJURY

Despite the developments in modern medicine, perinatal brain injury remains a common cause of morbidity and mortality. In particular, neonatal hypoxic-ischemic injury (HII) is one of the most important causes of neurologic disabilities, accounting for 15% to 28% of children with cerebral palsy.[3]

Global impairment in the exchange of respiratory gases occurring in the perinatal period causes deficit in oxygen supply, leading to neural tissue dysfunction and consequent hypoxic-ischemic encephalopathy in term and near-term neonates. Hypoxemia and mainly hypoperfusion are the two major pathogenic mechanisms. Because the neonatal brain is quite resistant to hypoxia in a setting of normal cerebral perfusion because of its ability to obtain energy from glucose and other substrates, most hypoxic ischemic brain injury likely results from a combination of both cerebral hypoxia and hypoperfusion.[4] Although hypoxia and hypoperfusion are thought to be primary factors, there are additional vulnerability factors such as inflammation, oxidative stress, and excitotoxicity that are thought to play a role in determining the extent and severity of brain injury, with different regions of brain having different susceptibility to injury at different maturational stages. For example, developing oligodendrocytes were found to be more susceptible to oxidative stress toxicity than mature oligodendrocytes, due to a depletion of intracellular glutathione in the oligodendrocyte progenitor cells and preoligodendrocytes.[5] These oligodendrocyte progenitor cells are also more vulnerable to glutamate excitotoxicity, because glutamate receptors are transiently expressed in this cell population but are downregulated in mature oligodendrocytes.[6] Inflammatory response may be critically important in the genesis of brain injury in the term as well as preterm newborn, even though in this population it may play more of a modulating role. Previous studies have suggested that chorioamnionites might be considered an independent risk factor for brain damage in term as well as preterm infants.[7]

Newborn HII may be associated with reperfusion before mitochondria are irreversibly damaged, preserving their ability to produce adenosine triphosphate (ATP). As a result, HII can trigger different pathways of cell death, both ATP-independent and ATP-dependent.[1] First, if an HI event is severe and prolonged enough to cause critical energy reduction then failure of the ATP-dependent Na^+/K^+ pump will occur, followed by NA^+, Cl^-, and water influx, cell swelling, and consequent immediate cell death by necrosis.[8] Second, if an HI event is less severe with blood flow and oxygen restored rapidly enough that transient energy recovery occurs, necrotic cell death is delayed. Finally, if an HI event is even less severe with blood flow and oxygen restored rapidly enough that transient energy recovery occurs and necrosis is averted, delayed cell death may still occur but by apoptotic or autophagic mechanisms.[1,9] Apoptosis occurs without significant inflammatory response, in contrast to cell necrosis in which strong inflammatory reaction usually occurs.[10] Autophagy is another pathway for the cell affected by asphyxia by mediating either successful repair or cell suicide.[9] After injury the cell may catabolize existing cytoplasmic components to maintain energy production, so that if reperfusion occurs the cell may survive. On the other hand, the cells can die if the apoptotic process cannot be interrupted.[10] Mixed patterns of cell death can also occur. A cell that has initiated apoptotic program may not have the necessary energy to finish the apoptotic process or may be irrevocably injured by prolonged overactivation of autophagy, and when this happens the process may progress toward necrosis.

Immediate necrosis is associated with immediate ADC decrease and delayed necrosis is associated with delayed ADC decrease. The ADC signatures of apoptotic and autophagic mechanisms have not been well described, but are unlikely to cause large ADC decreases. Therefore, the magnitude of ADC decrease is likely affected by delays in initiation of necrotic cell death as well as by the proportion of necrotic, apoptotic, and normal cells. It must be noted that a normal

DWI study does not exclude imminent necrotic cell death or ongoing apoptosis/autophagosis.

Most cases of HI encephalopathy are positive on DWI within the first day of life if therapeutic hypothermia has not been initiated. However, in milder cases or with therapeutic hypothermia, delays of at least 24 hours can occur before ADC decreases are evident or, if apoptosis dominates, ADC decreases may never occur. Therefore regions of decreased ADC may appear only after a few days and increase in volume over time as the injury evolves. Consequently, DWI performed in the first day of injury may be a poor predictor of the final extent of injury. A second MR image obtained between days 5 and 8 is beneficial in evaluating progression of injury. ADC pseudonormalization may occur around 7 to 10 days and could underestimate the extent; however, at this time abnormalities on conventional MR imaging sequences are typically amply evident.[11]

Global Arterial Ischemic Injury in Term Neonates

Arterial ischemic injury can be global or focal. Global injuries are often associated with encephalopathy, and have two major patterns that can coexist: a profound or central pattern and a peripheral or partial pattern.

The central or profound pattern is usually related to a sentinel event, such as placental abruption, severe maternal hypotension, twin-twin transfusion, or cardiac failure, causing global profound hypoxia and ischemia for a short period of time and without time to establish collateral blood flow, resulting in damage to the most metabolically active zones.[12] The affected regions on DWI correspond to zones of active myelination or high concentration of excitatory amino acids and corresponding receptors, therefore abnormalities can be observed in the ventrolateral thalamus, corticospinal tract in posterior limb internal capsule with or without involvement of the perirolandic cortex, other cortical areas, white matter, hippocampi, midbrain, dorsal brainstem, and superior vermis. Absent or less collateral blood flow in the basal ganglia, thalamus, and hippocampus make these regions more susceptible to injury when compared with cerebral cortex (**Fig. 1**).[13]

T1 shortening can be observed in areas of injury approximately 3 days after injury. However, subtle abnormalities may be difficult to detect because these areas correspond to the myelination zones with normal expected T1 shortening. T2 prolongation can also be seen in these areas with blurring of deep gray nuclei and cortical margins, but these findings are subtle and difficult to detect if one is unfamiliar with neonatal images. Abnormalities on DWI are seen earlier and are more conspicuous. Reduced diffusion may be evidenced on the first day and evolve over time because of delayed cell death, as stated earlier. Pseudonormalization on ADC maps occurs around 7 to 10 days, making diffusion imaging insensitive to recent injury after this time.[14–16] Vermeulen and colleagues,[17] studying 46 infants with neonatal HII, showed that low ADC values in the posterior limb of the internal capsule between 0 and 4 days of life were highly predictive of poor motor outcomes at 2 years of age. An increase in the lactate/choline ratio on MR spectroscopy on the first 72 hours after birth is also correlated with bad outcome.[11,18] However, the authors' group has seen several cases with no lactate in the first 24 to 48 hours that did not survive. In some of these cases arterial spin labeling images showed increased blood flow, which leads the authors to suspect that rebound hyperperfusion may correct the anaerobic metabolism but may not prevent delayed necrosis.

When extremely severe and prolonged hypoxia and ischemia occurs, diffuse damage to the brain with diffuse brain swelling and involvement of basal ganglia and thalami may take place, sparing only medulla oblongata and cerebellum. In this situation, where there is extensive supratentorial involvement, visual analyses of the DWI images can be challenging to the radiologist unfamiliar with normal studies, although the cerebellum, which is usually spared from the ischemia in term neonates, can be used as a reference.[19]

When the hypoxia and/or hypoperfusion is less profound but lasts hours or days, continuously or intermittently, blood flow is redistributed to regions with lower energy demands, sparing the highly metabolically active zones involved in the profound pattern. The resulting DWI pattern of injury is a partial or peripheral pattern of injury with variable regions of cortex and subcortical white matter involved, but with cortex at the sulcal depths often preferentially involved. T1 shortening can also be observed in the depth of sulci on T1-WI beginning around day 3 and cortical increased T2 signal or blurring of cortical margins on T2-WI detected beginning sometime between the acute and subacute phase.[14–16] DWI permits an earlier detection of injury, particularly in the first few days subsequent to injury (**Fig. 2**).

White matter injury can also occur in the absence of gray matter injury in term neonates. Li and colleagues[20] described term neonates with mild encephalopathy and without congenital heart disease, with focal white matter injury

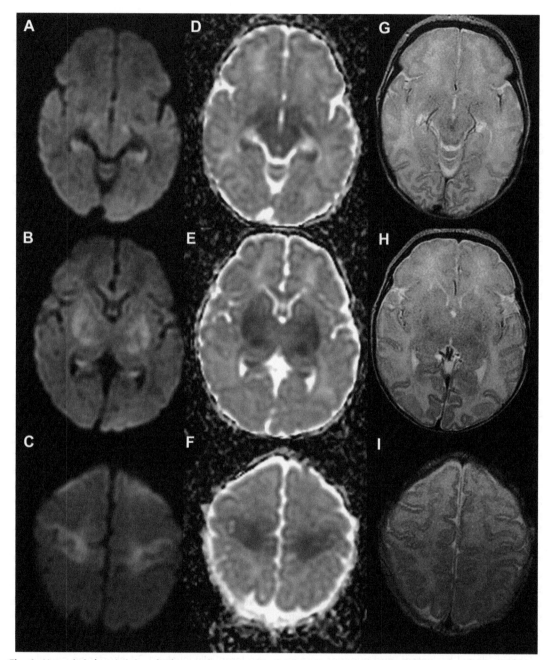

Fig. 1. Hypoxic-ischemic injury (HII) central pattern. (*A–C*) Echo planar imaging (EPI) diffusion-weighted imaging (DWI) 8300/98.5; (*D–F*) apparent diffusion coefficient (ADC) maps; (*G–I*) T2-spin echo (SE) 3916.66/105.98. Three-day-old female term baby with a history of hypoxic-ischemic encephalopathy and neonatal seizures. DWI and ADC maps show reduced diffusion bilaterally in the putamina, ventral lateral thalami, hippocampi, corticospinal tracts, and perirolandic cortex. T2-weighted imaging (T2-WI) and T1-WI demonstrate abnormal signal in these same distributions.

associated with decreased diffusion on the third day of life suggesting perinatal injury. The investigators hypothesized that the lesions could be attributed to heterogeneous oligodendrocyte progenitor cell maturation, as white matter lesions were commonly recognized in "early" term neonates rather than low birth weight neonates. However, in the author's experience similar lesions can also be seen in full-term infants in a pattern that suggests venous injury.[21]

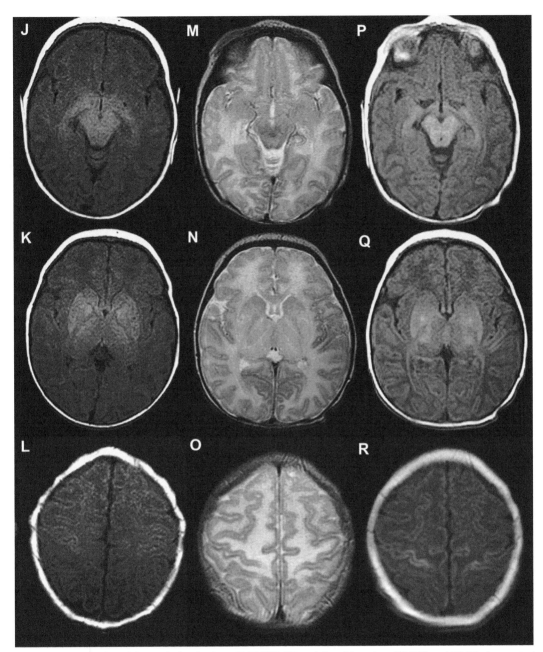

Fig. 1. Same three-day-old term baby, (*J–L*) T1-SE 500/10. T2-weighted imaging (T2-WI) and T1-WI demonstrate abnormal signal in these same distributions. (*M–O*) T2-SE 3800/104.69; (*P–R*) T1-SE 500/10. Follow-up examination at day 13 demonstrates evolution of the ischemic injury with perirolandic cortical increased T1 signal suggesting laminar necrosis and increased T1 signal basal ganglia and thalami bilaterally.

Encephalopathy of Prematurity

Advances in neonatal intensive care have increased the survival rates of preterm infants, including the ones with low birth weight. However, premature infants have a high incidence of cerebral palsy, cognitive impairment, visual loss, and epilepsy.[22] Although these disabilities were first described as secondary to white matter injury, recent imaging studies have shown abnormalities consistent with both white matter injury and apparent neuronal/axonal disease. Thus, the term "encephalopathy of prematurity" has been found to be more accurate to describe the complexity of findings in the injured premature brain.[23]

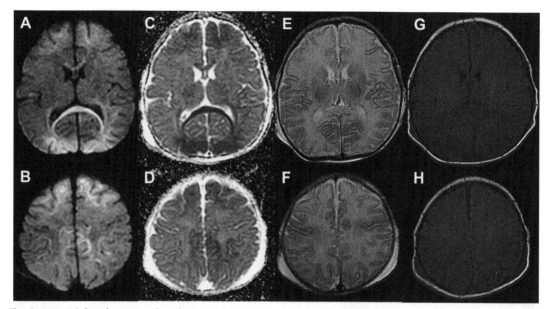

Fig. 2. HII peripheral pattern. (*A, B*) EPI DWI 7000/85.6; (*C, D*) ADC maps. Three-day-old girl with a history of nuchal cord and low Apgar scores. Multifocal areas of reduced diffusion are noted within the bilateral frontal and parieto-occipital regions, and in the splenium of the corpus callosum. (*E–G*): T2-WI 4616.66/104.16; (*G, H*) T1-WI 516.66/9. Conventional images show increased T2 and decreased T1 signal in the cortex in portions of the bilateral frontal, parietal, and occipital lobes and increased T2 signal within the areas of decreased diffusion. Subgaleal hematomas are also noted.

The pathophysiological basis of white matter injury on preterm newborns is not completely understood, although hypoperfusion and maternal infection or inflammation has been implicated in its development. In addition, vulnerability of specific cell populations, such as late oligodendrocyte progenitor cells and subplate neurons, and the complexity of developmental events make the immature white matter susceptible to damage.[22]

White matter injury has both focal and diffuse components. Focal areas of microscopic necrosis involve pre-oligodendrocytes, axons, and perhaps late-migrating interneurons. This condition can evolve to cystic cavities in deep cerebral white matter around the ventricles. The diffuse component comprises mainly the pre-oligodendrocytes, leading to impaired myelination and consequent axonal deficiency. Along with the white matter injury, volume loss of the cerebral cortex, thalamus, basal ganglia, brainstem, and cerebellum is also observed, likely secondary to injury to subplate neurons, and retrograde and anterograde (transsynaptic) effects.[23]

Signal abnormalities become evident first on DWI, being perceptible in the first week after birth. Both focal lesions and diffuse white matter decreases in diffusion have been reported.[24] In one study, reduced diffusion progressed to increased diffusion in about the second to the fourth week of life and finally disappeared around the fourth month.[25] Corresponding findings on conventional MR imaging are hyperintensity on T1-WI and hypointensity on T2-WI in the periventricular white matter. Susceptibility imaging may or may not show blooming indication that not all lesions are associated with hemorrhage.

The area of abnormal signal intensity seen on DWI is usually larger than the area of damage demonstrated on subsequent conventional MR imaging; however, Roelants-van Rijn and colleagues[26] demonstrated histopathological white matter injury beyond the area of DWI signal abnormality, suggesting that both DWI and conventional MR imaging underestimate the real extent of damage. On follow-up MR imaging examination gliosis, white matter volume loss, callosal thinning, irregularity of ventricular walls, and ventricular dilatation can be recognized. MR imaging analyses can also demonstrate a decreased volume of neuronal structures as early as term-equivalent age, as well as later in childhood, adolescence, and adulthood.

Another common type of brain injury in premature infants is germinal matrix hemorrhage. Damage to the germinal matrix along the ventricular wall typically has its onset within 5 hours of birth. Hemorrhage is thought to be secondary to vascular pressure changes within the fragile germinal matrix capillaries. It can also be seen within the external granular layer of the cerebellum, which represents the cerebellar germinal zone. Cranial ultrasonography can be used to assess these lesions; however, gradient echo T2-WI or susceptibility-weighted images have higher sensitivity, and improve detection of cerebellar hemorrhage and periventricular venous hemorrhagic infarctions (Fig. 3).[19]

Arterial Ischemic Stroke

Arterial strokes are more common in term neonates and have an incidence of approximately 1 in 4000 deliveries. Focal arterial occlusion occurs in an otherwise normal brain, unlike global HII where the entire brain is exposed to hypoxia and ischemia. The origin of the arterial occlusion in unknown, but potential causes includes emboli, thrombosis, or transient spasm.[16]

Early detection of neonatal ischemic stroke is challenging because these neonates typically appear healthy at birth and have normal Apgar scores. Moreover, clinical symptoms can be subtle, and typically present as symptomatic seizure around 48 hours after birth when cortical edema is already evident.

White matter and cortical hyperintensity on T2-WI result in the "missing cortex sign" in the first postnatal week. The cortex becomes hypointense during the second week while hyperintense signal persists in the white matter until 2 to 3 weeks. Reduced diffusion is observed on DWI when symptoms are evident, and is more marked during the first 4 days. ADC pseudonormalization takes places from the seventh day. Frequently the area of reduced diffusion tends to be larger than the area of signal abnormality seen on follow-up conventional MR imaging. This mismatch is likely due to early reperfusion when compared with adult stroke or later hypertrophy of adjacent cortical regions (Fig. 4).[27]

SINOVENOUS THROMBOSIS

An important cause of neurologic morbidity in the neonatal period is the occurrence of sinovenous thrombosis. This condition is generally identified in neonates with history of maternal infection or corioamnionitis, and less regularly in the presence of congenital heart disease or prothrombotic disorders. Most of the infants present with seizures between 36 hours and 28 days of life, although apnea, hypotonia, and lethargy can also occur.[28]

MR imaging may show diffuse parenchymal edema, intraventricular, subarachnoid, or intracerebral hemorrhage (can affect thalamus and caudate), ischemic injury with decreased diffusion on DWI, or signal abnormality in deep or superficial

venous system.[21] Intraluminal clot may be seen in the deep venous system but is rarely identified in the superficial system. MR venography can infrequently demonstrate decreased flow-related enhancement or abrupt change in caliber due to a superficial sinovenous thrombosis. However, changes in caliber of the superior sagittal sinus are most often caused by sutural diastasis at the lambdoid suture, a common sequela of delivery. The difficulty in finding an occlusion could be related to rapid dissolution of the clot or transient damage to the venous system resulting from mechanical forces during delivery.[21] An important number of neonates that undergo neuroimaging studies present with small parturitional hemorrhage along the tentorium, which should not be misinterpreted as venous thrombosis.[15]

DWI can exhibit reduced or increased diffusion, representing cytotoxic or vasogenic edema, respectively. Vasogenic edema occurs secondarily to minor blood-brain barrier breakdown in the setting of venous congestion, and usually resolves on follow-up examinations. Venous ischemic injuries show reduced diffusion in a venous drainage territory involving subcortical white matter that on follow-up, similar to arterial ischemic strokes, may undergo atrophy or almost completely resolve, likely depending on the severity and duration of the injury (Fig. 5).[15]

COOLING THERAPY

Despite being a major cause of death and disability, hypoxic-ischemic encephalopathy has had no specific therapy until recently. Selective head or whole-body cooling has been enthusiastically received by clinicians over the last few years. Despite not knowing the optimum target cooling temperature and duration of cooling, the interval between the primary injury and the secondary energy failure is thought to constitute a therapeutic window in which prolonged moderate hypothermia could act to prevent or reduce cerebral injury by suppressing some pathways to delayed cell death.[29] Although individual trials have failed to show undeniable proof of benefit from therapeutic hypothermia, meta-analysis including selective head cooling and whole-body cooling trials (Coolcap study group, National Institute of Child Health and Human Development study, and the Total Body Hypothermia trial [TOBY]) indicates a uniform reduction of the risk of death and neurologic impairment at 18 months of age. However, behavioral and cognitive problems, which require assessment later in childhood, were not evaluated by any of these trials.[30] Rutherford and colleagues,[31] analyzing conventional

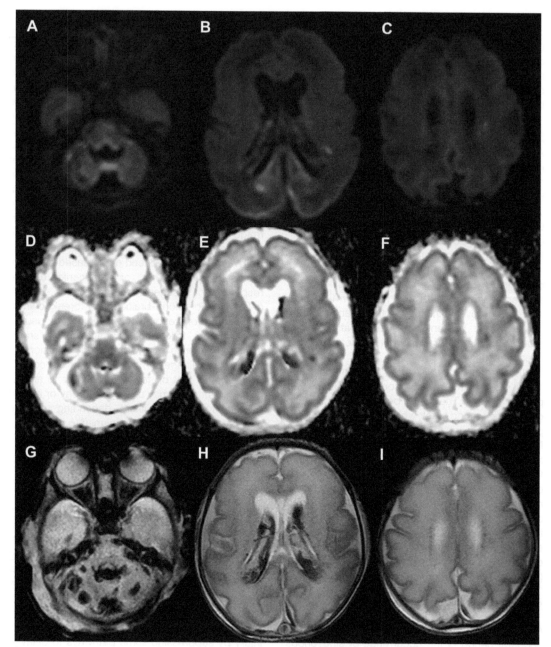

Fig. 3. Germinal matrix, intraventricular and cerebellar hemorrhage. White matter injury of prematurity. (A–C) DWI 633.33/10; (D–F) ADC maps; (G–I) T2-SE 3966.66/106.13. Four-day-old premature infant (32-week) with scattered foci of T1 signal shortening is seen within the periventricular white matter with associated reduced diffusion. Prominent hemorrhage is seen within the lateral, third, and fourth ventricles. Multifocal areas of parenchymal hemorrhage are observed within the cerebellum. Subdural blood is also noted in the parietal regions bilaterally along with subcutaneous fluid collection.

MR imaging scans obtained from infants recruited to the TOBY trial, observed that those who underwent moderate hypothermia had substantial reduction in abnormalities in the basal ganglia, thalami, and the white matter when compared with the noncooled group. In addition, the cooled group was more likely to have normal scans than the noncooled group. The authors also have

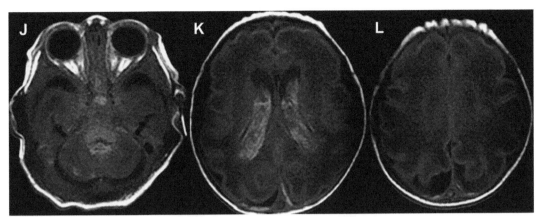

Fig. 3. Germinal matrix, intraventricular and cerebellar hemorrhage. White matter injury of prematurity. (J–L) T1-SE 633.33/10. Same four-day-old premature infant (32-week) with scattered foci of T1 signal shortening is seen within the periventricular white matter with associated reduced diffusion. Prominent hemorrhage is seen within the lateral, third, and fourth ventricles. Multifocal areas of parenchymal hemorrhage are observed within the cerebellum. Subdural blood is also noted in the parietal regions bilaterally along with subcutaneous fluid collection.

observed a decrease in the number of cases with positive findings since initiation of therapeutic hypothermia at their center.

OTHER CAUSES OF NEONATAL ENCEPHALOPATHY

Encephalopathy related to HII typically manifests in the first few hours after birth. For that reason, if encephalopathy occurs later in neonates with unremarkable delivery history and without an obvious reason, metabolic encephalopathy from hypoglycemia and inborn errors of metabolism, infection, and trauma must be considered.

Hypoglycemia

Hypoglycemia is a common event in the neonatal period, but only rarely is it severe and prolonged enough to result in brain injury. Unlike HII, parieto-occipital lobes are predominantly affected with relative sparing of the frontal lobes. Brain injury has been associated with a blood glucose level of less than 30 mg/dL and is usually symptomatic. Neonates present with stupor, jitteriness, respiratory disturbance, hypotonia, and seizure. Hypoglycemia can occur in association with other pathology, mainly hypoxia and ischemia, and in these cases may be a potentiating factor but in such situations the imaging pattern of HII dominates.

MR imaging performed in term neonates typically shows edema involving the parieto-occipital lobes and, less frequently, the basal ganglia. The extent of brain injury is more easily identified with

DWI, which demonstrates reduced diffusion in the affected areas in the first 6 days following the hypoglycemic event. Pseudonormalization occurs after this period, in a similar way as described for ischemic injury. These areas of reduced diffusion, probably attributable to excitocytotoxic cellular injury, correlate with areas of atrophy seen on follow-up examinations.[16,32] Neuronal injury is also identified on MR spectroscopy, which shows a decreased N-acetyl aspartate (NAA) peak, and increased lactate-lipid peak in the injured areas (**Fig. 6**).[32]

There is no substantial knowledge to explain why the posterior the pattern of brain injury occurs in hypoglycemic encephalopathy; however, it has been attributed to regional and developmental variation in glucose consumption between brain areas. Also, there is no explanation why the preterm brains are more infrequently affected by injury when compared with mature brain, but it has been hypothesized that developmental differences related to gestational ages, including variable regional energy requirement, blood flow, and vascular permeability, are involved.[33]

Inborn Errors of Metabolism

The possibility of inborn errors of metabolism must be considered when evaluating the encephalopathic neonate, principally when the history is not typical for HII. The main metabolic causes of neonatal encephalopathy are congenital lactic acidosis, urea cycle disorders, and amino acidurias.[19] Although the definitive diagnosis of metabolic disorders is based on biochemical

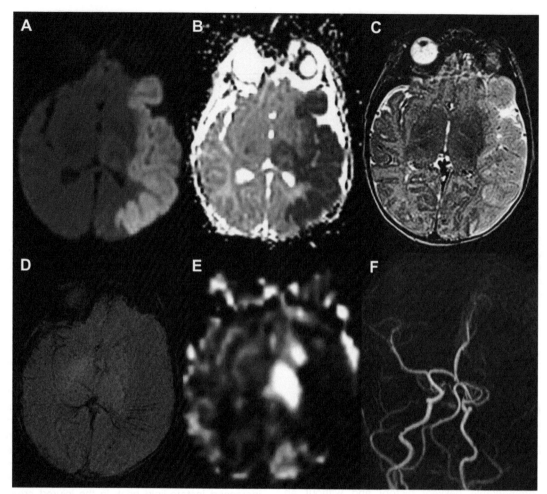

Fig. 4. Left middle cerebral artery infarct. (*A*) DWI 8400/84; (*B*) ADC maps; (*C*) T2-WI 16000/123; (*D*) susceptibility weighted imaging 28/15; (*E*) arterial spin labeling (ASL); (*F*) 3-dimensional time-of-flight (TOF) MR angiography (MRA). Reduced diffusion is seen within the left occipital lobe, temporal lobe, and insula in the distribution of the left middle cerebral artery territory. The thalamus also demonstrates reduced diffusion, which is supplied by posterior cerebral artery branches. There is mild associated mass effect with effacement of the cortical sulci. The susceptibility weighted images demonstrate asymmetric prominence of the deep medullary veins in the regions of infarct. ASL shows hyperperfusion within the left thalamus and basal ganglia. The MRA of the circle of Willis demonstrates diminished flow-related signal within the left supraclinoid internal carotid artery.

confirmation, brain MR imaging, including DWI and spectroscopy, forms part of the investigation, sometimes giving clues to diagnosis before the laboratory workup is completed.

Pyruvate dehydrogenase (PDH) deficiency is the most frequent cause of primary lactic acidosis and results from mutations in the mitochondrial PDH complex, an important enzyme for mitochondrial energy metabolism. Lactic and pyruvic acidosis, hyperalaninemia, and normal lactate/pyruvate ratios are typically verified.[34,35]

The brain malformations observed on routine MR imaging include enlarged ventricles, cerebral and cerebellar white matter involvement (including cystic changes), brainstem atrophy, absence of medullary pyramids, abnormal inferior olives, cerebellar dysplasia, partial or complete agenesis of the corpus callosum, and basal ganglia hyperintensities on T2-WI. Increased water diffusion in the white matter has been demonstrated in DWI studies and is thought to be predictive of progressive atrophy.[33] A large lactate doublet at 1.33 ppm and a narrow singlet at 2.37 ppm corresponding to pyruvate may be observed on MR spectroscopy (**Fig. 7**).[36]

Maple syrup urine disease (MSUD) is characterized by a deficiency of the catalytic components of the α-ketoacid–dehydrogenase complex, which is responsible for the catabolism of branched-chain amino acids (BCAAs), which results in the

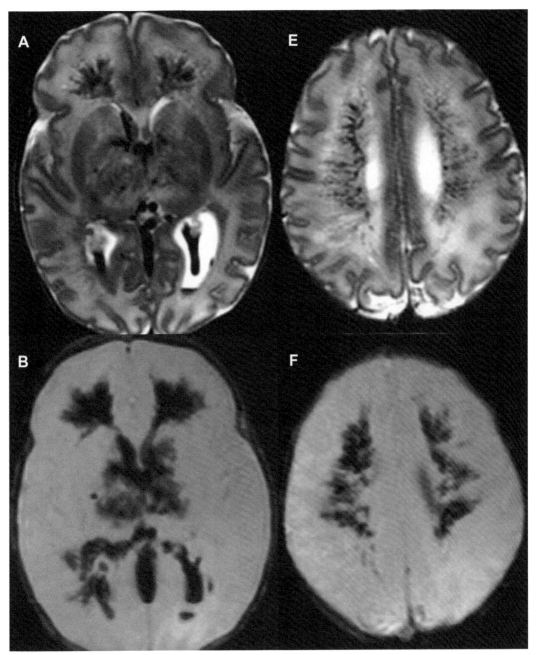

Fig. 5. Sinovenous thrombosis with associated venous edema, ischemia, and hemorrhage. (*A, E*) T2–turbo spin echo (TSE); (*B, F*) gradient echo (GRE).

accumulation of BCAAs, leucine, isoleucine, and valine as well as branched-chain α-ketoacids that can cause encephalopathy.

The maple syrup odor of the urine, increased levels of BCAAs in the plasma and urine, and the presence of α-hydroxyacid and branched-chain α-ketoacids in urine of an encephalopathic newborn make the clinical diagnosis of this disease. The presence of plasma L-alloisoleucine and urinary α-hydroxyisovalerate are pathognomonic for MSUD.[37]

Classic MSUD is characterized by a neonatal onset of encephalopathy, and is the most common and most severe form. Early diagnosis and treatment are essential to prevent significant sequelae and even death. Normal neurologic

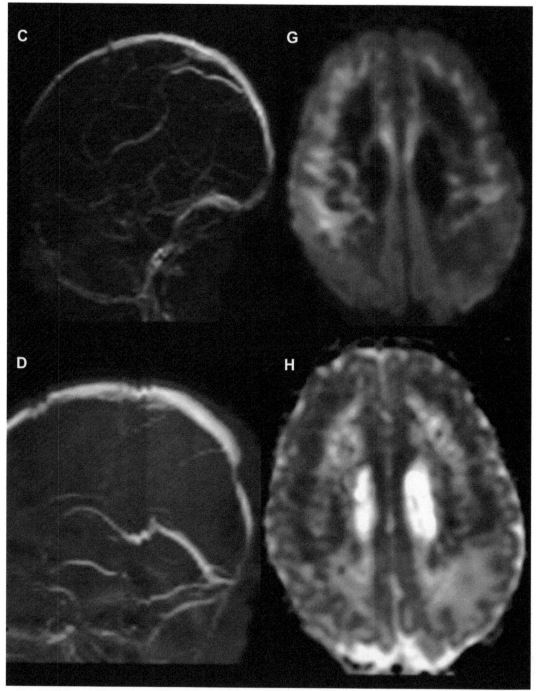

Fig. 5. Sinovenous thrombosis with associated venous edema, ischemia, and hemorrhage. (*C*) 2-dimensional (2D) TOF MR venography (MRV); (*D*) 2D TOF MRV in another neonate without deep venous thrombosis; (*G*) DWI; (*H*) ADC map. Eleven-day-old male with seizures. Deep venous thrombosis is noted by absence of flow-related enhancement in MRV (*C*) as compared to a normal MRV (*D*). T2 TSE and GRE images show venous stasis and hemorrhage in the medullary veins, deep venous system, and thalami in addition to intraventricular hemorrhage. DWI and ADC maps show decreased diffusion in the subcortical white matter due to venous ischemia, and increased diffusion in deeper white matter due to venous edema.

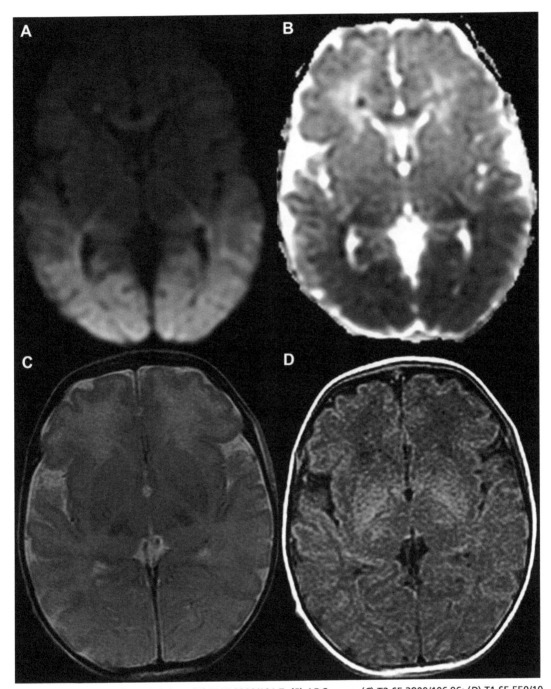

Fig. 6. Profound hypoglycemic injury. (*A*) DWI 8300/101.7; (*B*) ADC maps; (*C*) T2-SE 3800/106.96; (*D*) T1-SE 550/10. DWI demonstrates a large symmetric area of reduced diffusion involving both occipital and parietal lobes. There is reduced diffusion in the pulvinar thalami, splenium of the corpus callosum, and posterior limbs of both internal capsules. Diffuse loss of gray-white differentiation within the parietal and occipital lobes is appreciated on the axial T2-WI and T1-WI.

development can be achieved with successful treatment.[38]

MR imaging performed during the encephalopathy shows hyperintense areas on T2-WI involving the cerebellar white matter, dorsal brainstem, cerebral peduncles, thalamus, posterior limb of the internal capsule, globus pallidus, and the perirolandic cerebral white matter (**Fig. 8**). These areas

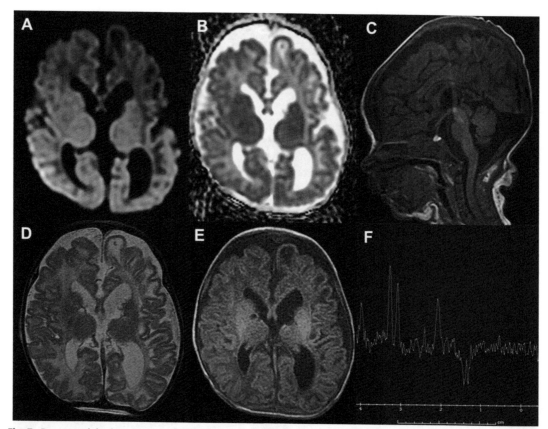

Fig. 7. Pyruvate dehydrogenase deficiency. (A) Axial DWI 8300/89.60; (B) axial ADC maps; (C) sagittal T1-SE 450/13; (D) axial T2-SE 3916.66/105.74; (E) axial T1-SE 500/10; (F) MR point-resolved spectroscopy (MRS PRESS) 144, voxel in the left basal ganglia. DWI demonstrates increased diffusion involving the subcortical and periventricular white matter left greater than right throughout both cerebral hemispheres, with associated with marked T2 and T1 prolongation. Diffuse volume loss is also observed. Sagittal T1 shows a thin and partially hypoplastic corpus callosum. MRS demonstrates an abnormal lactate peak at 1.33 ppm.

correspond to the areas of myelination in the normal full-term neonate and present reduced water diffusion on DWI corresponding to intramyelinic edema. In addition, areas with a T2 hyperintense signal can be identified in the unmyelinated white matter; however, these areas appear as low signal intensity areas on DWI and they have marked high values in ADC, indicating vasogenic edema. Therefore, DWI is better than conventional MR imaging because it can demonstrate brain abnormalities more evidently and may discriminate between two distinctive types of brain edema.[38,39]

Nonketotic hyperglycinemia is an autosomal recessive inborn error of metabolism caused by a defect in the glycine cleavage enzyme system, resulting in high glycine concentrations in urine, plasma, cerebrospinal fluid (CSF), and the brain. Nonketotic hyperglycinemia causes neurologic impairment with encephalopathy early in the neonatal period. Prognosis is poor, and most patients die in the first few weeks of life.[40]

Biochemical diagnosis is made when a raised CSF to plasma ratio of glycine is found. An abnormal peak at 3.56 parts per million seen in long-echo proton MR spectroscopy is also considered specific for nonketotic hyperglycinemia. However, the presence of blood in CSF and in the brain parenchyma can make the interpretation of the CSF sample and MR spectroscopy unreliable.[41]

Structural abnormalities observed on conventional MR imaging during the neonatal period include ventriculomegaly, absent corpus callosum, and posterior fossa cysts. Areas of T2 hyperintensity were described in the white matter tracts that should be myelinated at birth. On DWI these areas showed reduced water diffusion attributed to spongy myelinopathy, which is observed in neuropathologic studies.[40,42]

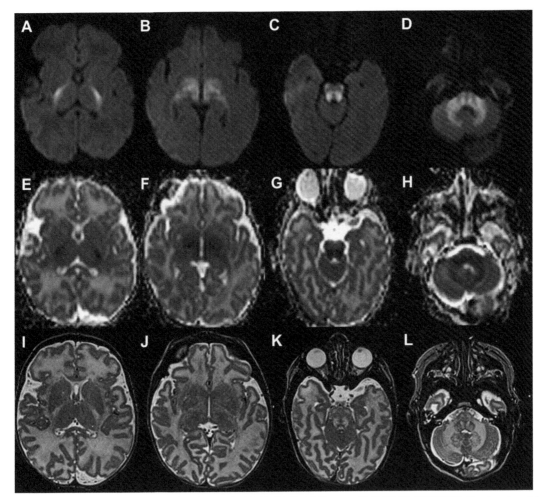

Fig. 8. Maple syrup urine disease. (*A–D*) DWI 8400/84; (*E–H*) ADC maps; (*I–L*) T2-SE 16000/123. Twelve-day-old male with history of bicycling movements of the lower extremities. Symmetrically abnormal reduced diffusion is present within the cerebellar white matter, brainstem, subthalamic regions, posterior limbs of the internal capsule, and corona radiata. Abnormal T2 prolongation is seen throughout the white matter of the brain, posterior limbs of internal capsules, cerebellum, and brainstem.

Isolated sulfite oxidase deficiency is a rare autosomal recessive disorder of the newborn that has a clinical and imaging appearance similar to those seen in severe ischemic encephalopathy. However, encephalopathy due to HII is present at birth and tends to clinically stabilize 1 to 2 weeks after delivery, whereas neonates with isolated sulfite oxidase deficiency may not become encephalopathic for a few days after birth and do not show improvement or stability in their clinical condition.[43] The presence of ectopia lentis, seizures, and progressive neurologic abnormalities should alert clinicians to the diagnosis.[44]

Initial MR imaging findings can look similar to those seen in the asphyxiated neonate, with diffuse loss of gray and white matter differentiation. However, caudate involvement can be noted while thalami are relatively spared, contrasting with what is observed in HII. Reduced diffusion can be apparent early on DWI throughout the entire cortex, subcortical white matter, and basal ganglia. Diffuse cystic lesions are demonstrated on follow-up examinations, appearing in a symmetric pattern in the frontal, parietal, and temporal lobes. MR spectroscopy shows large lactate peaks in multiple regions as well as decreased NAA to creatine ratio, and an increase in the ratio of choline to creatine (Fig. 9).[45]

Urea cycle disorders are important causes of neonatal metabolic encephalopathy. The inability to produce urea observed in these disorders leads to hyperammonemia and glutamine accumulation, causing astrocyte swelling and encephalopathy. The presence of progressive lethargy, hypothermia,

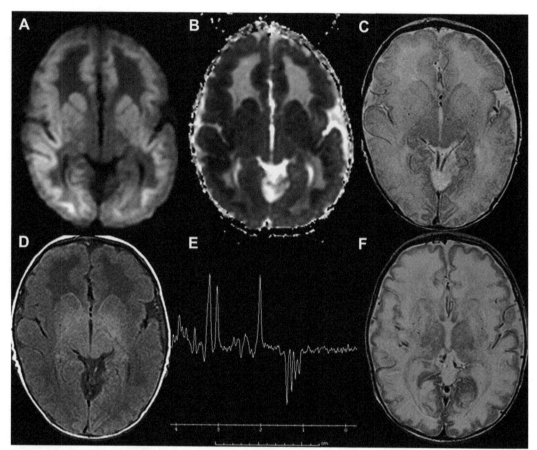

Fig. 9. Sulfide oxidase deficiency. (A) DWI 8300/93.4; (B) ADC maps; (C) T2-SE 3000/100.74; (D) T1-SE 550/10; (E) MRS PRESS 144 ms, voxel located in the left basal ganglia. Seven-day-old infant in status epilepticus. DWI shows diffuse reduced diffusion within the cortex, subcortical white matter, basal ganglia, and cerebral peduncles. There is hyperintense signal on T2 and hypointense signal on T1 diffusely within the cerebral white matter. Within the basal ganglia, MRS shows a large lactate peak. (F) T2-SE 3800/98.9. Follow-up examination on day 14 shows interval diffuse cerebral gray matter and deep gray nuclei volume loss, with associated diffuse abnormal T2 prolongation within the cerebral white and subcortical gray matter.

and apnea, accompanied by high blood ammonium levels in a full-term neonate with uneventful delivery and that appeared healthy in first 24 to 48 hours, should raise the suspicion for urea cycle disorders.[46]

Conventional MR imaging shows symmetric high signal intensity of the temporal, parietal, and occipital cortex, subcortical white matter, caudate nuclei, thalami, internal capsules, and globus pallidus on T2-WI. Reduced water diffusion is observed in these areas on DWI, consistent with cellular swelling (**Fig. 10**).[47]

Leukodystrophies comprise any inborn error of metabolism that interferes with the normal formation and/or maintenance of myelin, and therefore has the potential to cause hypomyelination, or dysmyelination with consequential demyelination.

Because ADC values show a gradual increase with gradual brain myelination, it is expected that diseases affecting this process may cause abnormal water diffusion.

Increased water content in the extracellular space is seen secondary to myelin instability and destruction, and results in increased diffusion. Decreased diffusion has been described in some leukodystrophies as well, and occurs in association with myelin vacuolization.[48]

In Canavan disease, an autosomal recessive inherited disorder characterized by a deficiency of the enzyme aspartoacylase leading to NAA accumulation through unknown mechanisms, reduced diffusion occurs within abnormal white matter, probably caused by the intramyelinic water accumulation (myelin vacuolization) (**Figs. 11 and 12**).[49,50]

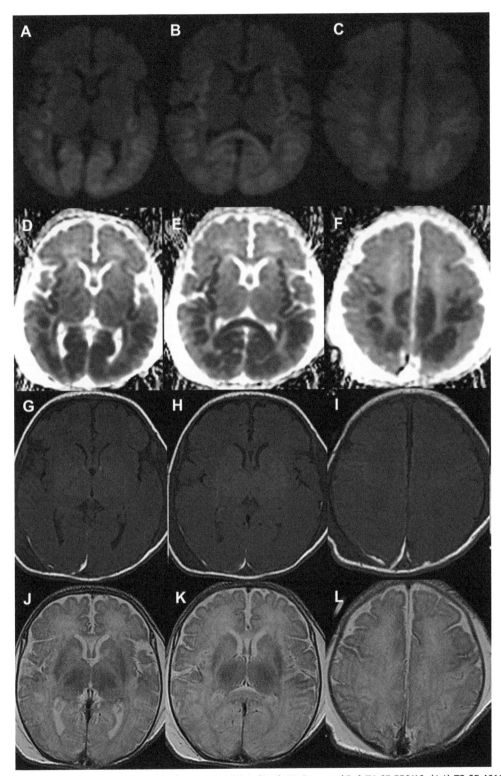

Fig. 10. Classic citrullinemia type I. (*A–C*) DWI 8300/89.1; (*D–F*) ADC maps; (*G–I*) T1-SE 550/10; (*J–L*) T2-SE 4616.66/105.50. Seven-day-old female with seizures and citrullinemia. Reduced diffusivity is seen predominantly in the cortex, in both cerebral hemispheres, and in the splenium of the corpus callosum with T1 and T2 prolongation in these same areas. Small bilateral parieto-occipital acute subdural hematomas and subgaleal hematomas with caput succedaneum are also observed.

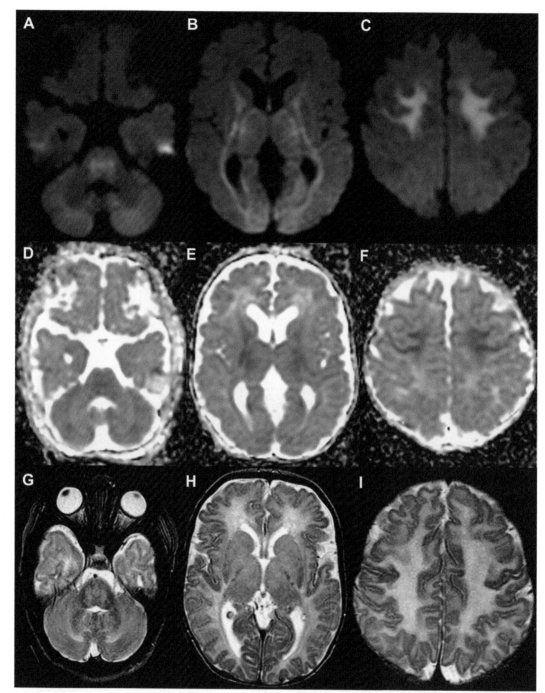

Fig. 11. Canavan disease. (*A–C*) DWI 8300/89; (*D–F*) ADC maps; (*G–I*) T2-SE 3500/104.78. Three-week-old male with a history of a large head. DWI shows reduced diffusion bilaterally within the perirolandic white matter, internal capsule, optic radiation, thalami, basal ganglia, and brainstem. Abnormal T2 prolongation is identified in the cerebellar hemispheres, brainstem, basal ganglia, thalami, and corona radiata of the cerebral hemispheres bilaterally.

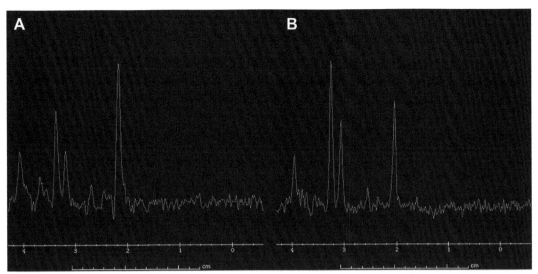

Fig. 12. Canavan disease versus normal. (A) Spectroscopy of a neonate with Canavan disease showing prominent N-acetyl aspartate peak, atypical for newborns. (B) Normal neonatal spectroscopy for comparison.

Infection

An important consideration regarding the encephalopathic neonate is infection. The imaging appearance of infection can represent the infectious process itself or its complications, such as infarction, and for that reason the diagnosis of infectious disease can be difficult.[51]

In the neonatal period, herpes encephalitis is usually a devastating disease, which is often part of a generalized infection, typically due to herpes simplex virus type 2. Eighty-five percent of cases occur during the peripartum period, 10% in the postnatal, and 5% in utero.[52] Herpes encephalitis is associated with high mortality and severe neurologic complications. Lesions may be multifocal or limited to the temporal lobes, cerebellum, or brainstem. Initially, brain edema is observed in white matter, which then progress to involve the cerebral cortex. Involvement of the deep gray nuclei and rapid brain necrosis with hemorrhage may ensue. DWI may depict decreased diffusion, and frequently demonstrates more extensive disease than conventional MR imaging sequences (Fig. 13). There may be meningeal enhancement after gadolinium administration. Rapid evolution to cystic encephalomalacia is commonly observed (Fig. 14).[19,52]

Bacterial meningitis is associated with high mortality and morbidity rates, and its central nervous system complications may contribute to the poor prognosis of neonatal meningitis. Although bacterial meningitis is most often a clinical diagnosis, complications attributed to arterial and venous infarcts caused by septic arteritis and phlebitis are evaluated by MR imaging. DWI is more sensitive in demonstrating these vascular consequences, as it can depict small cortical and deep white matter ischemic injuries that may not be recognizable on conventional MR imaging.[16,53]

Subdural empyema (SDE) is another important complication related to meningitis. It is particularly important to differentiate between SDE and reactive subdural effusion (RSE), because RSE tends to spontaneously regress whereas SDE commonly needs aggressive intervention.[54] DWI has an advantage over conventional MR imaging in performing this differentiation, as SDE shows high signal intensity on DWI and markedly diminished ADC, whereas RSE exhibits low signal intensity on DWI and only mild reduction of ADC.[53]

Neonatal brain abscesses are very rare and usually occur as a complication of bacterial meningitis or septicemia. The most common organism leading to meningitis complicated by abscess is Citrobacter.[55] Despite modern antibiotics, mortality and morbidity is still conspicuous.[56] MR is greatly helpful in delineating tissue involvement when an abscess is suspected. DWI shows reduced water diffusion first at the presuppurative cerebritis stage and then in the central purulent collection, making possible the differentiation between an abscess and a cystic necrotic tumor.[16,57]

Traumatic Brain Injury

The major causes of traumatic injury in neonates are related to birth trauma and can be represented by subarachnoid or intraparenchymal hemorrhages, but most commonly are subdural hematomas, the majority being infratentorial. Subdural hematomas are thought to result from tears in the tentorium, falx, or bridging veins during labor.[58]

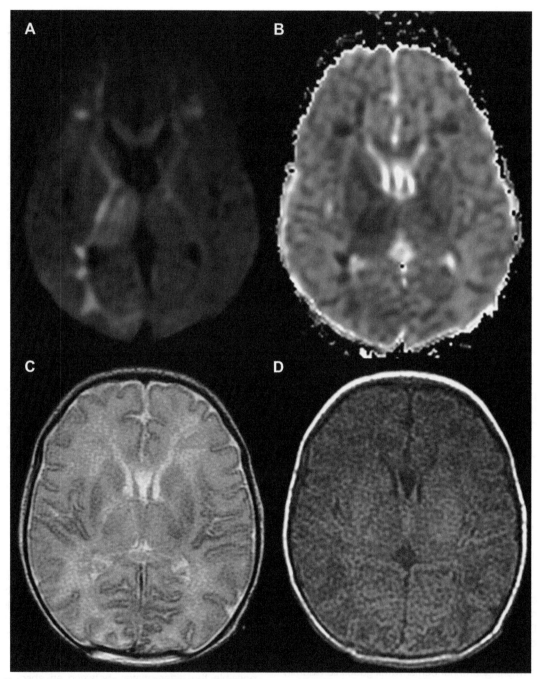

Fig. 13. HSV encephalitis. (*A*) DWI 7500/114.10; (*B*) ADC maps; (*C*) T2-SE 3916.66/104.32; (*D*) T1-SE 516.66/9. Extensive areas of reduced diffusion are identified involving the periventricular white matter with more confluent involvement of the deep white matter of the right frontal and occipital lobes, the right thalamus, and internal capsule bilaterally. Discrete abnormal T2 prolongation is observed in these same areas with no myelination seen within the posterior limb of the internal capsules on T1-WI.

Nonaccidental trauma

Abuse-related head injury is an important cause of trauma in infants, being a significant cause of neurologic and visual impairment. Despite the fact that the mechanism of injury is not fully understood because the executor hides the types of injury, several factors are expected to be involved, and include mechanical forces and hypoxia resulting from a decrease in cerebral perfusion secondary to violent shaking. Retinal

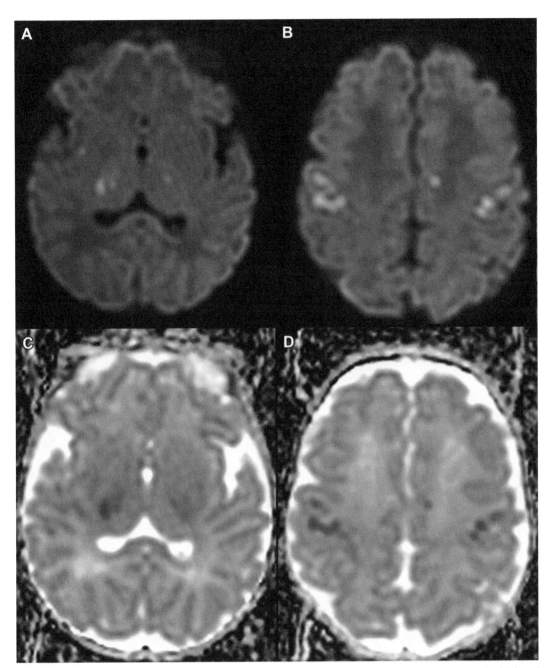

Fig. 14. Viral meningitis/meningoencephalitis. (A, B) DWI 8300/74.40; (C, D) ADC maps. Four-week-old female with left focal seizure and viral meningeal encephalitis. DWI shows multiple scattered foci of diffusion decrease within the subcortical white matter of the bilateral cerebral hemispheres and within the basal ganglia related to areas of secondary ischemic injury. Additional regions of abnormal T2 hyperintensity and increased ADC are seen within the white matter. Mild symmetric leptomeningeal enhancement in the bilateral perirolandic regions.

hemorrhage, and subdural and subarachnoid hemorrhages are commonly recognized. Because infants have relatively big heads and weak neck muscle tone, they are at a greater risk of presenting with brainstem damage caused by stretch injury at the craniocervical junction during shaking. Also, the smoothness of the skull base associated with the soft unmyelinated brain make skull fractures unlikely in this age group.[59]

The first examination performed in cases of suspected abuse-related head injury is computed tomography (CT); however, parenchymal lesions can be missed or underestimated on CT scans. DWI has been shown to be more sensitive and

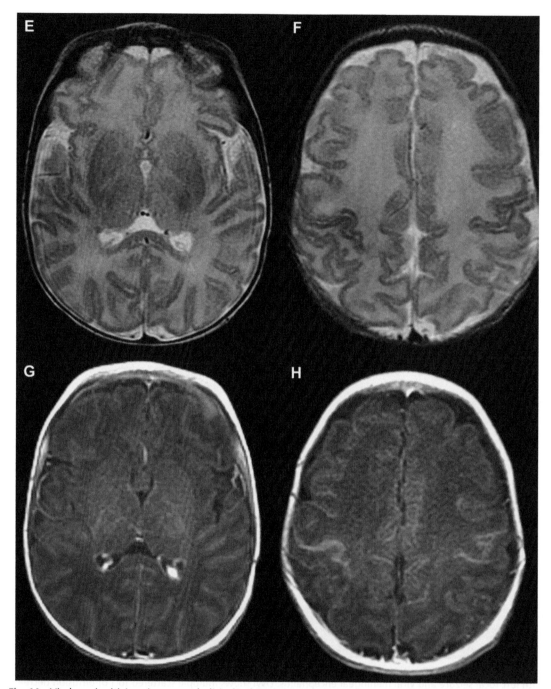

Fig. 14. Viral meningitis/meningoencephalitis. (*E*, *F*) T2-SE 4116.66/106.9; (*G*, *H*) T1-SE 516.66/9 postgadolinium of same four-week-old female.

can reveal ischemic/contusion injury hours to days before CT scanning or conventional MR imaging. Moreover, DWI can give better information with reference to the timing of cerebral ischemia, adding essential medicolegal information (**Fig. 15**).[60,61]

Parenchymal DWI abnormalities tend to be multifocal and involve multiple lobes of the brain, with predominance in the posterior portion of the hemispheres and relative sparing of anterobasal frontal lobes and anterior temporal lobes. Large

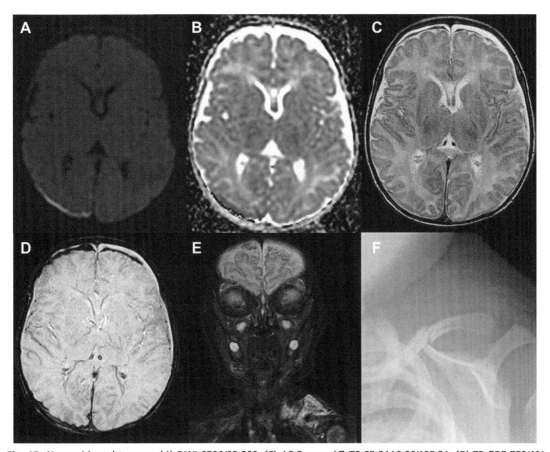

Fig. 15. Nonaccidental trauma. (A) DWI 6500/93.800; (B) ADC map; (C) T2-SE 3116.66/105.31; (D) T2-GRE 750/40/30; (E) short tau inversion recovery 4016.66/49.94; (F) plain radiograph. Three-week-old victim of alleged abuse with a shaking injury. DWI shows reduced diffusion in the occipital right subdural. Bifrontal subdural hemorrhages, characterized by T2 and T2*-GRE hypointense signal. On the coronal fast spin-echo inversion recovery images, note is made of abnormal signal within the soft tissues surrounding the left clavicle, consistent with the presence of fracture of the left clavicle seen on the skeletal survey.

DWI abnormalities are associated with a poor neurologic outcome in these patients.[60,61]

SUMMARY

DWI has become a valuable tool in the evaluation of the neonatal brain in the past decade. When interpreted concurrently with conventional MR imaging and other advanced MR imaging techniques, such as spectroscopy and arterial spin labeling, with an adequate clinical scenario, DWI can give clues in facilitating an accurate diagnosis, provide important information about pathophysiology and prognosis of the diseases, and guide adequate therapeutic modalities.

REFERENCES

1. Grant PE, Yu D. Acute injury to the immature brain with hypoxia with or without hypoperfusion. Radiol Clin North Am 2006;44:63–77, viii.

2. Dudink J, Larkman DJ, Kapellou O, et al. High b-value diffusion tensor imaging of the neonatal brain at 3T. AJNR Am J Neuroradiol 2008;29: 1966–72.

3. Counsell SJ, Tranter SL, Rutherford MA. Magnetic resonance imaging of brain injury in the high-risk term infant. Semin Perinatol 2010;34:67–78.

4. Barkovich AJ, Westmark KD, Bedi HS, et al. Proton spectroscopy and diffusion imaging on the first day of life after perinatal asphyxia: preliminary report. AJNR Am J Neuroradiol 2001;22:1786–94.

5. Baud O, Greene AE, Li J. Glutathione peroxidase-catalase cooperativity is required for resistance to hydrogen peroxide by mature rat oligodendrocytes. J Neurosci 2004;24(7):1531–40.

6. Deng W, Wang H, Rosenberg PA, et al. Role of metabotropic glutamate receptors in oligodendrocyte excitotoxicity and oxidative stress. Proc Natl Acad Sci U S A 2004;101(20):7751–6.

7. Ferriero DM. Neonatal brain injury. N Engl J Med 2004;351:1985–95.

8. Volpe JJ. Hypoxic-ischemic encephalopathy: biochemical and physiological aspects. In: Volpe JJ, editor. Neurology of the newborn. 5th edition. Philadelphia: Saunders; 2008. p. 247–324.

9. Chu CT. Eaten alive: autophagy and neuronal cell death after hypoxia-ischemia. Am J Pathol 2008; 172:284–7.

10. Balduini W, Carloni S, Buonocore G. Autophagy in hypoxia-ischemia induced brain injury: evidence and speculations. Autophagy 2009;5:221–3.

11. Triulzi F, Parazzini C, Righini A. Patterns of damage in the mature neonatal brain. Pediatr Radiol 2006; 36:608–20.

12. Okereafor A, Allsop J, Counsell SJ, et al. Patterns of brain injury in neonates exposed to perinatal sentinel events. Pediatrics 2008;121:906–14.

13. Takeoka M, Soman TB, Yoshii A, et al. Diffusion-weighted images in neonatal cerebral hypoxic-ischemic injury. Pediatr Neurol 2002;26:274–81.

14. Grant PE. Term hypoxic ischemic injury. In: Osborn AG, editor. Diagnostic imaging. Brain. 2nd edition. Altona (Germany): Amirys; 2010. p. I4-90–3.

15. Robertson RL, Glasier CM. Diffusion-weighted imaging of the brain in infants and children. Pediatr Radiol 2007;37:749–68.

16. Sagar P, Grant PE. Diffusion-weighted MR imaging: pediatric clinical applications. Neuroimaging Clin N Am 2006;16:45–74, viii.

17. Vermeulen RJ, van Schie PE, Hendrikx L, et al. Diffusion-weighted and conventional MR imaging in neonatal hypoxic ischemia: two-year follow-up study. Radiology 2008;249:631–9.

18. Zarifi MK, Astrakas LG, Poussaint TY, et al. Prediction of adverse outcome with cerebral lactate level and apparent diffusion coefficient in infants with perinatal asphyxia. Radiology 2002; 225:859–70.

19. Shroff MM, Soares-Fernandes JP, Whyte H, et al. MR imaging for diagnostic evaluation of encephalopathy in the newborn. Radiographics 2010;30: 763–80.

20. Li AM, Chau V, Poskitt KJ, et al. White matter injury in term newborns with neonatal encephalopathy. Pediatr Res 2009;65:85–9.

21. Eichler F, Krishnamoorthy K, Grant PE. Magnetic resonance imaging evaluation of possible neonatal sinovenous thrombosis. Pediatr Neurol 2007;37: 317–23.

22. Kidokoro H, Kubota T, Ohe H, et al. Diffusion-weighted magnetic resonance imaging in infants with periventricular leukomalacia. Neuropediatrics 2008;39:233–8.

23. Volpe JJ. Brain injury in premature infants: a complex amalgam of destructive and developmental disturbances. Lancet Neurol 2009;8:110–24.

24. Soul JS, Robertson RL, Tzika AA, et al. Time course of changes in diffusion-weighted magnetic resonance imaging in a case of neonatal encephalopathy with defined onset and duration of hypoxic-ischemic insult. Pediatrics 2001;108:1211–4.

25. Fu J, Xue X, Chen L, et al. Studies on the value of diffusion-weighted MR imaging in the early prediction of periventricular leukomalacia. J Neuroimaging 2009;19:13–8.

26. Roelants-van Rijn AM, Nikkels PG, Groenendaal F, et al. Neonatal diffusion-weighted MR imaging: relation with histopathology or follow-up MR examination. Neuropediatrics 2001;32:286–94.

27. Dudink J, Mercuri E, Al-Nakib L, et al. Evolution of unilateral perinatal arterial ischemic stroke on conventional and diffusion-weighted MR imaging. AJNR Am J Neuroradiol 2009;30:998–1004.

28. Wu YW, Miller SP, Chin K, et al. Multiple risk factors in neonatal sinovenous thrombosis. Neurology 2002; 59:438–40.

29. Shankaran S. Neonatal encephalopathy: treatment with hypothermia. J Neurotrauma 2009;26: 437–43.

30. Edwards AD, Brocklehurst P, Gunn AJ, et al. Neurological outcomes at 18 months of age after moderate hypothermia for perinatal hypoxic ischaemic encephalopathy: synthesis and meta-analysis of trial data. BMJ 2010;340:c363.

31. Rutherford M, Ramenghi LA, Edwards AD, et al. Assessment of brain tissue injury after moderate hypothermia in neonates with hypoxic-ischaemic encephalopathy: a nested substudy of a randomised controlled trial. Lancet Neurol 2010;9:39–45.

32. Kim SY, Goo HW, Lim KH, et al. Neonatal hypoglycaemic encephalopathy: diffusion-weighted imaging and proton MR spectroscopy. Pediatr Radiol 2006; 36:144–8.

33. Tam EW, Widjaja E, Blaser SI, et al. Occipital lobe injury and cortical visual outcomes after neonatal hypoglycemia. Pediatrics 2008;122:507–12.

34. Patay ZR, Robertson NJ, Cox IJ. Metabolic disorders in the neonate. In: Rutherford M, editor. MRI of the neonatal brain. London: W.B. Saunders; 2002. p. 315–47.

35. Soares-Fernandes JP, Teixeira-Gomes R, Cruz R, et al. Neonatal pyruvate dehydrogenase deficiency due to a R302H mutation in the PDHA1 gene: MRI findings. Pediatr Radiol 2008;38:559–62.

36. Zand DJ, Simon EM, Pulitzer SB, et al. In vivo pyruvate detected by MR spectroscopy in neonatal pyruvate dehydrogenase deficiency. AJNR Am J Neuroradiol 2003;24:1471–4.

37. Ferraz-Filho JR, Floriano VH, Quirici MB, et al. Contribution of the diffusion-weighted MRI in the diagnosis and follow-up of encephalopathy caused by maple syrup urine disease in a full-term newborn. Arq Neuropsiquiatr 2009;67:719–23.

38. Sakai M, Inoue Y, Oba H, et al. Age dependence of diffusion-weighted magnetic resonance imaging

findings in maple syrup urine disease encephalopathy. J Comput Assist Tomogr 2005;29:524–7.

39. Ha JS, Kim TK, Eun BL, et al. Maple syrup urine disease encephalopathy: a follow-up study in the acute stage using diffusion-weighted MRI. Pediatr Radiol 2004;34:163–6.

40. Khong PL, Lam BC, Chung BH, et al. Diffusion-weighted MR imaging in neonatal nonketotic hyperglycinemia. AJNR Am J Neuroradiol 2003;24:1181–3.

41. Manley BJ, Sokol J, Cheong JL. Intracerebral blood and MRS in neonatal nonketotic hyperglycinemia. Pediatr Neurol 2010;42:219–22.

42. Mourmans J, Majoie CB, Barth PG, et al. Sequential MR imaging changes in nonketotic hyperglycinemia. AJNR Am J Neuroradiol 2006;27:208–11.

43. Hoffmann C, Ben-Zeev B, Anikster Y, et al. Magnetic resonance imaging and magnetic resonance spectroscopy in isolated sulfite oxidase deficiency. J Child Neurol 2007;22:1214–21.

44. Eyaid WM, Al-Nouri DM, Rashed MS, et al. An inborn error of metabolism presenting as hypoxic-ischemic insult. Pediatr Neurol 2005;32:134–6.

45. Eichler F, Tan WH, Shih VE, et al. Proton magnetic resonance spectroscopy and diffusion-weighted imaging in isolated sulfite oxidase deficiency. J Child Neurol 2006;21:801–5.

46. Takanashi J, Barkovich AJ, Cheng SF, et al. Brain MR imaging in neonatal hyperammonemic encephalopathy resulting from proximal urea cycle disorders. AJNR Am J Neuroradiol 2003;24:1184–7.

47. Majoie CB, Mourmans JM, Akkerman EM, et al. Neonatal citrullinemia: comparison of conventional MR, diffusion-weighted, and diffusion tensor findings. AJNR Am J Neuroradiol 2004;25:32–5.

48. Engelbrecht V, Scherer A, Rassek M, et al. Diffusion-weighted MR imaging in the brain in children: findings in the normal brain and in the brain with white matter diseases. Radiology 2002;222:410–8.

49. Srikanth SG, Chandrashekar HS, Nagarajan K, et al. Restricted diffusion in Canavan disease. Childs Nerv Syst 2007;23:465–8.

50. Patay Z. Diffusion-weighted MR imaging in leukodystrophies. Eur Radiol 2005;15:2284–303.

51. Teixeira J, Zimmerman RA, Haselgrove JC, et al. Diffusion imaging in pediatric central nervous system infections. Neuroradiology 2001;43:1031–9.

52. Lo CP, Chen CY. Neuroimaging of viral infections in infants and young children. Neuroimaging Clin N Am 2008;18:119–32, viii.

53. Jan W, Zimmerman RA, Bilaniuk LT, et al. Diffusion-weighted imaging in acute bacterial meningitis in infancy. Neuroradiology 2003;45:634–9.

54. Wong AM, Zimmerman RA, Simon EM, et al. Diffusion-weighted MR imaging of subdural empyemas in children. AJNR Am J Neuroradiol 2004;25:1016–21.

55. Volpe JJ. Bacterial and fungal intracranial infections. In: Volpe JJ, editor. Neurology of the newborn. 5th edition. Philadelphia: Saunders; 2008. p. 851–915.

56. de Oliveira RS, Pinho VF, Madureira JF, et al. Brain abscess in a neonate: an unusual presentation. Childs Nerv Syst 2007;23:139–42.

57. de Vries LS, Verboon-Maciolek MA, Cowan FM, et al. The role of cranial ultrasound and magnetic resonance imaging in the diagnosis of infections of the central nervous system. Early Hum Dev 2006;82:819–25.

58. Looney CB, Smith JK, Merck LH, et al. Intracranial hemorrhage in asymptomatic neonates: prevalence on MR images and relationship to obstetric and neonatal risk factors. Radiology 2007;242:535–41.

59. Blumenthal I. Shaken baby syndrome. Postgrad Med J 2002;78:732–5.

60. Biousse V, Suh DY, Newman NJ, et al. Diffusion-weighted magnetic resonance imaging in shaken baby syndrome. Am J Ophthalmol 2002;133:249–55.

61. Suh DY, Davis PC, Hopkins KL, et al. Nonaccidental pediatric head injury: diffusion-weighted imaging findings. Neurosurgery 2001;49:309–18 [discussion: 318–20].

Diffusion MR Imaging for Monitoring Treatment Response

Antonio Carlos Martins Maia Jr, MD, PhD[a],*,
Bruno Vasconcelos Sobreira Guedes, MD[b],
Ademar Lucas Jr, MD[b], Antonio José da Rocha, MD, PhD[a]

KEYWORDS

• Treatment response • Diffusion MR • Stroke • Neoplasms

Magnetic resonance (MR) imaging is currently the most widely used tool for the evaluation of pathologic processes that affect the central nervous system (CNS), allowing the delineation of anatomic structures that are affected and, in many situations, an inference of the pathologic substrate. In this way, MR imaging can be used to identify inflammatory/infectious, demyelinating, neoplastic, and vascular diseases, among others. New image sequences have recently been developed; among these, there is particular interest in those based on the random motion of water molecules. These sequences allow the investigation of the hemodynamic, metabolic, functional, cellular, and cytoarchitectural status of brain tissue under different physiologic or pathologic settings, thus increasing the sensitivity and specificity of MR imaging studies. The biologic behavior of a particular disease can be measured by such methods, enabling confident diagnosis and appropriate approach, as well as the recognition of related prognostic factors. These techniques can also be used to monitor disease response to the therapeutic regimen.

The physical principles of the diffusion sequence are complex, and a detailed explanation of these principles is beyond the scope of this text. The contrast in tissues obtained from sequence diffusion-weighted imaging (DWI) is based on the stochastic displacement of water molecules, in different structures and tissues, which determines the attenuation of the MR imaging signal intensity in the presence of a strong magnetic field gradient.[1] The degree of attenuation depends on the strength of the gradient, the length of time for which it is applied, and the magnitude of water diffusion. The free movement of water molecules can be prevented by a decrease in the volume of the extracellular medium (increased cellularity), changes in the ion transport across membranes, and a decrease in intracellular water content (increase in the nucleus-to-cytoplasm ratio); thus, any of these situations can modulate the intensity of the signal sequence.

Normal brain characteristics can be modified under pathologic conditions and influenced by various therapies. The DWI is important in the study of many different CNS disorders; the objective of this article was to emphasize the use of DWI in the diagnosis and follow-up of several major disease contexts, as established in recent literature.

VASCULAR DISEASES
Stroke

The perfect function of ion channels is directly related to the free movement of water molecules

[a] Section of Neuroradiology, Centro de Medicina Diagnostica Fleury and Santa Casa de Misericordia de São Paulo, R. Cincinato Braga 282, Paraíso, São Paulo, SP, CEP 01333-910, Brazil
[b] Santa Casa de Misericórdia de São Paulo. R. Cesário Motta Junior, 112, São Paulo, SP, CEP 01221-020, Brazil
* Corresponding author.
E-mail address: Antonio.Maia@fleury.com.br

Neuroimag Clin N Am 21 (2011) 153–178
doi:10.1016/j.nic.2011.02.004
1052-5149/11/$ – see front matter © 2011 Elsevier Inc. All rights reserved.

through the cell membrane, which requires a constant input of energy. Thus, neuronal and glial metabolism requires an adequate supply of oxygen, glucose, and other nutrients, which, in turn, depends on an efficient circulatory system.

Ischemic or hemorrhagic stroke may ultimately cause irreversible injuries. However, an early diagnosis of the ischemic vascular event may allow appropriate therapy and prevent, or at least attenuate, a negative outcome. It is also critical to estimate the irreversibly involved area (ischemic core) and the potentially reversible area (penumbra), because there is a direct correlation between the proportional size of the core and the risk of hemorrhagic complication after thrombolytic therapy. These size estimates can be achieved by measuring the mismatch between the area of restricted diffusion and the area of perfusion deficit estimated in perfusion studies by MR imaging. Moreover, the scaling of the penumbra affects the likelihood of favorable clinical outcomes after

fibrinolytic treatment with partial or complete recovery of the impaired neurologic function.[2]

The ischemic core has experienced extreme energy deprivation and a consequent loss of cellular metabolism resulting from the dysfunction of the ATP-dependent Na^+ and K^+ pump. This leads to an intracellular influx of water and Na^+, which restricts the movement of water molecules and consequently creates a focal hyperintense signal on DWI sequence, which can be confirmed by the apparent diffusion coefficient (ADC) map. This region was once considered unrecoverable, although the hyperintense signal observed in the DWI sequence is a marker of a recent ischemic event (acute/subacute), ie, documented soon after the occurrence of cytotoxic edema. These signals are usually obtained before conventional MR sequence modification. The restriction decays gradually because of cell death and the subsequent increase in the free movement of water molecules in the affected area (**Fig. 1**).[2] However,

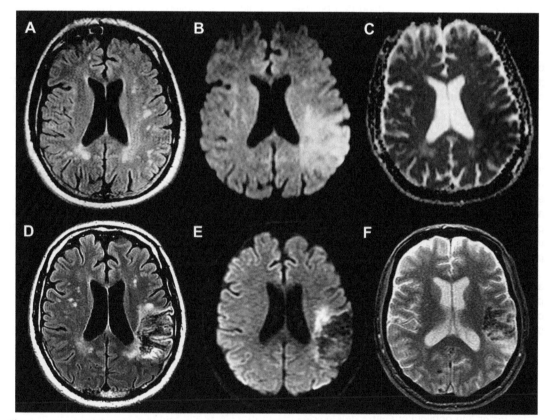

Fig. 1. Acute partial territorial ischemic infarct of the left middle cerebral artery in a 53-year-old male (*A–C*). The FLAIR image (*A*) shows microangiopathic foci in the white matter and a slight signal alteration in the left parietal lobe. The signal alteration and extension of the core is evident on DWI (b = 1000 sec/mm²) (*B*), and the cytotoxic nature of the area is confirmed by the ADC map (*C*). After 3 weeks (*D–F*), the gliotic area is now obvious on FLAIR image (*D*) and the same sequelae appear to have a low signal on DWI (*E*). The region with a strong signal in the more anterior segment of the lesion may result from hemorrhage, as shown with T2 * gradient-echo (*F*).

recent studies have suggested that damage to the area of restricted diffusion may be reversible in some situations.[3] The main argument is that the restriction of diffusion in animals extends beyond the area of ATP-dependent pump impairment, which also correlates with the reduction of pH associated with anaerobic neuronal and glial metabolism.[4] The diffusion tensor images (DTI) allow the visualization of areas suggestive of Wallerian degeneration in compromised brain regions, and is thus a promising technique for early estimates of reversibility.[5]

Hypoxic-Ischemic Encephalopathy

Through some related mechanisms, global cerebral anoxia can also be diagnosed early on, and its extension can be established with great sensitivity through the DWI sequence. This provides a basis for early prognosis as well as the clinical management of the patient.[6] Certain brain regions appear to be preferentially affected by anoxia, most likely owing to a mechanism of selective vulnerability rather than a segmental perfusion defect. The selective vulnerability of gray matter to anoxia can be attributed to its reduced blood flow, local basal metabolic rate, and the presence of receptors for excitatory amino acids.[6,7] Ischemia causes an excessive release of glutamate that, after binding to the N-methyl-D-aspartate (NMDA) receptors, promotes the influx of calcium into the cell, initiating several cytotoxic processes such as the production of free radicals. This damages the cell membrane, allowing water to enter the cell and ultimately causing cytotoxic edema. The changes observed in the DWI sequence correlate with sites that are prone to cytotoxic edema, which are generally rich in glutamate receptors. In a less severe event, the neurons survive the initial insult but eventually suffer apoptotic cell death.[8]

The MR imaging abnormalities found upon anoxia are variable and depend on several factors, including brain maturity, the severity and duration of the insult and the period of examination.[8,9] Severe insults in term newborns cause selective injury to the lateral regions of the thalamus, the posterior region of the putamens, the perirolandic region, and corticospinal tract. These changes are observed as areas of hyperintensity on DWI sequence within the first 24 hours after the injury, during which the conventional sequences remain normal.[6] However, during this period, the DWI usually underestimates the extent of anoxic injury, probably because of the apoptosis and delayed neuronal death that occurs later.[10] Abnormalities on DWI peak at 3 to 5 days and "pseudonormalize"

toward the end of the first week, reflecting the progressive increase in vasogenic edema and loss of cell membrane integrity.[11,12] This apparent resolution of the DWI signal does not imply any real improvement, making evaluation with conventional MR images important during this period.[13] Still, any negative DWIs performed within the first 24 hours after injury should be repeated at 2 to 4 days, when the restriction reaches its peak, for optimal interpretation. In term newborns, moderate anoxia causes injury in areas bordering the arterial irrigation and sites of minor perfusion, especially in the parasagittal regions. Again, DWI is the first sequence able to demonstrate the parenchymal abnormalities that appear within the first 24 hours, such as altered areas of hyperintensity in the cortex and subcortical regions of the affected site. However, we suggest that assessment with DWI should always be made in conjunction with conventional sequences and ADC values because restricted areas on the DWI may be masked because of the intrinsic high signal on T2 in the brain parenchyma observed in this age group. Areas of recent hemorrhage can also hamper the interpretation.[8]

In preterm neonates, serious insult causes damage in areas similar to those detected in term neonates, ie, the thalamus, hippocampus, and cerebellum; less severe injuries are observed in the putamens and perirolandic region.[8,9] Similarly, the DWI is altered early, typically with areas of hyperintensity, even though the conventional sequences still appear normal. The restriction zones reach a signal peak within 3 to 5 days, followed by pseudonormalization. The most common mild/moderate injuries in preterm neonates are periventricular leukomalacia and germinal matrix hemorrhage.[8] Fu and colleagues[14] have reported early findings of symmetric signal alteration of the periventricular white matter, similar to the findings observed in conventional sequences in the advanced stages of periventricular leukomalacia.

In older children and in adults, anoxia primarily affects the gray matter, mainly in the basal ganglia, thalamus, cortex, cerebellum, and hippocampus. Similarly, changes on DWI sequence occur early; hyperintensity can be observed before lesions appear on T1 and T2.

ADC maps and quantitative ADC of the whole brain parenchyma assist the assessment of brain damage and recovery potential in coma after cardiorespiratory arrest (CRA). A severe reduction in ADC in the first few days after global anoxia is highly indicative for permanent injury.[15] The ideal period for the assessment is between 49 and 108 hours after CRA.[16] A drop in the ADC over large regions of the parietal, temporal, and occipital lobes in the acute phase is associated with irreversible damage and the worst prognosis,[15,17] regardless of electrophysiological test results. Lesions restricted to the thalamus and selective cortical regions suggest mild hypoxia, with potential neurologic recovery.[17] Moreover, the ADC map can help to evaluate the benefit of various therapies; higher ADC values are observed in patients undergoing hypothermia.[15]

An intriguing entity known as postanoxic leukoencephalopathy occurs in 2% to 3% of patients after a diffuse cerebral hypoxic-ischemic event. It is characterized by a period of clinical stability or even improvement (lucid interval), followed by an acute neurologic decline, usually 2 to 3 weeks after the insult, involving delirium, personality changes, motor disturbances and, rarely, seizures.

Typically, DWI sequence fails to reveal abnormalities at the time of the insult, but instead shows diffuse and confluent areas of restricted diffusion in the cerebral white matter at the end of the lucid interval, followed by a decrease in ADC values and signal change in T2 (Fig. 2).[8] Good clinical outcomes, as usual, are accompanied by the reduction of signal changes observed on DWI sequence and a progressive increase in ADC values. Presumably, postanoxic leukoencephalopathy may be caused by oligodendrocyte apoptosis (induced by previous anoxia) followed by diffuse demyelination.[18]

Posterior reversible encephalopathy syndrome (PRES) may be triggered by acute decompensation of blood pressure levels (eclampsia), immunosuppressive drugs (cyclosporine, tacrolimus), renal failure, systemic lupus erythematosus, and

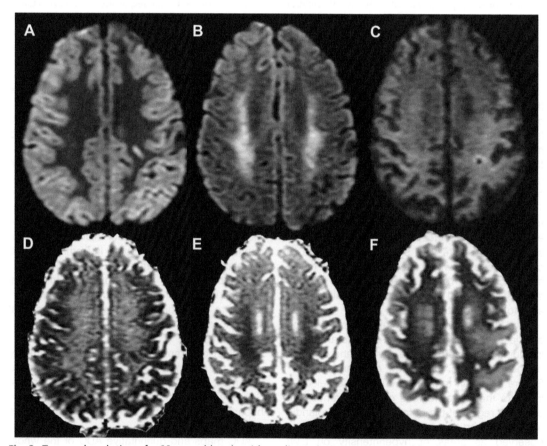

Fig. 2. Temporal evolution of a 66-year-old male with cardiorespiratory arrest caused by decompensation of the underlying cardiovascular disease. DWI (b = 1000 sec/mm²) (A) and ADC map (D) in the acute phase show restriction throughout the cerebral cortex, as well as a small focus of lacunar hyperintensity in the left semioval center, probably of embolic etiology. (B, E) Signs of postanoxic leucoencephalopathy, with restricted diffusion in the deep white matter and disappearance of the cortical change, can be observed after 2 weeks. During the chronic phase (C, F), the hyperintense signal in the white matter on DWI disappears (C), concurrent with the appearance of high signal intensity on the ADC map (F) and the occurrence of parenchymal atrophy. (Courtesy of L.T. Lucato, MD, PhD, São Paulo, Brazil).

thrombocytopenia, among others.[19] PRES is clinically characterized by altered consciousness, variable visual impairment, seizures, and headache. Its pathogenesis is not fully understood, but is known to be related to lower sympathetic tone of the brain vasculature in posterior regions (parieto-occipital) and endothelial microinjury, allowing macromolecule leakage during hyperperfusion that results in cortical and subcortical edema. This leads to an increase in interstitial pressure and a discrete compressive effect on the CNS, including small arteries. Reflexive vascular spasm is associated with this hemodynamic status. Rarely, vasospasm related to subarachnoid hemorrhage can also occur.[20] The DWI sequence is especially relevant here, since this etiology can lead to reduced blood supply, resulting in tissue ischemia and subsequent cytotoxic edema. Thus, the presence of confirmed abnormalities on DWI sequence and ADC map indicate poor prognosis, ie, clinical and radiological irreversibility, whereas an abnormality on fluid-attenuated inversion recovery (FLAIR) with normal DWI defines a favorable clinical outcome (**Fig. 3**).[21] The reduction in fractional anisotropy (FA) might be caused by vasogenic edema, and should be used to indicate a favorable prognosis and reversibility.[22,23]

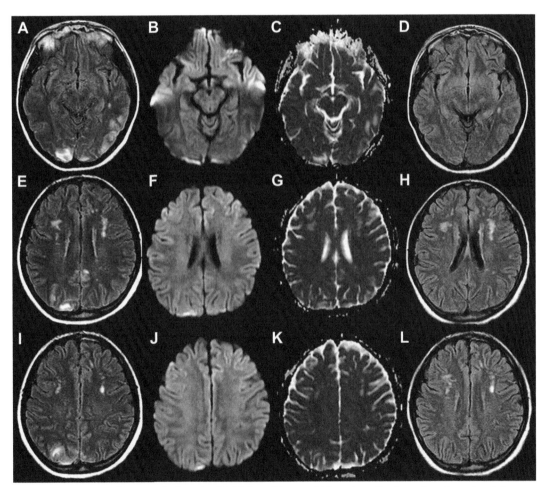

Fig. 3. Posterior reversible encephalopathy (PRES) in a 15-year-old female patient, carrier of a systemic lupus erythematosus, treated with cyclophosphamide. Acute phase: FLAIR images (A, E, I) show focal signal abnormalities in the bilateral parietal white matter that extend to the cortex, most evident at the right, in addition to other foci of high signal in the frontal white matter. DWI (B, F, J) and correlated ADC map (C, G, K) do not confirm any restricted diffusion, only show vasogenic edema (T2 shine-through effect). Eight days after the withdrawal of cyclophosphamide (and with a good clinical outcome), FLAIR (D, H, L) showed a reversal of the parietal cortical edema but the continued presence of hyperintense foci in the frontal white matter, confirming that these sequelae are secondary in nature to the underlying disease (SLE).

NEOPLASMS
Glioma

Neoplasms of the CNS are a major cause of morbidity worldwide despite advances in surgical techniques and adjuvant treatment. The choice of therapeutic approach (and therefore its effectiveness) is directly related to the degree of tumoral differentiation, which cannot be established precisely by conventional imaging methods, especially in tumors that do not display classic signs of anaplasia, such as gadolinium enhancement or macroscopic necrosis.

The diffusion-weighted sequence can be used to estimate the degree of tumoral differentiation. High-grade tumors generally have a high nucleus/cytoplasm ratio, resulting in a reduction of the free movement of water molecules. Moreover, the size of the tumor, presence of residual tumor tissue after treatment, and even changes induced by treatment (eg, actinic ischemic sequelae) can be identified by DWI. Tracing the movement of water molecules through FA can be used to delineate the brain tracts, allowing a relatively accurate estimation of regional tumoral involvement/extension.[24] This is possible because the high-grade tumors have expansive potential, which groups tracts of normal-appearing peritumoral white matter and simultaneously infiltrates this site, resulting in the interposition of tumor and necrotic cell/tumor cysts between these fibers, resulting in reduction of FA.

Tumors also release chemical mediators (eg, tumor necrosis factor) that increase regional vascular permeability, establishing the peritumoral edema. This edema further reduces anisotropy values and is easily identifiable in the reconstruction color maps as a reduction in the intensity of the colors of the affected fibers. Unlike high-grade tumors, low-grade neoplasms have a compressive effect only on the adjacent brain parenchyma and the corresponding fibers and tracts, but are not associated with the infiltration and peritumoral edema that increase regional anisotropy. This differential profile, in combination with apparent diffusion coefficients and conventional imaging with intravenous contrast, can contribute to a presumptive analysis of tumor grade.[25]

The utility of the ADC is not limited to diagnosis or to post-therapeutic monitoring. A recent study reported that neoplasms with low ADCs responded better to pretreatment than did lesions with high ADCs (related to tumoral necrosis).[26] Experimental studies evaluating early treatment response used chemotherapy subdoses, noting changes in the ADC and even slight decreases in

the viable tumor cell populations, which may be a biomarker of early response.[27,28] Therefore, an early increase in ADC after or during chemotherapy or radiotherapy indicates a positive therapeutic response (**Fig. 4**).

Tumor cells respond to invasive treatment by undergoing apoptosis, which releases intracellular water into the local environment. Cysts arising from tissue necrosis, especially in high-grade tumors, lead to significant heterogeneity in the neoplasm, and an extremely dynamic profile over the long periods of therapy. The calibration of the ADC by the ROI standard summarizes the mean and median of these values throughout the tumor but does not distinguish between areas of heterogeneity or characterize the tumor response at a particular location, which can yield an erroneous estimate of the therapeutic response. An alternative strategy is to evaluate the tumor voxel by voxel, a concept described as a functional diffusion map (fDM). These 3-dimensional maps allow superimposition of the ADC maps taken before treatment with those obtained during or after treatment, allowing a very precise delineation of the evolutionary changes in the tumor and thus its susceptibility to treatment. It is also possible to overlay these images with volumetric images taken with postparamagnetic contrast, increasing the sensitivity and specificity of the method.[28]

The relative stability of ADC values in gliomas treated with corticotherapy after surgery belies changes in enhancement parameters (break of the blood-brain barrier), edema, permeability, and blood volume.[29] This emphasizes the importance of monitoring tumors with diffusion-weighted images,[30] which can differentiate between tumor progression and pseudoprogression. The presence of viable tumor cells leads to reduction of ADC values, unlike the vasogenic edema present in pseudoprogression (**Figs. 5 and 6**).[31] False-positive results can occur when tumor development is assessed by diffusion alone, for example, when there is significant leukocyte infiltration that increases regional cellularity and consequently reduces the ADC.

Lymphoma

Primary lymphoma of the central nervous system (PCNSL) represents 1% of all lymphomas, about 5% of non-Hodgkin lymphomas and 2% to 3% of CNS tumors.[32] The most common histologic type of PCNSL is diffuse large B-cell lymphoma. The incidence of PCNSL differs between immunocompetent and immunocompromised individuals, as do the MR imaging characteristics of the disease. In immunocompetent patients, PCNSL

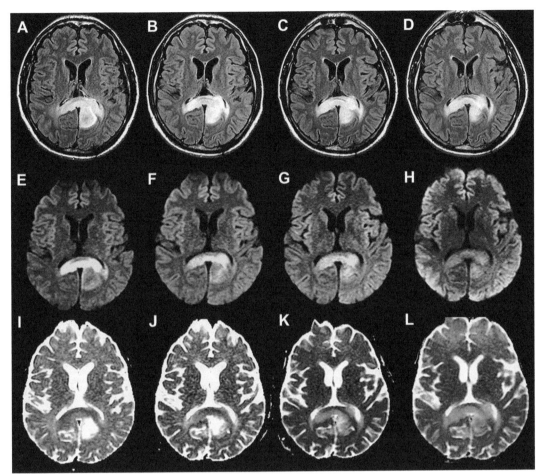

Fig. 4. A 43-year-old male patient with grade II glioma dedifferentiated in the splenium of the corpus callosum; positive response to chemotherapy and radiotherapy inferred by DWI sequence. Baseline images depict infiltrative lesion with restricted diffusion characterized by a hyperintense signal on the FLAIR (A) and DWI (E) (b = 1000 sec/mm^2) and a evident low signal on the ADC map (I), with an ADC value measured at 0.81×10^{-3}. After treatment institution, in comparative images (B, F, J after 1 month, C, G, K after 3 months, and D, H, L after 6 months), a progressive reduction of signal on the DWI sequence is observed, correlated with an elevation of ADC values to 1.05×10^{-3} and 1.44×10^{-3} at 3 and 6 months, respectively.

is composed primarily of solid lesions, generally with homogeneous enhancement, and often without areas of necrosis. This presentation is unusual in immunocompromised patients, where the disease tends to affect the basal ganglia and the periventricular region and may contain foci of central necrosis or, less commonly, calcification and hemorrhage.[33] The high cellularity of the PCNSL in both solid areas of viable tumor cells and necrotic foci (large populations of nonviable lymphocytes) restricts the free movement of water molecules in both segments,[34] features that are important in differentiating the disease from an infection and in therapeutic follow-up (Fig. 7). During treatment, the reduction of ADC values

may indicate a good response, whereas the maintenance or elevation of this index suggests treatment failure or cancer progression.[35]

Some recent studies have provided prospective quantitative assessments that promise to provide better detail of the microstructural disorganization of white matter involved in the neoplastic process (or its treatment) relative to its FA.[36]

Infections of the Central Nervous System

Infections of the CNS are potentially fatal, occur in all age groups, and have varied clinical presentation and varied imaging characteristics and different etiologic agents. These diseases pose

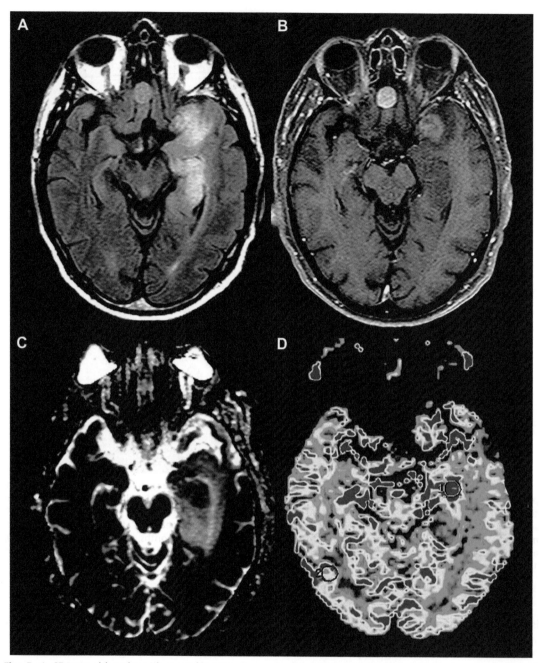

Fig. 5. A 67-year old male with an infiltrative tumor in the left temporal lobe (glioblastoma multiforme) confirmed on conventional images FLAIR (*A*) and T1 after gadolinium (Gd) administration (*B*). ADC map (*C*) confirms focal area of hypointensity on the mesial temporal structures strictly correlated to the hyperperfused area on perfusion-weighted imaging (PWI) (*D*).

a diagnostic challenge for clinicians and neuroradiologists. MR imaging is a very sensitive tool for detecting early changes in this context.

The DWI has added specificity in some major classes of neural infections. Several studies have proven the effectiveness of this technique in differentiating between cerebral abscess and necrotic or cystic tumors. As a complement to the diagnosis, the assessment of therapeutic response, whether conservative or surgical, can be adequately estimated through follow-up with DWIs and ADC values.[37] Here, we discuss the use of DWI and ADC in the diagnosis and follow-up of pyogenic, granulomatous, viral, and prion infections.

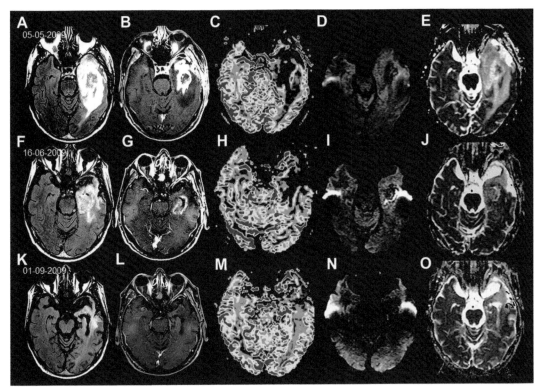

Fig. 6. The same patient as in Fig. 5 after surgical resection of tumor and adjuvant treatment with temozolomide. First row exhibit control images after 4 months. FLAIR image (*A*), T1 post-Gd (*B*), PWI (*C*), DWI (*D*), and ADC map (*E*) show an extensive area of signal alteration in the left temporal lobe, with a focal area of Gd enhancement that was found to represent tumoral pseudoprogression. Note the absence of DWI abnormalities. Comparative images show progressive reduction of this lesion in the 40-day (*F–J*) and 5-month (*K–O*) studies.

Pyogenic infections

The abscess is the most common focal CNS infection. It is often observed on hematogenous spread from distant foci, on direct inoculation (via trauma or surgery), on spread from an extracranial site, or as a complication of meningitis. The main signs and symptoms of the abscess result from expansive effects owing to the growth of the lesion: headache, altered mental state, focal deficits, seizures, nausea, and vomiting. Only 40% to 50% of patients are febrile in the early stages of neural infection.[38] Abscess formation follows a predictable path that can be divided into 4 sequential stages: early cerebritis (1 to 3 days), late cerebritis (4 to 9 days), early capsule (10 to 14 days), and late capsule (beyond the 14th day).

In conventional MR imaging, the abscess appears as a lesion with ring enhancement and a thin and regular capsule. The capsule may present hypersignal on T1 and a hyposignal on T2, whereas the lesional content displays a hyposignal on T1 and a hypersignal on T2 because of perilesional vasogenic edema.[39] Moreover, the presence of brain lesions with these

characteristics does not ensure a diagnosis of the abscess; these must always be differentiated from primary or metastatic necrotic neoplasms and other infectious lesions. The first description of DWI used in this context was published by Ebisu and colleagues in 1996.[40] These investigators observed high signal intensity within the abscess using this MR imaging sequence, associated with low ADC values, suggesting a real restriction of the free movement of water molecules, unlike what is observed in neoplastic lesions. The hypersignal intensity probably results from the physical and biochemical properties of the abscessed cavity. The presence of pus or mucus containing inflammatory cells, necrotic tissue, bacteria, and proteinaceous fluid gives the content high viscosity,[38] with markedly restricted diffusibility. The signal abnormalities observed on DWI sequence are attributed to this set of conditions.

The treatment of pyogenic abscess varies and generally depends on the evolution of the lesion. Stereotactic aspiration followed by antibiotic therapy has been the method of choice for single or multiple abscesses, although aspiration may

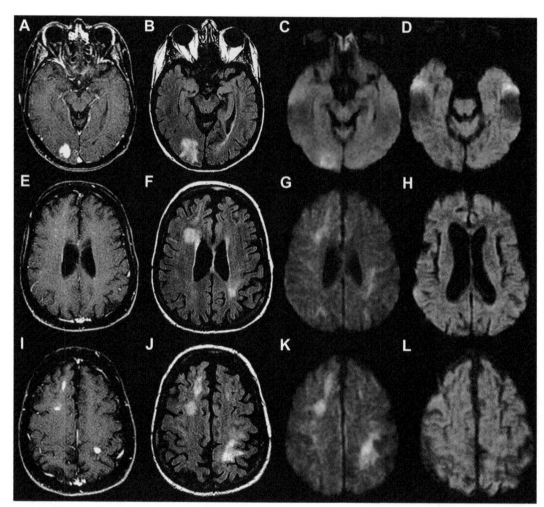

Fig. 7. A 74-year-old male. Comparative images on T1 after-Gd (*A, E, I*), FLAIR (*B, F, J*), initial DWI (*C, G, K*), and after treatment DWI (*D, H, L*). Note that DWI sequence (b = 1000 sec/mm^2) shows multiple areas of signal hyperintensity scattered throughout the cerebral hemispheres, simulating ischemic events, with hypoperfusion on PWI (not shown), but related to abnormal enhancement after Gd administration. Brain biopsy confirmed the diagnosis of primary lymphoma of large B cells with intravascular component. After chemotherapy, DWI shows brain atrophy and disappearing of the abnormal areas.

be declined in favor of broad-spectrum intravenous antibiotics in some situations (eg, lesions smaller than 2.5 cm). A second surgical drainage is recommended if the abscess increases in size after 2 weeks of treatment, or fails to respond within 3 to 4 weeks. The need for reoperation is relatively common, occurring in approximately 62% of cases.[41]

All of the previously mentioned measures require reliable parameters for monitoring, so imaging methods that are able to confirm the stage of the abscess and reliably monitor its progress during and after the initiation of therapy are necessary.[42] The literature has described MR spectroscopy as a potential tool for this purpose[43]: the disappearance of pyogenic abscess peak markers (cytosolic amino acids, acetate, alanine, succinate) and presence of a single lactate peak imply successful treatment and a positive outcome. Still, the diffusion sequence seems even more promising in this context. Cartes-Zumelzu and colleagues[37] have demonstrated the value of DWI in monitoring the therapeutic course applied to the abscess. These investigators reported a good correlation between the persistence or reappearance of a hyperintense signal on DWI and low ADC values after treatment (either surgical or clinical only) with pus reaccumulation within the lesion (**Fig. 8**). Conventional MR sequences, when used in isolation, are not sufficient to predict the evolution of the lesion. The visual inspection of T1-weighted sequences after

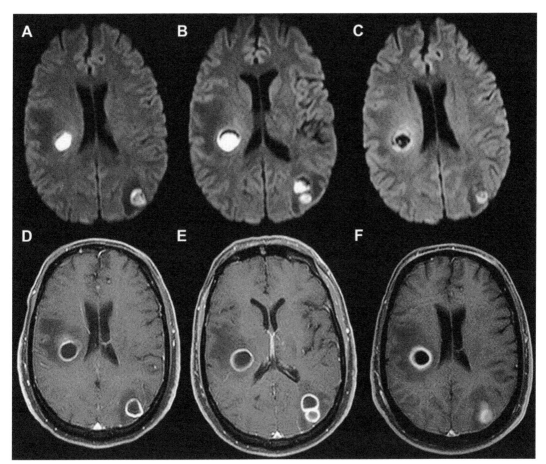

Fig. 8. A 45-year-old male with 2 cerebral pyogenic abscesses, in treatment. (A–C) DWI temporal evolution (b = 1000 sec/mm²). Baseline image on DWI (A) shows a large right periventricular lesion with restricted diffusion and another left occipital lesion of smaller dimensions. (B) After 8 days of empirical antibiotic therapy, there is little reduction of the hyperintense component, formation of a gravity-dependent meniscus and no clear evidence of clinical improvement. (C) After 21 days, comparative image on DWI demonstrated complete disappearance of the hyperintense signal within the right periventricular lesion and significant reduction of the occipital one. (D–F) The T1-weighted post-Gd administration showed no significant changes during therapy.

contrast may show a reduction in the size of the abscess, but this finding does not necessarily allow the inference of an appropriate response. Although the use of DWI to follow-up on abscess treatment is promising, some questions about its sensitivity and specificity for this purpose remain and further studies are required.

However, the interpretation of all these image signals must be made with caution, because the hyperintense signal on DWI of lesions with capsular enhancement is not pathognomonic for abscess. There are reports of metastatic adenocarcinoma or squamous cell carcinoma, and even radionecrotic lesions that present identically in the MR imaging.[44,45]

Other applications of DWI in the context of neural infection include cerebritis, ventriculitis, and the empyemas. Cerebritis is the earliest manifestation of a cerebral infection, occurring about 2 to 3 days after pathogen inoculation, and may progress to abscess formation. An ill-defined area of coagulative necrosis is generated in response to the infectious agent, exhibiting extravasation of polymorphonuclear cells in the necrotic center and adjacent parenchymal edema with perivascular exudate. There are few studies demonstrating imaging of cerebritis, because most patients with cerebritis do not receive medical care during this stage. The several studies that do exist report low signal on T1 and a poorly delineated hyperintense signal on T2; perilesional vasogenic edema can be observed in the absence of evident parenchymal enhancement. However, the restriction of diffusion is also described in this phase, most likely a result of ischemia, hyper-cellularity, or cytotoxic edema, as there is still no purulent fluid. The diffusion resembles bacterial or fungal cerebritis.[46,47] We were not able to find any report of the monitoring of cerebritis treatment using this MR method.

Pyogenic ventriculitis is an uncommon compli-cation of intracranial infections in adults, but it is often found in pediatric patients with meningitis. Ventriculitis may be the source of persistent infec-tion and treatment failure in the management of meningitis, usually caused by gram-negative bacteria. The imaging finding most characteristic of ventriculitis is the presence of irregular intra-ventricular debris. This can be identified in computed tomography (CT) and conventional MR sequences, but is more conspicuous in diffusion-weighted sequences.[48] The high signal in this sequence is related to real restriction, as evi-denced by low ADC values, unless only a small amount of diluted pus is present in the cerebro-spinal fluid (CSF) (this is insufficient to reduce the ADC).[49–51]

Hong and colleagues[51] examined the impor-tance of the ADC measured in the lower portions of the ventricles (CSF-dependent) in the evolution of ventriculitis in 12 patients and its correlation with CSF analysis. These investigators concluded that there is an inverse relationship between ADC values and pleocytosis or spinal fluid protein concentration; when the ADC values increased within the ventricle, both protein levels and pleocy-tosis decreased. These findings show that ADC values may be used in follow-up of these patients.

The epidural and subdural empyemas may be clinically differentiated based on the more insid-ious signs of focal expansive lesion and the absence of systemic manifestations in patients with epidural empyema. In contrast, subdural empyema is an acute condition that rapidly progresses to toxemia and neurologic abnor-malities requiring immediate surgery. These infec-tions are correlated with the presence of sinusitis and mastoiditis. Empyemas are best seen with a FLAIR sequence, but the purulent nature of the injury, as well as the presence of abscesses, is clearly confirmed in the diffusion-weighted sequence.[52,53]

Granulomatous infections

The fungal cerebral abscesses are well-known entities in immunosuppressed individuals. Although the central restriction on DWI is present in nearly all pyogenic abscesses, these nonpyo-genic infectious lesions have less specific char-acteristics. A homogeneous central restriction pattern identical to that seen in bacterial abscess can also be found in the fungal abscesses, reflect-ing the proteinaceous fluid and hypercellularity, as well as hematic content, that are common in infec-tions caused by aspergillus. Therefore, this possi-bility should be considered and antifungal drugs should be included in the therapeutic regimen for such lesions, especially in immunocompromised individuals, when biopsy is impossible or results have not yet been received.[54] Heterogeneous restriction patterns have also been described for fungal abscess, with restriction predominantly occurring on the walls and solid peripheral projec-tions in these collections. It is assumed that these different patterns are generated by the complete or partial filling of the cavity by inflammatory cells and hyphae in the late capsular stage, giving the appearance of homogeneous or heterogeneous restriction, respectively.[55] Importantly, Luthra and colleagues[55] found lower ADC values in the restriction sites of the fungal abscess than in pyogenic lesions.

CNS infection is one of the more serious forms of *Mycobacterium tuberculosis* and is character-ized by high morbidity and mortality. The AIDS pandemic has resulted in a significant increase of neural tuberculosis around the world. Tuberculous meningitis is characterized by the triad of cisternal meningeal enhancement, hydrocephalus, and deep infarcts, secondary to vasculitis of the medial lenticulostriate-striatal arteries and thalamic-perforating arteries ("medial TB zone"). Infarcts can be detected early by the DWI sequence as areas of high signal and low ADC values. In another form of CNS tuberculosis, the tuberculo-mas present a varied MR imaging signal according to their evolutionary characteristics and the pres-ence of solid or liquid caseous necrosis. DWIs show restriction in tuberculomas with liquefied necrosis and no restriction in those with solid necrosis. Restriction of the diffusion in the pres-ence of a low signal on T2 can contribute to the differentiation between lymphoma and tuberculo-ma in the context of brain focal lesions in patients with AIDS. The tuberculous abscess is a rare condition caused by *M tuberculosis*, constituting 4% to 7% of the total number of cases of neural tuberculosis in developing countries.[56] The use of DWI in the diagnosis of such abscesses, as well as in pyogenic abscesses, reveals restriction with low ADC values, probably because of the presence of intact inflammatory cells in the pus.[55,56] The evaluation of this sequence alone makes it difficult to differentiate between pyogenic and tuberculous etiologies.

Neurocysticercosis is the most important para-sitic disease that affects the CNS and is a public health problem in developing countries. The cysts have a signal intensity similar to or slightly higher than CSF in all sequences, including DWI.[57] The calculated ADC is high, with published values ranging from 1.55 to 2.25 $\times$ 10^{-3} with slight variations according to the evolutionary stage of the parasite. These data make it possible to safely differentiate between neurocysticercosis and abscesses, whether pyogenic or tuberculous.[57,58] Eccentric hyperintense signal in the DWI sequence at the location of the scolex in other sequences was described in at least 1 lesion of 7 cases with scolex studied by Raffin and colleagues.[57] The ADC map showed a signal similar to that of CSF, and ADC measurement was not possible because of the small size of the nodule.[57]

Viral encephalitis

The prototypical case of viral encephalitis is caused by herpes simplex. The herpes simplex virus type 1 (HSV-1) is the principal cause of fatal sporadic encephalitis, mainly producing focal encephalitis. The mortality rate reaches 70% in patients who received no treatment or incomplete treatment. The main features of this disease are signs and symptoms of focal encephalopathy, including headache, fever, neck stiffness, changes in personality and mental status, convulsions, and an acute decrease in consciousness associated with focal neurologic signs such as weakness, sensibility disorders, aphasia, defects in visual fields, and cranial nerve palsies.[59] A polymerase chain reaction (PCR)-based technique is the method of choice for diagnosis, with sensitivity and specificity similar to those found for brain biopsies.[60]

MR imaging, especially with diffusion-weighted sequence, is quite sensitive for the early diagnosis of herpes encephalitis, and can be used within the first 72 hours when PCR assays can yield false-negative results.[61] The lesions are consistent with edema and inflammation, with low signal on T1-weighted and hypersignal on T2-weighted sequences. Lesions typically involve the medial aspect of the temporal lobes and inferior frontal lobes, asymmetrically, sparing the lentiform and extending to the insula within the first 48 hours. The lesions are usually not enhanced or exhibit a minimum enhancement after gadolinium administration, and may have a hemorrhagic component. Hemorrhagic lesions can easily be detected using T1 sequences or T2 gradient-echo. The DWI sequence is more sensitive than T2 or FLAIR for the early detection of necrotizing encephalitis.[59] At this stage, 2 different patterns in the spread can occur. In the first, the spread of water is reduced as a result of cytotoxic edema, seen as hyperintense signal on DWI and

hypointensity on the ADC map, usually reflecting irreversible neuronal damage and bad prognosis. The acute phase involves areas of congestion, perivascular infiltrate, and pathologic thrombi. These changes may lead to cytotoxic edema, primarily in gray matter neurons. Therefore, the change in DWI is the most precocious cell abnormality and can confirm the acute clinical symptoms of those patients. In some patients, this sequence is the only one that is altered.[62] The second pattern of spread may indicate a subacute phase of the disease and involves an increase in water molecule diffusion owing to vasogenic edema, with reduced congestion and perivascular infiltrate seen as areas of hypersignal in DWI and the ADC map. This stage is also accompanied by the formation of vasogenic or interstitial fluid collections, with lesions evident on T2 sequences. The evolution of the spectrum of pathologic findings from cytotoxic edema to cell lysis and necrosis causes a change in the free movement of water, similar to the pseudonormalization found in stroke.[59] Prakash and colleagues[63] highlighted the superiority of the T2 sequence over DWI in 2 patients with encephalitis who received MR imaging between 3 and 7 weeks after the onset of symptoms. Sener[64] reported 2 patients with simultaneous patterns of cytotoxic and vasogenic edema and suggested that the cytotoxic edema indicated fulminant necrosis and poor prognosis. However, an understanding of all the mechanisms involved in the different stages of development of herpes simplex encephalitis still requires more detailed studies with larger and more representative samples. It is possible that very early diagnosis and the institution of appropriate therapy enable effective treatment, preventing irreversible damage or even allowing the reversal of some changes. Differentiation from neoplastic processes can be achieved based on differences in the ADC values, which are lower in herpes lesions than in normal parenchyma (from 0.48 $\times$ 10^{-3} to 0.66 $\times$ 10^{-3}).[59]

Herpes simplex type 2 (HSV-2) causes genital herpes and can infect the mouth and face via sexual transmission. In the CNS, HSV-2 may be transmitted from mother to child during passage through the birth canal and causes neonatal encephalitis. Outside of the neonatal period, the virus causes HSV-1-like frontotemporal encephalitis in immunocompetent patients. The imaging findings are also similar to those in HSV-1, with areas of water molecule restriction. In immunocompromised patients, the lesions are present in a more diffuse and multifocal way, with strong signals in T2 and DWI, and are difficult to differentiate from other forms of encephalitis.[59]

Human herpesvirus 6 (HHV-6) has 2 variants: HHV-6A and HHV-6B. Subtype B causes roseola in children, infecting virtually all children younger than 3 years. Subtype A is acquired later and displays specific neurotropic properties. HHV-6A is associated with febrile seizures, subacute and fulminant encephalitis, meningitis, meningoencephalitis, myelitis, and chronic fatigue syndrome.[65] The cerebral infection may also selectively involve the temporal lobe, similar to limbic encephalitis, with inflammation of the uncus, amygdale, and the hippocampus body, typically sparing the parahippocampal gyrus.[66] With the advent of DWI, characteristic findings such as irregular restriction (patchy) of diffusion may be evident before any change is visible in conventional sequences. The lesions appear hyperintense on DWI and with low ADC values in the early stages. However, follow-up in patients with unfavorable outcomes revealed an increase of ADC values, representing the T2 shine-through effect owing to the development of vasogenic edema and encephalomalacia.[65] Another entity related to HHV-6, probably of a postinfectious nature, is acute necrotizing encephalopathy. This typically presents with changes affecting the thalami, basal ganglia, cerebellar hemispheres, and brainstem. The ADC map reveals specific findings of high central signal, indicating necrosis and hemorrhage, low central peripheral signal, related to cytotoxic edema, and high signal in the adjacent tissue, suggesting perifocal vasogenic edema. This is described as a tricolor pattern (**Fig. 9**).[65]

Although infection by herpes simplex is the major form of viral encephalitis, other nonherpetic infections should be considered in the diagnosis of acute viral encephalitis. In immunocompromised patients, the spectrum of possibilities is even greater. Recently, the use of techniques such as DWI has provided additional information for differential diagnosis; however, the definitive diagnosis depends on the detection of viral DNA or specific serologic markers in the CSF.[67] Among the nonherpetic viral infections, an important group of diseases are related to arbovirus, including Japanese encephalitis, West Nile encephalitis, St Louis and Murray Valley encephalitis, and dengue virus encephalitis. However, the imaging findings in these disorders are nonspecific and overlapping, which hinders the diagnosis based on an isolated evaluation of the MR imaging. Changes in imaging tests show preferences for the thalami, basal ganglia, mesial temporal lobe structures, cortex, brainstem, substantia nigra, cerebellum, and, in some cases, the cervical cord. As with other types of viral encephalitis, the DWI is useful for the detection of lesions at early stages during which

conventional MR imaging appears virtually normal.[68]

The JC virus, which has become more prevalent in recent decades with the emergence of the AIDS epidemic, causes a subacute opportunistic infection of the CNS called progressive multifocal leukoencephalopathy (PML). The virus infects the oligodendrocyte and promotes myelin breakdown with the consequent formation of infectious lesions with demyelinated substrate. The lesions are usually multifocal and can occur anywhere, most often in the parieto-occipital region. The thalami are usually affected, as are the cerebellum and the brainstem. On T2 sequences, the lesions are patchy, scalloped, and feature a high signal intensity in the white matter and extending along the white fibers that tend to cross through the splenium of the corpus callosum. PML also features the involvement of subcortical regions, minimum expansive effect and, rarely, thin peripheral enhancement.[69] The evaluation of these lesions by diffusion-weighted sequence has proved to be a useful method of evaluating and monitoring the disease, as well as establishing differential diagnosis.[70] The patterns of lesions in the diffusion-weighted sequence depend on the stage of the lesion. Acute lesions or the margins of large lesions (leading edges) show reduced ADC values and hypersignal on DWI. Advanced lesions and the central regions of large lesions have a high ADC and consequently low signal on DWI (**Fig. 10**).[71,72] Histopathological examination shows that the extended extracellular space is enlarged, with sparse oligodendrocytes and macrophages in the central region (where the ADC is high) and myelin loss and enrichment in the number of macrophages and oligodendrocytes with intranuclear inclusions in the periphery of the lesion.[71] Usiskin and colleagues[73] have demonstrated the effectiveness of the diffusion-weighted sequence by following a patient treated with HAART (highly active antiretroviral therapy regimen). After 6 months of treatment with good clinical evolution, the DWI showed less hypointensity of the central signal, with a significant decrease in ADC values and an absence of the peripheral hyperintensity signal observed in the first examination, notably with the use of a b-value of 3000.

Prionic infections

Creutzfeldt-Jakob disease and other transmissible spongiform encephalopathies are characterized by progressive dementia, neurologic abnormalities, and eventually death. The disease is caused by an infectious protein particle (prion) and early diagnosis is essential for the prevention of human-to-human transmission. DWIs have been

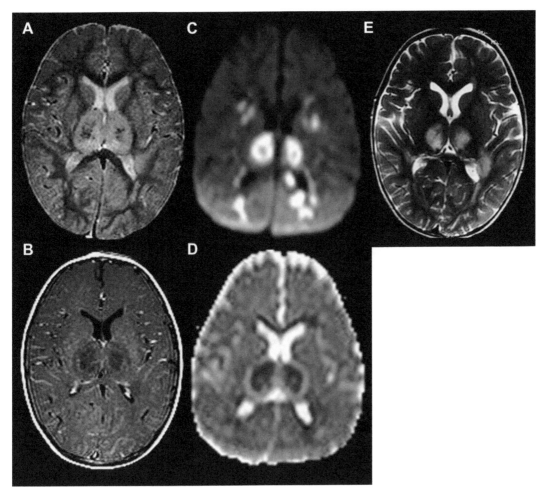

Fig. 9. Female child, 2 years of age, exhibited decreased level of consciousness, with an MR imaging diagnosis of acute necrotizing encephalopathy (ANE). (A) The axial T2-weighted sequence shows an increase in volume and changes in the thalami both bilaterally and symmetrically, with a slightly peripheral enhancement on T1 post-Gd sequence (B). (C, D) DWI sequence (b = 1000 sec/mm²) (C) and ADC map (D) show signal abnormalities that represent the characteristic pattern of the disease, ie, high ADC values in the central portion of the thalamus, low peripheral ADC values, and high values in areas adjacent to the thalamus and in periventricular white matter (tricolor pattern in the ADC map). (E) Axial T2-weighted image. This pattern confirms an unfavorable prognosis and this child died a few days later.

used to reveal lesions in the early stages of the disease.[74]

Approximately 90% of the cases of human prion disease are classified as sporadic Creutzfeldt-Jakob of unknown etiology. In the initial phase, these patients report fatigue, behavioral disorders, visual disturbances, depression, and insomnia. After a few weeks, patients experience a rapidly progressing dementia, followed by pyramidal and extrapyramidal changes and a final stage characterized by akinetic mutism.[75] The electroencephalogram (EEG) shows the classic finding of periodic synchronous discharges (periodic pattern), but this is a late finding and is sometimes absent. The detection of the 14-3-3 protein in the

cerebrospinal fluid was considered an important biomarker of the disease, although it is not pathognomonic of Creutzfeldt-Jakob disease and currently plays a limited role in diagnosis. The definitive diagnosis is confirmed by histopathological study. However, because of the risk inherent in the procedure, this is not performed in many patients.[74]

The MR imaging abnormalities described in Creutzfeldt-Jakob disease include signal abnormalities in the cerebral cortex and basal ganglia, associated with progressive cerebral atrophy. The DWI sequences may reveal early changes, such as a characteristic elevation of the signal intensity in the cerebral cortex, caudate nuclei,

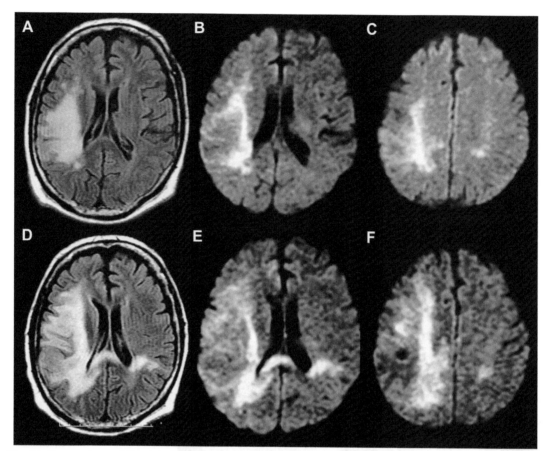

Fig. 10. Progressive multifocal leukoencephalopathy (PML) in a patient with systemic lymphoma. Axial FLAIR image (*A*) reveals a right subcortical signal abnormality that extends to the periventricular area. Note the absence of any expansive effect or enhancement (not shown), with small rounded peripheral hyperintense foci, especially at its anterior edge. (*B, C*) The DWI overtly demonstrates a hyperintense signal at the margins of the lesion and in peripheral foci in the anterior portion. There is a similar small lesion in the left semioval center. (*D–F*) After 1 month, volume of the lesion increased and now it crosses the splenium of the corpus callosum and extends to the contralateral cerebral hemisphere. The increase of the hyperintense signal in the growing margins of the DWI sequence (b = 1000 sec/mm²) is highlighted. Brain biopsy represented by the focus of markedly hypo-intense signal in the right cerebral hemisphere (*F*) confirmed the presence of the JC virus.

putamens, and thalami, in regions outside of arterial territories. Early stages are dominated by the cortical hyperintensity signal, which may be focal or diffuse, or symmetric or asymmetrical on DWI. Low ADC values are observed in these areas, implying a true restriction of the free movement of water molecules. These changes most often precede abnormalities on the EEG and conventional MR imaging sequences, including FLAIR. These sites of restricted diffusion represent areas of neuropil vacuolization secondary to spongiform degeneration. If these vacuoles are smaller than 20 μm, gliosis or astro-cytosis lead to restricted diffusion in the affected tissue.[74]

With the evolution of the disease, findings become evident on T2, and especially on FLAIR sequence. The signal abnormality on DWI, initially limited to the cortex and caudate nucleus, can progress to the anterior putamen, and lesions that initially involved only the anterior portion of the putamen extend to involve the entire region of the basal ganglia (Fig. 11). These findings imply that the proteinaceous infectious particles initially accumulate in the caudate nucleus and subse-quently progress to the putamen through the gray lenticulostriate branches. In the final stages of Creutzfeldt-Jakob disease, the hyperintense DWI signals in the cortical and basal ganglia may disappear in some cases; this abnormality is

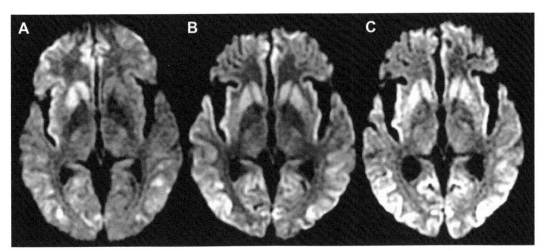

Fig. 11. Creutzfeldt-Jakob disease, inexorable evolution monitored by DWI (b = 1000 sec/mm²) at quarterly intervals. (*A*) In the initial examination, hyperintensity on DWI is observed in the right frontal cortex, and in the ipsilateral striatum. Note also a subtle abnormality in the right occipito-temporal cortex. (*B*) Observe that abnormal hyperintensity symmetrically extended to the bilateral striatum and to the posterior cortex. (*C*) Six months later, there is an increase in signal in the regions mentioned previously, which also markedly affects the cortex of the medial occipital gyri. Obvious parenchymal atrophy is also present, mainly in the right frontal cortex.

attributed to changes in the tissue as mild spongiform degeneration becomes status spongiosus.[76]

DEMYELINATING DISEASES

Multiple sclerosis (MS) is the archetypical idiopathic inflammatory demyelination. It is characterized by an immune-mediated acute inflammatory process that causes focal demyelination of the brain and the spinal cord. MS also involves axonal loss, whose evolution is characterized by spatial and temporal spread and a clinical course with alternating periods of relapse and remission. The relapsing remitting (RR) and secondary progressive (SP) forms of MS are the most common.[77]

The use of conventional MR imaging sequences in the diagnosis of MS is well established.[78] Recently, new tools have been emphasized in the literature, expanding the scope of MR imaging studies to magnetization transfer ratio (MTR), diffusion and diffusion tensor (DTI), spectroscopy, and perfusion and functional MR imaging, especially in the evaluation of normal-appearing white matter (NAWM).[78]

Studies conducted using diffusion sequences to evaluate demyelinating plaques revealed highly variable ADC values, consistent with the histopathological heterogeneity of MS lesions.[79] In general, the demyelinating lesions have higher mean diffusivity (MD) and ADC values and lower FA values than do contralateral NAWM or normal white matter,[80] indicating disorganized myelin or axonal structure and increased extracellular space. The highest MD values are found in hypointense lesions (black holes) on T1 relative to lesions with enhancement, or isointense lesions[81] representing destructive long-term damage.[82] However, the literature descriptions of differences in ADC values found in lesions with enhancement and no enhancement are inconsistent,[81,83] although the FA is invariably found to be lower in lesions with enhancement.[80,84,85] This finding suggests that the inflammatory process (edema) has a more variable impact on ADC and MD than on FA.[86] These observations demonstrate the potential of DWI to provide quantitative measures for monitoring irreversible tissue damage in multiple sclerosis.

DTI studies in NAWM also showed decreased FA and increased MD in different regions,[80] in agreement with studies of MTR that suggest subtle microstructural changes in NAWM, and also with the resolution of conventional sequences. These abnormalities tend to be more severe in periplaque regions.[87] Some studies have shown early significant changes in water diffusion in normal-appearing corpus callosum in the context of MS, even in the absence of DTI abnormalities in other regions (NAWM), suggesting preferential occult injury in the corpus callosum.[88–90] In line with this finding, a more recent study using weekly DWI has shown that an increase in ADC can be detected in NAWM starting as early as 6 weeks before the appearance of new lesions.[91]

Nusbaum and colleagues[92] demonstrated that whole-brain MR diffusion histograms may quantitate overall cerebral lesion load in patients with MS (**Fig. 12**) and may be able to discern differences between clinical subgroups. Mean whole-brain MR ADC in patients with MS is usually elevated and histograms are shifted to higher values compared with healthy control subjects. Mean whole-brain ADC of secondary progressive patients is shifted to higher values compared with relapsing–remitting patients.[92]

Although acute demyelinating lesions usually show an increase in diffusibility, credited to the expansion of the extracellular space,[81,93] a decrease in ADC values during a short early phase, especially in large lesions, has also been reported. Rovira and colleagues[94] described 2 large demyelinating lesions, which showed mean ADC values of 22% and 33% compared with contralateral side at the initial examination, demonstrating an injury with truly restricted diffusion. This pattern persisted for a few weeks, during which inflammation was also present. Despite the

differential diagnosis ruling out acute infarction, the decline in the ADC values was less than expected for the infarction core (40% to 50% in the first days). The investigators proposed that the restriction of diffusion in pseudotumoral lesions might be a result of intramyelinic edema, cytotoxic edema secondary to a reduction in the vascular supply, or dense inflammatory infiltrate inhibiting effective movement of molecules in the extracellular environment (**Fig. 13**).

Acute disseminated encephalomyelitis (ADEM) is an acute demyelinating inflammatory disease, usually monophasic, that is temporally related to a previous infectious episode or vaccination. Conventional MR imaging studies show hyperintense lesions on FLAIR and T2 that are asymmetrically distributed in the white and gray matter. Similar to other demyelinating lesions, these lesions often have strong signals in the DWI sequence and high ADC values, presumably because of the expansion of the extracellular

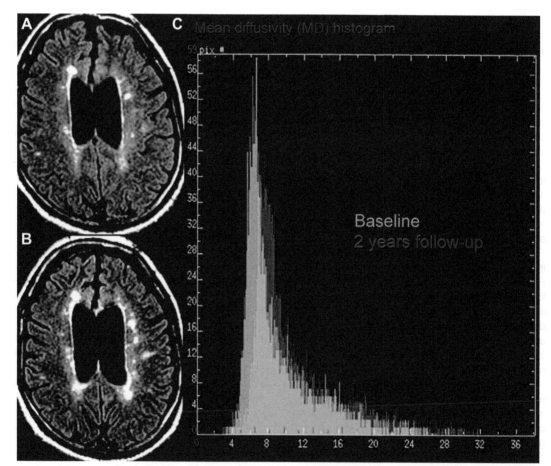

Fig. 12. Multiple sclerosis. The baseline study (*A*) and 2-year follow-up (*B*) showing atrophic changes and increase of the number of the lesions on FLAIR. Mean diffusivity (MD) histogram (*C*). In comparison with baseline (*yellow*), the follow-up curve (*blue*) shows a reduction of the MD histogram peak height, which reflects the amount of truly normal tissue.

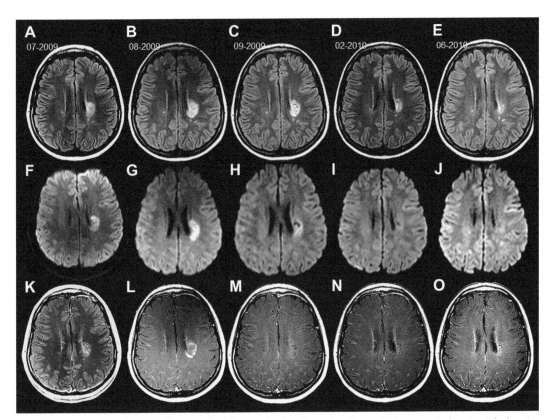

Fig. 13. Female, 24 years of age, diagnosed with tumefactive demyelination, which promoted acute right hemiparesis. Monthly comparative images on FLAIR (*A–E*), DWI (b = 1000 sec/mm²) (*F–J*), and T1 post-Gd (*K–O*) show an acute pseudotumoral lesion in the left periventricular region with restricted diffusion, particularly in the peripheral region. Note that diffusion abnormality enlarged in the first month, but in the next months after the introduction of therapy demonstrates the gradual reduction. The post-Gd T1 sequences follow the evolution of diffusion.

space concomitant with axonal loss, demyelination, and edema.[95] Meanwhile, patients examined during the early stages of the disease, like patients with pseudotumoral lesions, may also exhibit a drop in ADC (acute stage), suggesting reduced diffusivity, with ADC elevation observed later (subacute stage) (**Fig. 14**).[96,97]

Other Clinical Situations

Partial seizures and status epilepticus are associated with changes in local blood perfusion and neuronal metabolism, as clearly demonstrated by numerous positron emission tomography (PET) and single-photon emission computed tomography (SPECT) studies.[98–100] Increased cerebral blood flow and metabolic consumption occur in the epileptogenic focus region, proportional to the frequency and duration of the episode.[101] There is a transient alteration in the blood-brain barrier, causing increased vascular permeability and subsequent cerebral edema. The hematoencephalic barrier may be impaired in different

ways, explaining the MR imaging findings described in the literature, which range from signal changes caused by vasogenic or cytotoxic edema, to secondary enhancement and barrier breakage.[102] During the peri-ictal period, DWI shows a transient increase in signal intensity in the cortex and subcortical white matter of the lobe focus noticed on EEG, with several reports of an ADC decline followed by an increase to normal or elevated ADC levels within minutes, hours, or days.[103] These findings cannot be attributed to ischemic brain damage, although they are similar to those observed in ischemia, because the ADC change in cases of epilepsy is a result of cell damage induced by high blood perfusion during epileptic activity, rather than by hypoxia or reduction of cerebral blood flow as is observed in heart attacks.[104]

There is a strong association between the degree of ADC reduction and a favorable or unfavorable disease course; tissues in which ADC is reduced by 10% to 15% become necrotic, whereas an ADC drop below 10% is associated

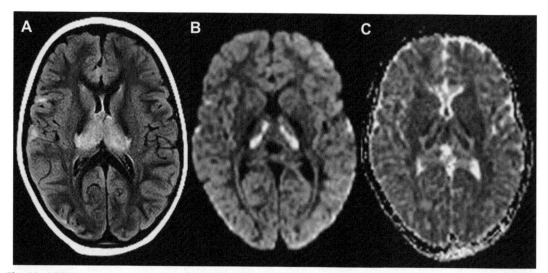

Fig. 14. ADEM. Age 4 years, 15 days after vaccination. (*A*) Axial FLAIR demonstrates hyperintense and symmetric bilateral thalamic signals, as well as scattered hyperintense foci in the cortical gray matter. (*B, C*) The DWI and ADC map (b = 1000 sec/mm²) show a restriction zone in the central thalamus, with a halo of high ADC values that do not form concentric lamellae. This particular pattern might favor good prognosis of ADEM in an appropriate clinical setting.

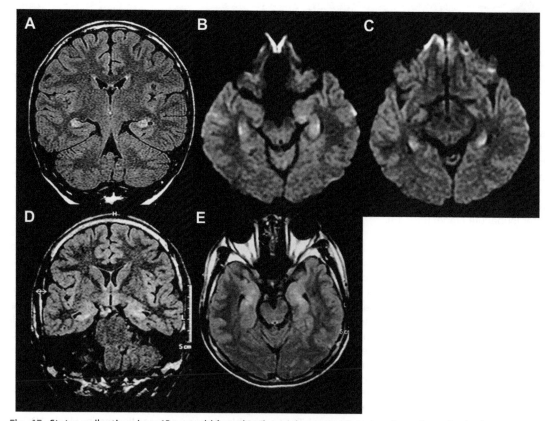

Fig. 15. Status epilepticus in a 13-year-old boy. (*A–C*) Initial examination showing edema in the hippocampus with hyperintensity on coronal FLAIR (*A*) and signal abnormality in the axial DWI (b = 1000 sec/mm²) (*B, C*). (*D, E*) After 5 months, imaging follow-up confirmed mesial temporal sclerosis on FLAIR.

with tissue recovery in rat models of ischemia.[105] Kim and colleagues[103] reported 2 cases of status epilepticus in which ADC was reduced by 10%, which resolved either completely or partially. Conversely, a drop of more than 10% was observed in 3 patients and was associated with hippocampal atrophy and partial seizures in 2 of the 3 patients. These findings suggest that cytotoxic edema induced by prolonged status epilepticus may be a first step toward the development of cerebral damage secondary to seizures, progressing to hippocampal sclerosis in relatively short periods (in one example, 4 months).[103] Several studies have demonstrated the development of hippocampal atrophy evident after a status epilepticus episode (Fig. 15).[106,107] In the interictal period, when hippocampal sclerosis occurs, ADC values are predominantly elevated, secondary to neuronal loss and gliosis.[106] It is important to note that these changes are found in regions that often appear normal in conventional studies, although they are identified clinically and by EEG as truly epileptogenic regions. Therefore, MR imaging diffusion appears to be sensitive enough to detect the physiologic effects of epilepsy in brain tissue, and may, in some cases, provide unique information regarding the location of the epileptogenic focus.

Transient global amnesia (TGA) is a benign syndrome that manifests itself in sudden-onset behavioral changes and temporary dysfunction of the anterograde and retrograde recent memory.[108] The pathophysiological basis of this disease is still unclear, and may be caused by ischemia in the territory bordering the hippocampus, spreading depression, epilepsy, secondary venous congestion to the Valsalva maneuver, or metabolic changes related to apoptosis and excess

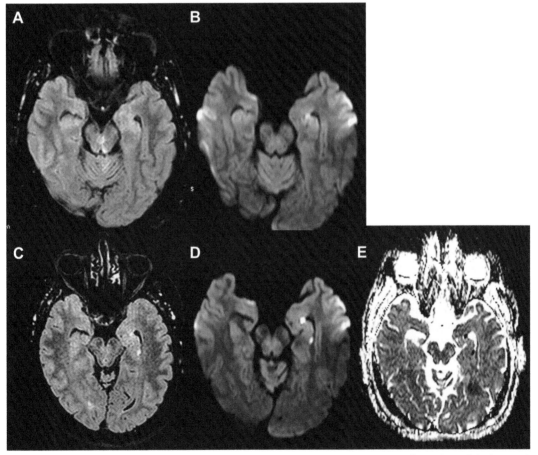

Fig. 16. A 49-year-old male with sudden onset of anterograde amnesia, suggestive of transient global amnesia. (A, B) Axial FLAIR (A) and DWI (b = 1000 sec/mm²) (B) performed 10 hours after symptom onset reveals a faint focus of signal change at the head of the left hippocampus, without any abnormality on FLAIR. (C–E) After 2 days, now with complete clinical resolution, FLAIR image (C) depicted 2 hyperintense foci in the left hippocampus; these are more evident on DWI (D) and ADC map (E).

glutamate.[109] It is usually unilateral, affecting the left hippocampus, but more rarely may be bilateral or affect the right hippocampus.[110] DWI has adequate sensitivity to diagnose TGA by imaging in the acute phase, as it detects focal points of increased signal intensity on the lateral aspect of the hippocampus, the CA-1 sector of the cornu ammonis (Sommer), with corresponding lesions with low signal on the ADC map indicating restricted water diffusion.[108] After the initial description of this finding, some investigators have reported that this method has only low diagnostic sensitivity.[111,112] Meanwhile, Sedlaczek and colleagues[110] have shown that DWI changes are observed only in the 24 to 48 hours after symptom onset (Fig. 16). Sedlaczek and colleagues[110] argue that the delayed ischemic mechanism and high metabolic rates leads to relative hypoperfusion in the Sommer sector of the hippocampus. The reversibility of the DWI abnormality is uniform and complete, and structural sequelae are absent after 4 to 6 months.[109] Therefore, the DWI should be routinely used when TGA is suspected, but only at the appropriate time and with acquisitions targeted to hippocampus (axial and coronal) to demonstrate the characteristic findings described.

FINAL CONSIDERATIONS

The diffusion-weighted sequence is not only a tool that allows more accurate diagnosis than the isolated use of conventional MR sequences, but is also an important auxiliary method for the evaluation of affected areas during and after treatment. However, concomitant analysis with other conventional and functional MR sequences is indispensable for the correct interpretation of any imaging findings.

The DWI sequence is particularly promising for a better understanding and monitoring of various morbid processes that affect the CNS. We believe that its use is currently safe and the parameters for its interpretation are relatively clear. However, many of the topics mentioned stem from preliminary findings, and numerous further studies will add to our knowledge of the real utility of this MR technique.

REFERENCES

1. Pagani E, Bammer R, Horsfield MA, et al. Diffusion MR imaging in multiple sclerosis: technical aspects and challenges. AJNR Am J Neuroradiol 2007; 28(3):411–20.
2. Srinivasan A, Goyal M, Al Azri F, et al. State-of-the-art imaging of acute stroke. Radiographics 2006; 26(Suppl 1):S75–95.
3. Kranz PG, Eastwood JD. Does diffusion-weighted imaging represent the ischemic core? An evidence-based systematic review. AJNR Am J Neuroradiol 2009;30(6):1206–12.
4. Kohno K, Hoehn-Berlage M, Mies G, et al. Relationship between diffusion-weighted MR images, cerebral blood flow, and energy state in experimental brain infarction. Magn Reson Imaging 1995;13(1): 73–80.
5. Lovblad KO, Baird AE. Actual diagnostic approach to the acute stroke patient. Eur Radiol 2006;16(6): 1253–69.
6. Arbelaez A, Castillo M, Mukherji SK. Diffusion-weighted MR imaging of global cerebral anoxia. AJNR Am J Neuroradiol 1999;20(6):999–1007.
7. Ferriero DM. Neonatal brain injury. N Engl J Med 2004;351(19):1985–95.
8. Huang BY, Castillo M. Hypoxic-ischemic brain injury: imaging findings from birth to adulthood. Radiographics 2008;28(2):417–39 [quiz: 617].
9. Chao CP, Zaleski CG, Patton AC. Neonatal hypoxic-ischemic encephalopathy: multimodality imaging findings. Radiographics 2006;26(Suppl 1):S159–72.
10. Robertson RL, Ben-Sira L, Barnes PD, et al. MR line-scan diffusion-weighted imaging of term neonates with perinatal brain ischemia. AJNR Am J Neuroradiol 1999;20(9):1658–70.
11. Provenzale JM, Sorensen AG. Diffusion-weighted MR imaging in acute stroke: theoretic considerations and clinical applications. AJR Am J Roentgenol 1999;173(6):1459–67.
12. Copen WA, Schwamm LH, Gonzalez RG, et al. Ischemic stroke: effects of etiology and patient age on the time course of the core apparent diffusion coefficient. Radiology 2001;221(1):27–34.
13. Forbes KP, Pipe JG, Bird R. Neonatal hypoxic-ischemic encephalopathy: detection with diffusion-weighted MR imaging. AJNR Am J Neuroradiol 2000;21(8):1490–6.
14. Fu J, Xue X, Chen L, et al. Studies on the value of diffusion-weighted MR imaging in the early prediction of periventricular leukomalacia. J Neuroimaging 2009;19(1):13–8.
15. Wu O, Sorensen AG, Benner T, et al. Comatose patients with cardiac arrest: predicting clinical outcome with diffusion-weighted MR imaging. Radiology 2009;252(1):173–81.
16. Wijman CA, Mlynash M, Caulfield AF, et al. Prognostic value of brain diffusion-weighted imaging after cardiac arrest. Ann Neurol 2009;65(4): 394–402.
17. Topcuoglu MA, Oguz KK, Buyukserbetci G, et al. Prognostic value of magnetic resonance imaging in post-resuscitation encephalopathy. Intern Med 2009;48(18):1635–45.
18. Kim HY, Kim BJ, Moon SY, et al. Serial diffusion-weighted MR imaging in delayed postanoxic

encephalopathy. A case study. J Neuroradiol 2002; 29(3):211–5.

19. Schwartz RB, Mulkern RV, Gudbjartsson H, et al. Diffusion-weighted MR imaging in hypertensive encephalopathy: clues to pathogenesis. AJNR Am J Neuroradiol 1998;19(5):859–62.

20. Casey SO, McKinney A, Teksam M, et al. CT perfusion imaging in the management of posterior reversible encephalopathy. Neuroradiology 2004; 46(4):272–6.

21. Covarrubias DJ, Luetmer PH, Campeau NG. Posterior reversible encephalopathy syndrome: prognostic utility of quantitative diffusion-weighted MR images. AJNR Am J Neuroradiol 2002;23(6):1038–48.

22. Mukherjee P, McKinstry RC. Reversible posterior leukoencephalopathy syndrome: evaluation with diffusion-tensor MR imaging. Radiology 2001; 219(3):756–65.

23. Lamy C, Oppenheim C, Meder JF, et al. Neuroimaging in posterior reversible encephalopathy syndrome. J Neuroimaging 2004;14(2):89–96.

24. Sorensen AG, Wu O, Copen WA, et al. Human acute cerebral ischemia: detection of changes in water diffusion anisotropy by using MR imaging. Radiology 1999;212(3):785–92.

25. Ferda J, Kastner J, Mukensnabl P, et al. Diffusion tensor magnetic resonance imaging of glial brain tumors. Eur J Radiol 2010;74(3):428–36.

26. Mardor Y, Roth Y, Ochershvilli A, et al. Pretreatment prediction of brain tumors' response to radiation therapy using high b-value diffusion-weighted MRI. Neoplasia 2004;6(2):136–42.

27. Chenevert TL, Stegman LD, Taylor JM, et al. Diffusion magnetic resonance imaging: an early surrogate marker of therapeutic efficacy in brain tumors. J Natl Cancer Inst 2000;92(24):2029–36.

28. Hall DE, Moffat BA, Stojanovska J, et al. Therapeutic efficacy of DTI-015 using diffusion magnetic resonance imaging as an early surrogate marker. Clin Cancer Res 2004;10(23):7852–9.

29. Bastin ME, Carpenter TK, Armitage PA, et al. Effects of dexamethasone on cerebral perfusion and water diffusion in patients with high-grade glioma. AJNR Am J Neuroradiol 2006;27(2):402–8.

30. Young GS. Advanced MRI of adult brain tumors. Neurol Clin 2007;25(4):947–73, viii.

31. Matsusue E, Fink JR, Rockhill JK, et al. Distinction between glioma progression and post-radiation change by combined physiologic MR imaging. Neuroradiology 2010;52(4):297–306.

32. Mohile NA, Abrey LE. Primary central nervous system lymphoma. Neurol Clin 2007;25(4): 1193–207, ix.

33. Haque S, Law M, Abrey LE, et al. Imaging of lymphoma of the central nervous system, spine, and orbit. Radiol Clin North Am 2008;46(2): 339–61, ix.

34. Zacharia TT, Law M, Naidich TP, et al. Central nervous system lymphoma characterization by diffusion-weighted imaging and MR spectroscopy. J Neuroimaging 2008;18(4):411–7.

35. Dong Q, Welsh RC, Chenevert TL, et al. Clinical applications of diffusion tensor imaging. J Magn Reson Imaging 2004;19(1):6–18.

36. Lu S, Ahn D, Johnson G, et al. Diffusion-tensor MR imaging of intracranial neoplasia and associated peritumoral edema: introduction of the tumor infiltration index. Radiology 2004;232(1):221–8.

37. Cartes-Zumelzu FW, Stavrou I, Castillo M, et al. Diffusion-weighted imaging in the assessment of brain abscesses therapy. AJNR Am J Neuroradiol 2004; 25(8):1310–7.

38. Kim YJ, Chang KH, Song IC, et al. Brain abscess and necrotic or cystic brain tumor: discrimination with signal intensity on diffusion-weighted MR imaging. AJR Am J Roentgenol 1998;171(6):1487–90.

39. Ferreira NP, Otta GM, do Amaral LL, et al. Imaging aspects of pyogenic infections of the central nervous system. Top Magn Reson Imaging 2005; 16(2):145–54.

40. Ebisu T, Tanaka C, Umeda M, et al. Discrimination of brain abscess from necrotic or cystic tumors by diffusion-weighted echo planar imaging. Magn Reson Imaging 1996;14(9):1113–6.

41. Mamelak AN, Mampalam TJ, Obana WG, et al. Improved management of multiple brain abscesses: a combined surgical and medical approach. Neurosurgery 1995;36(1):76–85 [discussion: 85–6].

42. Chen SC, Chung HW. Diffusion-weighted imaging parameters to track success of pyogenic brain abscess therapy. AJNR Am J Neuroradiol 2004; 25(8):1303–4.

43. Burtscher IM, Holtas S. In vivo proton MR spectroscopy of untreated and treated brain abscesses. AJNR Am J Neuroradiol 1999;20(6):1049–53.

44. Tung GA, Evangelista P, Rogg JM, et al. Diffusion-weighted MR imaging of rim-enhancing brain masses: is markedly decreased water diffusion specific for brain abscess? AJR Am J Roentgenol 2001;177(3):709–12.

45. Hartmann M, Jansen O, Heiland S, et al. Restricted diffusion within ring enhancement is not pathognomonic for brain abscess. AJNR Am J Neuroradiol 2001;22(9):1738–42.

46. Hollinger P, Zurcher R, Schroth G, et al. Diffusion magnetic resonance imaging findings in cerebritis and brain abscesses in a patient with septic encephalopathy. J Neurol 2000;247(3):232–4.

47. Tung GA, Rogg JM. Diffusion-weighted imaging of cerebritis. AJNR Am J Neuroradiol 2003;24(6): 1110–3.

48. Fukui MB, Williams RL, Mudigonda S. CT and MR imaging features of pyogenic ventriculitis. AJNR Am J Neuroradiol 2001;22(8):1510–6.

49. Pezzullo JA, Tung GA, Mudigonda S, et al. Diffusion-weighted MR imaging of pyogenic ventriculitis. AJR Am J Roentgenol 2003;180(1):71–5.

50. Han KT, Choi DS, Ryoo JW, et al. Diffusion-weighted MR imaging of pyogenic intraventricular empyema. Neuroradiology 2007;49(10):813–8.

51. Hong JT, Son BC, Sung JH, et al. Significance of diffusion-weighted imaging and apparent diffusion coefficient maps for the evaluation of pyogenic ventriculitis. Clin Neurol Neurosurg 2008;110(2):137–44.

52. Ramsay DW, Aslam M, Cherryman GR. Diffusion-weighted imaging of cerebral abscess and subdural empyema. AJNR Am J Neuroradiol 2000;21(6):1172.

53. Bernardini GL. Diagnosis and management of brain abscess and subdural empyema. Curr Neurol Neurosci Rep 2004;4(6):448–56.

54. Gaviani P, Schwartz RB, Hedley-Whyte ET, et al. Diffusion-weighted imaging of fungal cerebral infection. AJNR Am J Neuroradiol 2005;26(5):1115–21.

55. Luthra G, Parihara A, Nath K, et al. Comparative evaluation of fungal, tubercular, and pyogenic brain abscesses with conventional and diffusion MR imaging and proton MR spectroscopy. AJNR Am J Neuroradiol 2007;28(7):1332–8.

56. Trivedi R, Saksena S, Gupta RK. Magnetic resonance imaging in central nervous system tuberculosis. Indian J Radiol Imaging 2009;19(4):256–65.

57. Raffin LS, Bacheschi LA, Machado LR, et al. Diffusion-weighted MR imaging of cystic lesions of neurocysticercosis: a preliminary study. Arq Neuropsiquiatr 2001;59(4):839–42.

58. Gupta RK, Prakash M, Mishra AM, et al. Role of diffusion weighted imaging in differentiation of intracranial tuberculoma and tuberculous abscess from cysticercus granulomas—a report of more than 100 lesions. Eur J Radiol 2005;55(3):384–92.

59. Bulakbasi N, Kocaoglu M. Central nervous system infections of herpesvirus family. Neuroimaging Clin N Am 2008;18(1):53–84, viii.

60. Rowley AH, Whitley RJ, Lakeman FD, et al. Rapid detection of herpes-simplex-virus DNA in cerebrospinal fluid of patients with herpes simplex encephalitis. Lancet 1990;335(8687):440–1.

61. Akyldz BN, Gumus H, Kumandas S, et al. Diffusion-weighted magnetic resonance is better than polymerase chain reaction for early diagnosis of herpes simplex encephalitis: a case report. Pediatr Emerg Care 2008;24(6):377–9.

62. Kiroglu Y, Calli C, Yunten N, et al. Diffusion-weighted MR imaging of viral encephalitis. Neuroradiology 2006;48(12):875–80.

63. Prakash M, Kumar S, Gupta RK. Diffusion-weighted MR imaging in Japanese encephalitis. J Comput Assist Tomogr 2004;28(6):756–61.

64. Sener RN. Diffusion MRI in Rasmussen's encephalitis, herpes simplex encephalitis, and bacterial meningoencephalitis. Comput Med Imaging Graph 2002;26(5):327–32.

65. Sauter A, Ernemann U, Beck R, et al. Spectrum of imaging findings in immunocompromised patients with HHV-6 infection. AJR Am J Roentgenol 2009;193(5):W373–80.

66. Wainwright MS, Martin PL, Morse RP, et al. Human herpesvirus 6 limbic encephalitis after stem cell transplantation. Ann Neurol 2001;50(5):612–9.

67. Gupta RK, Jain KK, Kumar S. Imaging of nonspecific (nonherpetic) acute viral infections. Neuroimaging Clin N Am 2008;18(1):41–52, vii.

68. Maschke M, Kastrup O, Forsting M, et al. Update on neuroimaging in infectious central nervous system disease. Curr Opin Neurol 2004;17(4):475–80.

69. Thurnher MM, Sundgren PC. Imaging of slow viruses. Neuroimaging Clin N Am 2008;18(1):133–48, ix.

70. Yoon JH, Bang OY, Kim HS. Progressive multifocal leukoencephalopathy in AIDS: proton MR spectroscopy patterns of asynchronous lesions confirmed by serial diffusion-weighted imaging and apparent diffusion coefficient mapping. J Clin Neurol 2007;3(4):200–3.

71. Henderson RD, Smith MG, Mowat P, et al. Progressive multifocal leukoencephalopathy. Neurology 2002;58(12):1825.

72. Bergui M, Bradac GB, Oguz KK, et al. Progressive multifocal leukoencephalopathy: diffusion-weighted imaging and pathological correlations. Neuroradiology 2004;46(1):22–5.

73. Usiskin SI, Bainbridge A, Miller RF, et al. Progressive multifocal leukoencephalopathy: serial high-b-value diffusion-weighted MR imaging and apparent diffusion coefficient measurements to assess response to highly active antiretroviral therapy. AJNR Am J Neuroradiol 2007;28(2):285–6.

74. Ukisu R, Kushihashi T, Tanaka E, et al. Diffusion-weighted MR imaging of early-stage Creutzfeldt-Jakob disease: typical and atypical manifestations. Radiographics 2006;26(Suppl 1):S191–204.

75. Caramelli M, Ru G, Acutis P, et al. Prion diseases: current understanding of epidemiology and pathogenesis, and therapeutic advances. CNS Drugs 2006;20(1):15–28.

76. Ukisu R, Kushihashi T, Kitanosono T, et al. Serial diffusion-weighted MRI of Creutzfeldt-Jakob disease. AJR Am J Roentgenol 2005;184(2):560–6.

77. Noseworthy JH, Lucchinetti C, Rodriguez M, et al. Multiple sclerosis. N Engl J Med 2000;343(13):938–52.

78. McDonald WI, Compston A, Edan G, et al. Recommended diagnostic criteria for multiple sclerosis: guidelines from the International Panel on the diagnosis of multiple sclerosis. Ann Neurol 2001;50(1):121–7.

79. Lassmann H, Bruck W, Lucchinetti C. Heterogeneity of multiple sclerosis pathogenesis: implications for diagnosis and therapy. Trends Mol Med 2001;7(3):115–21.

80. Filippi M, Inglese M. Overview of diffusion-weighted magnetic resonance studies in multiple sclerosis. J Neurol Sci 2001;186(Suppl 1):S37–43.

81. Roychowdhury S, Maldjian JA, Grossman RI. Multiple sclerosis: comparison of trace apparent diffusion coefficients with MR enhancement pattern of lesions. AJNR Am J Neuroradiol 2000;21(5):869–74.

82. Castriota Scanderbeg A, Tomaiuolo F, Sabatini U, et al. Demyelinating plaques in relapsing-remitting and secondary-progressive multiple sclerosis: assessment with diffusion MR imaging. AJNR Am J Neuroradiol 2000;21(5):862–8.

83. Droogan AG, Clark CA, Werring DJ, et al. Comparison of multiple sclerosis clinical subgroups using navigated spin echo diffusion-weighted imaging. Magn Reson Imaging 1999;17(5):653–61.

84. Werring DJ, Clark CA, Barker GJ, et al. Diffusion tensor imaging of lesions and normal-appearing white matter in multiple sclerosis. Neurology 1999;52(8):1626–32.

85. Castriota-Scanderbeg A, Fasano F, Hagberg G, et al. Coefficient D(av) is more sensitive than fractional anisotropy in monitoring progression of irreversible tissue damage in focal nonactive multiple sclerosis lesions. AJNR Am J Neuroradiol 2003;24(4):663–70.

86. Ge Y. Multiple sclerosis: the role of MR imaging. AJNR Am J Neuroradiol 2006;27(6):1165–76.

87. Guo AC, MacFall JR, Provenzale JM. Multiple sclerosis: diffusion tensor MR imaging for evaluation of normal-appearing white matter. Radiology 2002;222(3):729–36.

88. Ge Y, Law M, Johnson G, et al. Preferential occult injury of corpus callosum in multiple sclerosis measured by diffusion tensor imaging. J Magn Reson Imaging 2004;20(1):1–7.

89. Saindane AM, Law M, Ge Y, et al. Correlation of diffusion tensor and dynamic perfusion MR imaging metrics in normal-appearing corpus callosum: support for primary hypoperfusion in multiple sclerosis. AJNR Am J Neuroradiol 2007;28(4):767–72.

90. Rueda F, Hygino LC Jr, Domingues RC, et al. Diffusion tensor MR imaging evaluation of the corpus callosum of patients with multiple sclerosis. Arq Neuropsiquiatr 2008;66(3A):449–53.

91. Rocca MA, Cercignani M, Iannucci G, et al. Weekly diffusion-weighted imaging of normal-appearing white matter in MS. Neurology 2000;55(6):882–4.

92. Nusbaum AO, Tang CY, Wei C, et al. Whole-brain diffusion MR histograms differ between MS subtypes. Neurology 2000;54(7):1421–7.

93. Werring DJ, Brassat D, Droogan AG, et al. The pathogenesis of lesions and normal-appearing white matter changes in multiple sclerosis: a serial diffusion MRI study. Brain 2000;123(Pt 8):1667–76.

94. Rovira A, Pericot I, Alonso J, et al. Serial diffusion-weighted MR imaging and proton MR spectroscopy of acute large demyelinating brain lesions: case report. AJNR Am J Neuroradiol 2002;23(6):989–94.

95. Harada M, Hisaoka S, Mori K, et al. Differences in water diffusion and lactate production in two different types of postinfectious encephalopathy. J Magn Reson Imaging 2000;11(5):559–63.

96. Kuker W, Ruff J, Gaertner S, et al. Modern MRI tools for the characterization of acute demyelinating lesions: value of chemical shift and diffusion-weighted imaging. Neuroradiology 2004;46(6):421–6.

97. Balasubramanya KS, Kovoor JM, Jayakumar PN, et al. Diffusion-weighted imaging and proton MR spectroscopy in the characterization of acute disseminated encephalomyelitis. Neuroradiology 2007;49(2):177–83.

98. Juhasz C, Scheidl E, Szirmai I. Reversible focal MRI abnormalities due to status epilepticus. An EEG, single photon emission computed tomography, transcranial Doppler follow-up study. Electroencephalogr Clin Neurophysiol 1998;107(6):402–7.

99. Lee BI, Markand ON, Wellman HN, et al. HIPDM-SPECT in patients with medically intractable complex partial seizures. Ictal study. Arch Neurol 1988;45(4):397–402.

100. Theodore WH, Newmark ME, Sato S, et al. [18F]fluorodeoxyglucose positron emission tomography in refractory complex partial seizures. Ann Neurol 1983;14(4):429–37.

101. Jackson GD, Connelly A, Cross JH, et al. Functional magnetic resonance imaging of focal seizures. Neurology 1994;44(5):850–6.

102. El-Koussy M, Mathis J, Lovblad KO, et al. Focal status epilepticus: follow-up by perfusion- and diffusion MRI. Eur Radiol 2002;12(3):568–74.

103. Kim JA, Chung JI, Yoon PH, et al. Transient MR signal changes in patients with generalized tonicoclonic seizure or status epilepticus: periictal diffusion-weighted imaging. AJNR Am J Neuroradiol 2001;22(6):1149–60.

104. Helpern JA, Huang N. Diffusion-weighted imaging in epilepsy. Magn Reson Imaging 1995;13(8):1227–31.

105. Nedelcu J, Klein MA, Aguzzi A, et al. Biphasic edema after hypoxic-ischemic brain injury in neonatal rats reflects early neuronal and late glial damage. Pediatr Res 1999;46(3):297–304.

106. Wieshmann UC, Woermann FG, Lemieux L, et al. Development of hippocampal atrophy: a serial

magnetic resonance imaging study in a patient who developed epilepsy after generalized status epilepticus. Epilepsia 1997;38(11):1238–41.

107. Nohria V, Lee N, Tien RD, et al. Magnetic resonance imaging evidence of hippocampal sclerosis in progression: a case report. Epilepsia 1994;35(6): 1332–6.

108. Felix MM, Castro LH, Maia AC, et al. Evidence of acute ischemic tissue change in transient global amnesia in magnetic resonance imaging: case report and literature review. J Neuroimaging 2005;15(2):203–5.

109. Bartsch T, Alfke K, Stingele R, et al. Selective affection of hippocampal CA-1 neurons in patients with transient global amnesia without long-term sequelae. Brain 2006;129(Pt 11):2874–84.

110. Sedlaczek O, Hirsch JG, Grips E, et al. Detection of delayed focal MR changes in the lateral hippocampus in transient global amnesia. Neurology 2004;62(12):2165–70.

111. Gass A, Gaa J, Hirsch J, et al. Lack of evidence of acute ischemic tissue change in transient global amnesia on single-shot echo-planar diffusion-weighted MRI. Stroke 1999;30(10):2070–2.

112. Huber R, Aschoff AJ, Ludolph AC, et al. Transient global amnesia. Evidence against vascular ischemic etiology from diffusion weighted imaging. J Neurol 2002;249(11):1520–4.

Diffusion Tensor Imaging for Evaluation of the Childhood Brain and Pediatric White Matter Disorders

Jared Isaacson, BS[a],*, James Provenzale, MD[b,c,d,e]

KEYWORDS

- Diffusion tensor imaging • Childhood brain
- Pediatric white matter disorders
- Magnetic resonance imaging

Magnetic resonance (MR) imaging has been used by investigators and clinicians alike to assess the development of the brain in childhood to understand both patterns of normal growth and patterns by which a maturing brain may deviate from normal. Advanced MR techniques such as diffusion tensor imaging (DTI) have gained prominence as a means of assessing brain development. This review explains the sequence of brain maturation and the means by which DTI can be used to assess it in normal children.

DEVELOPMENT CHANGES DURING EARLY BRAIN MATURATION

Maturation of the white matter (WM) tracts of the brain occurs in an orderly and predictable fashion, beginning during intrauterine development and continuing into early adulthood. This maturation process is governed by several complex processes, including myelination and changes in axonal numbers (including not only increases of numbers of axons in many regions but also decreases in a process termed axonal pruning).

Such changes are delineated in postmortem studies, which have shown that myelination typically occurs in a standard fashion in the prenatal and neonatal brain (**Fig. 1**).[1–3] Such fixed-tissue studies have helped identify the microstructural changes (eg, axonal proliferation and the process of myelination), which imaging studies are designed to depict. As a general rule, maturation of the WM occurs in 2 major patterns: (1) beginning within deep central structures and proceeding peripherally and (2) proceeding from posterior structures anteriorly.[3]

CONVENTIONAL MR IMAGING ASSESSMENT

When interpreting MR imaging studies of the newborn infant brain, one often wishes to assess whether WM development is occurring at a normal

[a] Duke University School of Medicine, 2301 Erwin Road, Durham, NC 27710, USA
[b] Department of Radiology, Duke University Medical Center, 2301 Erwin Road, Durham, NC 27710, USA
[c] Department of Radiology, Emory University School of Medicine, 1364 Clifton Road Northeast, Atlanta, GA 30304, USA
[d] Department of Oncology, Emory University School of Medicine, 1364 Clifton Road Northeast, Atlanta, GA 30304, USA
[e] Department of Biomedical Engineering, Emory University School of Medicine, 1364 Clifton Road Northeast, Atlanta, GA 30304, USA
* Corresponding author.
E-mail address: jared.isaacson@duke.edu

Neuroimag Clin N Am 21 (2011) 179–189
doi:10.1016/j.nic.2011.02.005
1052-5149/11/$ – see front matter © 2011 Published by Elsevier Inc.

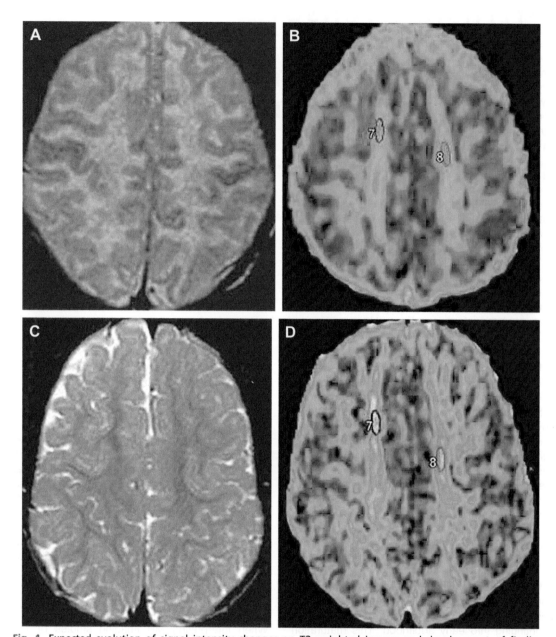

Fig. 1. Expected evolution of signal intensity changes on T2-weighted images and development of findings reflecting brain maturation on FA maps in an infant with Krabbe disease who underwent unrelated hematopoietic stem cell transplantation at a few weeks of age, before symptoms developed. The child was identified from an older sibling with Krabbe disease, which prompted testing for the missing enzyme in the infant shown here. (A) Axial T2-weighted images of the subcortical WM at age 3 weeks shows the expected relatively high signal intensity of WM, which is brighter than brain cortex on this image. Note that on this image, the entire WM appears relatively featureless. (B) Axial color-coded FA map (in which regions of low FA are coded as blue and regions of high FA are coded as orange) obtained during the same MR examination as (A) shows only small regions of high FA within WM. Representative ROIs have been placed within WM. (C) Axial T2-weighted images of the subcortical WM at age 57 weeks shows that the WM now has uniformly low signal, consistent with myelination. (D) Axial color-coded FA map obtained during the same MR examination as (C) shows only that the regions of high FA are now widely distributed within WM, consistent with WM maturation and reflecting the WM maturational changes depicted in (C). (Adapted from McGraw PM, Liang L, Escolar M, et al. Krabbe disease treated with hematopoietic stem cell transplantation: serial assessment of anisotropy measurements in Krabbe disease patients treated with hematopoietic stem cell transplantation-initial experience. Radiology 2005; 236:225; with permission.)

rate. Conventional MR imaging can allow this assessment of the newborn brain, but only within certain limits. For instance, on a T2-weighted image, the newborn brain appears largely diffusely hyperintense. In general, it is recognized that T1-weighted images are more valuable in determining brain maturation during the first 6 months or so of life; thereafter T2-weighted images seem to be more valuable.[4]

In the newborn, one can reliably attend to only a few specific landmarks (eg, middle cerebellar peduncle and posterior limb of internal capsule) to determine whether age-appropriate development has occurred.[5] In these regions, normal maturation is determined based on whether hyperintense signal has begun to appear in these regions on T1-weighted images by the time of birth. However, assessment of the remainder of the brain is more difficult because such landmarks are generally not present. Similarly, on T2-weighted images of the newborn infant (see **Fig. 1**), some of these same landmark regions appear hypointense relative to the (almost uniformly) hypointense background of WM.[5] However, early in postnatal life, these regions are few in number; most infant brain structures cannot be adequately assessed on conventional MR images because they appear relatively isointense to one another (see **Fig. 1**).

MR signal changes within the developing WM are considered to occur because of several factors. One major factor is change in brain water content. Specifically, the infant brain contains high water content compared with the adult brain. The high water content in early life produces an increase in T1 relaxation time that corresponds to hypointense signal on a T1-weighted image; similarly, the increased water content results in an increased T2 relaxation time and hyperintense signal within WM on T2-weighted images.[6] With the onset of brain maturation (which is manifested by increases in myelination and axonal numbers), the ratio of water to macromolecules decreases, producing an increase in signal intensity on T1-weighted images and a decrease in signal intensity on T2-weighted images (see **Fig. 1**). Other factors influencing this change in appearance include increased numbers of cells and their components (eg, axons, dendrites, cell membranes, and intracellular organelles) and increased amounts of myelin.[7] During this process, major compact WM structures (eg, the corpus callosum) undergo standard and predictable changes in signal intensity, which can serve as milestones that can be used by the radiologist to determine whether brain maturation is proceeding at the expected rate throughout the remainder of the first year of life.

The signal intensity changes in the corpus callosum can serve as an example of this maturational process. At birth, the entire corpus callosum appears relatively isointense with surrounding cerebral WM tracts at birth on both T1-weighted and T2-weighted pulse sequences.[8] At approximately 4 months after birth the splenium and the adjacent posterior body of the corpus callosum begin to appear hyperintense relative to adjacent WM on T1-weighted images. As maturation proceeds from posterior to anterior, the genu of the corpus callosum appears hyperintense relative to nearby WM at approximately 4 to 6 months of life. Similarly, on T2-weighted images, the splenium of the corpus callosum begins to appear hypointense at approximately age 4 to 6 months, and the genu appears hypointense at approximately 5 to 8 months of life. These changes have the advantage of being evident on visual inspection (and hence seen without the need for computational analysis). Nonetheless, they are solely qualitative (as opposed to quantitative) in nature and are subject to substantial interobserver variability. Furthermore, as outlined earlier, the number of regions in which such pronounced changes are seen in the infant brain (which can serve as markers of brain development) are few in number. Hence, the development of quantitative methods that are less observer dependent and which can be applied to the entire WM (such as diffusion imaging and DTI) are expected to be of great value in understanding brain maturation.

DIFFUSION IMAGING AND DTI

The primary advanced MR imaging techniques used for assessing brain development are diffusion-weighted imaging (DWI) and DTI. DWI is based on application of diffusion gradients in 3 orthogonal directions; this technique allows measurement of rate of water motion, which is needed for measurement of the apparent diffusion coefficient (ADC) value.[9] In many studies, ADC values have been found to be useful as a marker to assess WM maturation.[10,11]

Whereas DWI typically uses 3 orthogonal diffusion gradient directions, DTI uses diffusion gradients in at least 6 orthogonal directions. This increase in number of encoding gradients allows estimation of the diffusion tensor, which is a mathematical representation of directionality of microscopic water motion within each pixel. Once the diffusion tensor can be estimated, the degree of anisotropy (ie, tendency of microscopic water motion to proceed in a single direction, as opposed to randomly) and the predominant direction of water diffusion can be determined. Such information is typically depicted by means of a fractional anisotropy (FA) map, from which representation of WM pathways can be visualized via a process termed tractography (**Fig. 2**). DTI has been used successfully to quantitatively evaluate milestones in brain development.[12,13]

Both DWI and DTI are sensitive to microstructural changes such as increases in cell density and development of myelination. These techniques can show WM changes that are inapparent on conventional MR imaging (discussed later).[14]

USES OF DWI TO STUDY NORMAL BRAIN MATURATION

DWI has been used to image the maturing brain. For instance, in 1 study of 30 infants and children between the ages of 1 month and 17 years, the investigators used DWI to study D_{av} (which is a measure of isotropic water diffusion within voxels and is a similar measurement to ADC) in the developing brain.[15] The study found that the average diffusion constant, D_{av}, decreased as age increased. This finding occurred throughout the whole brain, the genu and splenium of the corpus callosum, and the periventricular WM, with D_{av} decreasing fastest during the first 2 years of life. This period of rapid ADC decrease correlates with the known period of rapid water content decrease within brain tissue.[16] Other studies have shown that ADC values decrease over time in various WM regions throughout infancy and childhood and that the correlation of ADC decrease with age is strong, although dependent on the

structure studied.[11,17] For instance, the correlation of ADC decrease with age in 1 study was strongest in the subcortical WM, and the correlation in deep compact WM regions (eg, the posterior limb of internal capsule) was only moderately strong.[17] Whereas the correlation within WM regions was generally good, the correlation was weak in gray matter regions.[17]

Because comparing both ADC values and values obtained from DTI (eg, FA) against a reference standard (eg, histologic determination of degree of myelination) has not been widely performed, the merit of each type of measurements relative to one another is difficult to fully determine.

ASSESSMENT OF THE BRAIN USING DTI

Our group has assessed the use of DTI to assess normal brain maturation in several studies. In 1 study of 53 normal infants in the first year of life who underwent DTI, we analyzed effect of age on FA and ADC values.[13] We studied these values in 3 deep WM regions (genu and splenium of the corpus callosum and posterior limb of the internal capsule) and 2 peripheral WM regions (ie, the subcortical WM underlying the prefrontal and posterior parietal cortex). We then plotted mean ADC and FA values for deep and peripheral WM against gestational age normalized to term. Using linear regression models, we found that the data were fit best by a broken line with a breakpoint at 100 days. We used the slope of the linear fits to determine the rate of WM maturation in both

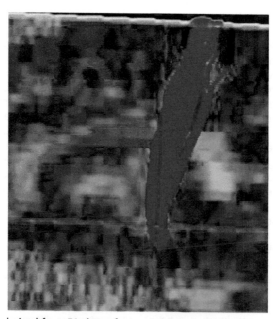

Fig. 2. Tractography image derived from FA data of a normal 6-year-old boy. FA map of brain is shown in background and corticospinal tract is depicted in red along its craniocaudad course.

the early (ie, before day 100) and the late periods. We used multivariate analysis of variance tests to compare deep and peripheral WM structures at term and at various early and late ages (eg, days 30 and 200) and to compare rates of ADC and FA maturation.

As expected, we found that at birth peripheral WM was significantly less mature than deep WM (Fig. 3). The mean ADC value in peripheral WM was 163% of adult values and that of deep WM was 143% of adult values. Similarly, mean FA value of peripheral WM was 32% of adult values and that of deep WM was 54% of adult values. These findings are consistent with the known characteristics of these regions from histologic studies.[1–3] Specifically, at term, the central WM is believed to be well established because of development of dense axonal fascicles during the second trimester of gestation, whereas the frontal and parietal peripheral WM contains only sparse myelination and few associational axons.[18,19]

We found discordant results in changes in ADC values and changes in FA values in deep WM and peripheral WM during the first 100 days of life. During the first 100 days of postnatal life, the rate of ADC decrease (which indicates maturation) in peripheral WM was significantly greater (ie, approximately twice) than for deep WM. However, opposite findings were seen for FA changes; the rate of FA increase (which indicates WM maturation) in peripheral WM was approximately half as great as that of deep WM. These findings suggest that FA and ADC depict distinct aspects of WM maturation in the developing brain. Throughout the remainder of the first year, the rates of change in FA values and in ADC values were similar between peripheral WM and deep WM. This study supported a role for DTI as a sensitive means of analyzing the microstructure of the infant brain during a critical period of brain development. The age-related changes in FA values continue throughout childhood and eventually attain values

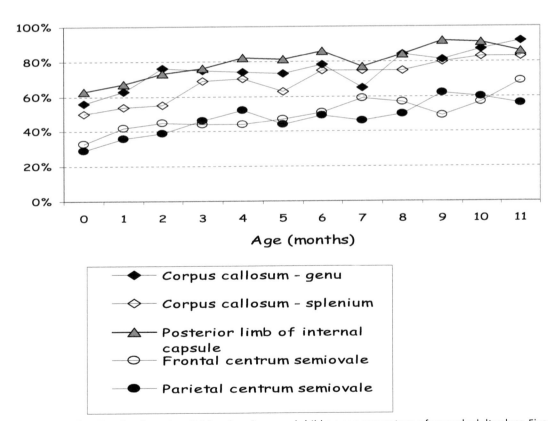

Fig. 3. Increasing FA values in various WM regions in normal children as a percentage of normal adult values. Five WM regions are represented, with 3 being from compact regions in deep WM (genu and splenium of the corpus callosum and posterior limb of the internal capsule) and 2 being from noncompact, peripheral WM regions (subcortical WM of the frontal lobe and parietal lobe). Note that FA values increase with age within each region. However, the FA values in the deep WM regions at the earliest ages shown are substantially higher than peripheral WM regions. In addition, at the end of the first decade of life, the FA values in the deep WM regions are at a higher proportion of adult values than those in the peripheral WM.

that are close to those of adult values (see **Fig. 3**). By early adolescence, FA values in the deep WM regions such as the corpus callosum and the posterior limb of the internal capsule are close to those of adults (see **Fig. 2**). On the other hand, by early adolescence, FA values in peripheral WM regions, such as the subcortical WM regions of the frontal and parietal lobes, are substantially lower than adult values (see **Fig. 3**).

In the past few years, increased attention has been paid to analysis of the 3 principal eigenvalues from which FA values are calculated as a mean to more sensitively assess changes in WM.[20] The standard designations for the major eigenvalue is λ_1 whereas λ_2 and λ_3 fare the standard designations or the minor principal eigenvalues (which are perpendicular to the major eigenvalue and to each other) (**Fig. 4**). The average of the 2 minor eigenvalues ($\lambda_2 + \lambda_3/2$) is usually analyzed rather than the 2 values separately. Many investigators refer to λ_1 by the term axial diffusivity (indicating that it likely represents water diffusion occurring along the long axis of axons) and ($\lambda_2 + \lambda_3/2$) by the term radial diffusivity (suggesting that it represents water diffusion perpendicular to axons and myelin sheaths).

Investigators have postulated that changes in myelination are reflected in changes in radial diffusivity, and changes in axonal integrity are reflected by changes in axial diffusivity.[20] Specifically, the assertion is that increases in myelination are reflected in decreases in radial diffusivity because of an increase in barriers to water diffusion posed by additional myelin. Thus, with brain maturation, λ_2 and λ_3 values are expected to decrease (see **Fig. 4**). Conversely, decreases in myelination are believed to be reflected in increases in radial diffusivity (and, hence, increases in λ_2 and λ_3). Radial diffusivity and axial diffusivity are independent of

one another (ie, a change in one is not necessarily reflected in a change in the other).

Based on the earlier discussion, changes in radial diffusivity might serve as a potential means of monitoring myelination in normal brain development and disorders of myelination in leukodystrophies. More specifically, such changes might be more sensitive to myelination than FA values. One recent study tested this hypothesis in young children.[21] The study found that during the first year of life, statistically significant increases in FA and decreases in both axial diffusivity and radial diffusivity were present. However, during the second year of life (when the brain is considered to be still undergoing prominent developmental changes), solely decreases in radial diffusivity were found to be statistically significant. The investigators considered these findings to represent evidence that radial diffusivity is more sensitive to increases in myelination than FA and axial diffusivity.

The researchers pointed out that contributions of microglia, astrocytes, and cell surface markers should also be considered as contributions to increased water restriction orthogonal to the primary diffusion direction. Specifically, during the first year of life radial diffusivity decreased more quickly than axial diffusivity, which the researchers suggested indicates a greater degree of myelination during the first year of brain development than axonal growth. This finding correlates with pathologic studies using specimen staining that show that a large degree of myelination occurs in the first year of life.[22] In the second year of life, radial diffusivity was found to decrease in all regions except for the splenium of the corpus callosum, possibly because the splenium had already attained a high degree of myelination at 1 year. In contrast to the splenium of the corpus callosum, the frontal and

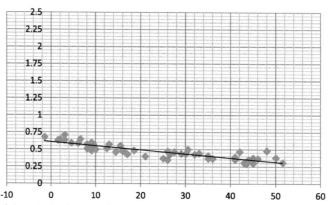

Fig. 4. Decreases in 1 of the principal eigenvalues (λ_3) in the posterior limb of the internal capsule during the first year of life. Age (in weeks) is represented on the x-axis and (λ_3) values are represented on the y-axis.

parietal WM showed a significant decrease in radial diffusivity and axial diffusivity after the first year of life, indicating that this region continues to undergo myelination and axonal development between the first and second year of life.

ASSESSMENT OF BRAIN MATURATION IN GENETIC WM DISORDERS

In addition to assessing WM tracts during normal brain development, DTI can also be used to assess WM in disease states. In such studies, it is important to have a control group of normal infants with whom the DTI values in abnormal brain can be compared. Because Duke University Medical Center is a major center for use of hematopoietic stem cells for treatment of various genetic WM disorders (ie, leukodystrophies), much of our experience is in the form of assessment of infants and children with such disorders.

We have extensively studied the use of DTI to evaluate WM in β-galactocerebrosidase deficiency (ie, Krabbe disease), a rare enzyme deficiency disorder that causes failure of development of normal myelin in infants and children.[23] Studies have shown benefit of hematopoietic stem cell transplantation in this otherwise almost uniformly fatal disorder in infants.[24] Our studies have focused on assessing response to therapy in children with Krabbe disease who have undergone transplantation. In almost all infants with Krabbe disease who come to the attention of a physician because of neurologic disability, the diagnosis is not established until after a few months of life, when clinical findings and MR imaging abnormalities are present (Fig. 5). Therefore, in those particular children, transplantation cannot be performed until the infant is a few months old. We have studied such infants using DTI.[25] However, another cohort of infants with Krabbe disease is available for assessment, namely the asymptomatic younger siblings of clinically affected infants. These unaffected infants come to the attention of the physician because, from having a clinically affected brother or sister, they undergo testing for the enzyme deficiency soon after birth. They thus have an opportunity to undergo transplantation before obvious clinical symptoms develop. Furthermore, they can also undergo DTI at an early stage of the disease and form a natural comparison group for infants who are clinically affected. Yet a third group of infants with Krabbe disease can be studied: those who never undergo transplantation and in whom the natural history of the disease can be studied clinically and using DTI.

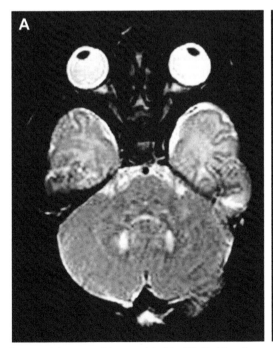 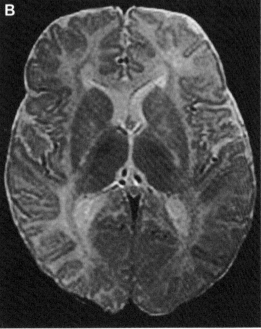

Fig. 5. MR images of 1-year-old girl with Krabbe disease who was treated with stem cell therapy at age 4 months after clinical symptoms and signs were already present. These images show that, although stem cell transplantation ameliorates disease to some extent, prominent MR imaging findings remain. (A) Axial T2-weighted MR image shows abnormal hyperintense signal within deep gray nuclei of cerebellum. (B) Axial T2-weighted image shows abnormal hyperintense signal within posterior limb of internal capsule.

In 1 study, we compared FA values in 2 groups of children with Krabbe disease (ie, those who did not undergo transplantation and those who underwent transplantation).[25] The children used in the study ranged in age from 3 weeks to 3 years and were assessed at a single time point. The untreated children typically died within the first few years of life. Treated infants were all clinically affected to some degree at the time of transplantation; after treatment, they had a longer lifespan than untreated children. FA values were assessed in numerous WM regions of interest (ROIs) in each child and were compared against FA values in the same regions in a control population of normal children who also underwent DTI. The results of the study were as follows. FA values in untreated children with Krabbe disease were markedly lower than in the control group. However, FA values in treated children were typically intermediate between normal children and untreated children with Krabbe disease. This finding suggested to us that the partial clinical benefit seen in treated patients was reflected in some degree of amelioration of decrease in FA values in the same patients.

Early in our experience, the initial group of infants underwent transplantation after clinical symptoms were already present; these clinical symptoms were the basis for their diagnosis. It soon became apparent that although the rate of clinical deterioration was slowed in such children and life span was increased, the maximal benefit of transplantation would likely be found if infants underwent transplantation early in life (ie, in the first few weeks after birth). With this in mind, transplantation was performed in asymptomatic infants with Krabbe disease soon after birth; these infants were typically the siblings of untreated or treated patients with Krabbe disease. As mentioned earlier, such asymptomatic infants underwent testing for the deficient enzyme soon after birth. We then turned our attention to studying DTI examinations in such children who underwent early transplantation to determine whether their FA values differed from those of children who underwent late transplantation and whether their FA values reflected their clinical course.[24]

In our study of DTI in infants who underwent transplantation at different times after birth, we performed a comparison of FA values in a small group of 3 infants with Krabbe disease after early transplantation (ie, stem cell transplantation in the first of life) and 4 infants who underwent transplantation between the age of 5 months and 8 months of life.[24] As mentioned earlier, the early-transplantation group was asymptomatic and identified from low β-galactocerebrosidase levels detected at birth; the average age of this group

of infants at the time of imaging was 13 days. The late transplantation group was symptomatic and diagnosed a few months after birth; the average age at the time of imaging was 5.5 months. All infants in both groups underwent MR imaging using DTI on initial diagnosis (ie, before transplantation) and at least 1 subsequent MR imaging examination with DTI was performed at least 10 months after stem cell transplantation. We performed follow-up MR imaging after transplantation on return clinical visits, which were variable in time (as opposed to being at set intervals).

We assessed both conventional MR images and DTI images. We initially reviewed conventional MR images for evidence of hyperintense signal within WM on T2-weighted images. Those (asymptomatic) infants who underwent early transplantation were found to have solely mild hyperintense signal abnormalities on T2-weighted images. However, the late-transplantation (symptomatic) infants had larger regions of abnormal signal intensity, predominantly in the periventricular WM of the frontal and parietal lobes, centrum semiovale, and dentate nucleus of the cerebellum. For all DTI scans, a single observer placed ROI measurements on FA maps. Measurements were made in the peripheral frontal lobe WM, 2 regions in the corpus callosum (ie, genu and splenium of the corpus callosum), and the posterior limb of the internal capsule. FA values for all patients with Krabbe disease were expressed as a ratio of FA values in age-matched control infants.

We hypothesized that baseline FA ratios (ie, before transplantation) would be decreased for patients with Krabbe disease. We did find this hypothesis to be the case for infants who underwent transplantation at ages 5 to 8 months (ie, the late-transplantation group). The mean pretransplantation FA ratios in the late-transplantation group were between 55% and 74%, reflecting substantial decreases compared with normal infants. However, the mean pretransplantation FA value for all 4 WM ROIs for early-transplantation (asymptomatic) infants ranged between 97% and 117%. Assuming that FA values are a good reflection of degree of myelination, these findings suggest that myelination is relatively normal in infants with Krabbe disease at the time of birth. Furthermore, by the age of 6 months or so, both conventional MR images and DTI images are substantially abnormal. These findings suggest that an intermediate phase may exist in which conventional MR images appear normal or near normal and FA values are abnormal. However, it is also possible that subtle histologic abnormalities are present but cannot be adequately depicted using FA values. Thus, it is possible that FA values do not strongly reflect demyelination; as of this writing few histologic studies have been performed that correlate microstructural features with FA values.

On subsequent imaging at 1 year and 2 years after initial imaging, the ratio of FA values to normal values in the early-transplantation children did not substantially change but remained in about the 80% to 85% range (Fig. 6). Again, if FA values are considered to reflect myelination, these findings suggest that brain myelination was occurring in these infants. This supposition was supported by the conventional MR imaging findings, which showed relatively good progression of hypointense signal on T2-weighted images throughout much of the WM. However, we found moderate or marked decreases in FA values in late-transplantation children; this finding correlated with many WM regions that failed to attain hypointense signal on T2-weighted images.

Another disease that can be assessed and monitored using DTI is X-linked adrenoleukodystrophy, which is a rare congenital disease that causes demyelination in the central nervous system of affected individuals. This disease is believed to be caused by a defect in the ALD transporter gene that transports very long chain fatty acids into peroxisomes. As a result of this defect, very long chain fatty acids accumulate within cells, which are believed to contribute to demyelination. X-linked

adrenoleukodystrophy has a highly variable clinical course. Several treatments are available, including hematopoietic stem cell transplantation.[26] Attention has focused on both conventional and advanced MR imaging techniques to provide markers that might correlate with clinical function so that optimal timing of therapy can be determined and results of such therapy monitored.

At our institution, we have used conventional MR imaging in an attempt to predict clinical outcome after stem cell transplantation.[26] In that study, we compared a scoring system based on hyperintense signal in important WM regions and degree of atrophy (termed the Loes scale) to predict outcome of patients undergoing hematopoietic stem cell transplantation. MR findings were compared against noninvasive electrophysiologic tests (ie, brainstem evoked potentials, visual evoked potentials, nerve conduction velocities, and electroencephalography).[26] That study found that MR findings better predicted patient outcome with regard to posttransplant cognitive and motor function. Another study provided an even simpler method for predicting outcome by examining whether presence of contrast enhancement of WM lesions was associated with poor outcome.[27] That study differed from our study using Loes scores in that the study did not specifically examine outcome after transplantation; instead

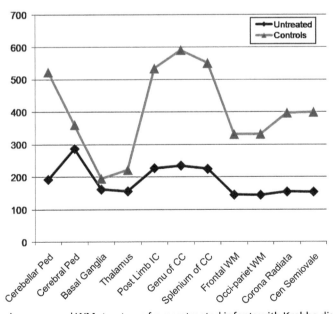

Fig. 6. FA values for various gray and WM structures from untreated infants with Krabbe disease (*blue*) compared with normal age-matched control infants (*orange*). FA values in WM structures in normal infants are substantially higher than in gray matter structures in the same individuals. They are also markedly higher than in WM structures in untreated infants with Krabbe disease. Note that in the infants with Krabbe disease, the FA values in WM are similar to those in gray matter. (*Data from* Guo AC, Petrella JR, Kurtzberg J, et al. Evaluation of WM anisotropy in Krabbe disease with diffusion tensor MR imaging: initial experience. Radiology 2001;218:814.)

the outcome measure was disease progression during a period when the patients were being considered for transplantation. The study found that the presence of contrast enhancement was a predictor of disease progression.

DTI has been used to assess patients with adrenoleukodystrophy. For example, 1 DTI study examined FA and isotropic coefficient values in 3 children with X-linked adrenoleukodystrophy and 7 age-matched normal control children.[28] The study found that FA values in hyperintense WM regions contained higher diffusion coefficient values and lower FA values compared with control subjects.

SUMMARY

DTI can be used in several ways to evaluate the infant brain in both normal development and disease states. This review has highlighted some of the more commonly used techniques and the most frequently used metrics of development, such as ADC and FA. However, the meaning of these metrics is still open to debate; the histologic correlations of these parameters in human brain tissue have not yet been performed in a truly meaningful manner. Nonetheless, the insights provided by DTI studies into the infant brain have shown great promise for future analyses.

REFERENCES

1. Yakovlev P, Lecours A. The myelogenetic cycles of regional maturation of the brain. In: Minkowski A, editor. Regional development of the brain in early life. Oxford (UK): Blackwell Scientific; 1967. p. 3–70.
2. Brody BA, Kinney HC, Kloman AS, et al. Sequence of central nervous system myelination in human infancy. I. An autopsy study of myelination. J Neuropathol Exp Neurol 1987;46(3):283–301.
3. Kinney HC, Brody BA, Kloman AS, et al. Sequence of central nervous system myelination in human infancy. II. Patterns of myelination in autopsied infants. J Neuropathol Exp Neurol 1988;47(3):217–34.
4. Barkovich AJ. MR of the normal neonatal brain: assessment of deep structures. AJNR Am J Neuroradiol 1998;19(8):1397–403.
5. Barkovich AJ, Kjos BO, Jackson DE Jr, et al. Normal maturation of the neonatal and infant brain: MR imaging at 1.5 T. Radiology 1988;166(1 Pt 1):173–80.
6. Holland BA, Haas DK, Norman D, et al. MRI of normal brain maturation. AJNR Am J Neuroradiol 1986;7(2):201–8.
7. Huppi PS, Maier SE, Peled S, et al. Microstructural development of human newborn cerebral white matter assessed in vivo by diffusion tensor magnetic resonance imaging. Pediatr Res 1998;44(4):584–90.
8. Ballesteros MC, Hansen PE, Soila K. MR imaging of the developing human brain. Part 2. Postnatal development. Radiographics 1993;13(3):611–22.
9. Le Bihan D, Moonen CT, van Zijl PC, et al. Measuring random microscopic motion of water in tissues with MR imaging: a cat brain study. J Comput Assist Tomogr 1991;15(1):19–25.
10. Lobel U, Sedlacik J, Gullmar D, et al. Diffusion tensor imaging: the normal evolution of ADC, RA, FA, and eigenvalues studied in multiple anatomical regions of the brain. Neuroradiology 2009;51(4):253–63.
11. Snook L, Paulson LA, Roy D, et al. Diffusion tensor imaging of neurodevelopment in children and young adults. Neuroimage 2005;26(4):1164–73.
12. Lovblad KO, Schneider J, Ruoss K, et al. Isotropic apparent diffusion coefficient mapping of postnatal cerebral development. Neuroradiology 2003;45(6):400–3.
13. Provenzale JM, Liang L, DeLong D, et al. Diffusion tensor imaging assessment of brain white matter maturation during the first postnatal year. AJR Am J Roentgenol 2007;189(2):476–86.
14. Girard N, Confort-Gouny S, Schneider J, et al. MR imaging of brain maturation. J Neuroradiol 2007;34(5):290–310.
15. Zhang L, Thomas KM, Davidson MC, et al. MR quantitation of volume and diffusion changes in the developing brain. AJNR Am J Neuroradiol 2005;26(1):45–9.
16. Dobbing J, Sands J. Quantitative growth and development of human brain. Arch Dis Child 1973;48(10):757–67.
17. Forbes KP, Pipe JG, Bird CR. Changes in brain water diffusion during the 1st year of life. Radiology 2002;222(2):405–9.
18. Rakic P, Yakovlev PI. Development of the corpus callosum and cavum septi in man. J Comp Neurol 1968;132(1):45–72.
19. Price DJ, Kennedy H, Dehay C, et al. The development of cortical connections. Eur J Neurosci 2006;23(4):910–20.
20. Song SK, Yoshino J, Le TQ, et al. Demyelination increases radial diffusivity in corpus callosum of mouse brain. Neuroimage 2005;26(1):132–40.
21. Gao W, Lin W, Chen Y, et al. Temporal and spatial development of axonal maturation and myelination of white matter in the developing brain. AJNR Am J Neuroradiol 2009;30(2):290–6.
22. Haynes RL, Borenstein NS, Desilva TM, et al. Axonal development in the cerebral white matter of the human fetus and infant. J Comp Neurol 2005;484(2):156–67.
23. Provenzale JM, Escolar M, Kurtzberg J. Quantitative analysis of diffusion tensor imaging data in serial assessment of Krabbe disease. Ann N Y Acad Sci 2005;1064:220–9.
24. Escolar ML, Poe MD, Provenzale JM, et al. Transplantation of umbilical-cord blood in babies with infantile Krabbe's disease. N Engl J Med 2005;352(20):2069–81.

25. Guo AC, Petrella JR, Kurtzberg J, et al. Evaluation of white matter anisotropy in Krabbe disease with diffusion tensor MR imaging: initial experience. Radiology 2001;218(3):809–15.

26. Beam D, Poe MD, Provenzale JM, et al. Outcomes of unrelated umbilical cord blood transplantation for X-linked adrenoleukodystrophy. Biol Blood Marrow Transplant 2007;13(6):665–74.

27. Melhem ER, Loes DJ, Georgiades CS, et al. X-linked adrenoleukodystrophy: the role of contrast-enhanced MR imaging in predicting disease progression. AJNR Am J Neuroradiol 2000;21(5):839–44.

28. Schneider JF, Il'yasov KA, Boltshauser E, et al. Diffusion tensor imaging in cases of adrenoleukodystrophy: preliminary experience as a marker for early demyelination? AJNR Am J Neuroradiol 2003;24(5):819–24.

Index

Note: Page numbers of article titles are in **boldface** type.

Neuroimag Clin N Am 21 (2011) 191–195
doi:10.1016/S1052-5149(11)00033-5

Printed and bound by CPI Group (UK) Ltd, Croydon, CR0 4YY

03/10/2024

01040359-0010